Romanticism and Colonial Disease

MEDICINE & CULTURE

Sander L. Gilman
SERIES EDITOR

Robert Michaels, M.D., Linda Hutcheon, Ph.D., and
Michael Hutcheon, M.D.
EDITORIAL BOARD

Georges Minois, *History of Suicide: Voluntary Death in Western Culture,*
trans. Lydia G. Cochrane

Jacques Jouanna, *Hippocrates,* trans. M. B. DeBevoise

Laura Otis, *Membranes: Metaphors of Invasion in
Nineteenth-Century Literature, Science, and Politics*

Alan Bewell, *Romanticism and Colonial Disease*

Romanticism and Colonial Disease

ALAN BEWELL

The Johns Hopkins University Press

BALTIMORE AND LONDON

© 1999 The Johns Hopkins University Press
All rights reserved. Published 1999

Printed in the United States of America on acid-free paper
2   4   6   8   9   7   5   3   1

The Johns Hopkins University Press
2715 North Charles Street
Baltimore, Maryland 21218-4363
www.press.jhu.edu

Library of Congress Cataloging-in-Publication Data will be
found at the end of this book.
A catalog record for this book is available from the
British Library.

ISBN 0-8018-6225-6

For Sharon

CONTENTS

ILLUSTRATIONS

In 1898 H. G. Wells published *The War of the Worlds,* a novella that powerfully encapsulates two of the primary concerns of this book—the emergence of a British understanding of the fundamental relation between imperialism and disease and the anxiety that accompanied that recognition. The ostensible focus of Wells's narrative is the invasion of earth by alien beings. The octopus-like Martians, inhabitants of a dying planet, seek to establish a new colony on earth. The violence of these events is graphically described. With absolute lack of concern for people, the Martians systematically destroy the human social order. Wells shrewdly notes that colonization is not just a military undertaking but also a profoundly biological and ecological event, something that British colonists recognized but that has largely been ignored by criticism. The Martians employ a poison, the "black smoke," to depopulate Earth. Although others have noted Wells's prediction of gas warfare during World War I, his glance extends backward too. The "black smoke" is also "miasma," the atmospheric poison that was frequently believed to cause epidemics, and its name summons up the massive depopulation caused by the Black Death. Disease is but one element in these outsiders' arsenal. Migrating along with them is a new plant, the "red weed," that quickly overruns the planet just as European flora and fauna overran so many colonial regions. The narrator describes how strange it is to walk through a world that has become foreign: "I had expected to see Sheen in ruins—I found about me the landscape, weird and lurid, of another planet" (114). The world produced by human beings interacting with their environment has disappeared; earth is becoming another red planet, another Mars. "When I had last seen this part of Sheen in the daylight it had been a straggling street of comfortable white and red houses, interspersed with abundant shady trees. Now I stood on a mound of smashed brickwork, clay and gravel, over which spread a multitude of red cactus-shaped plants, knee-high, without a solitary terrestrial growth to dispute their footing. The trees near me were dead and brown, but farther, a network of red threads scaled the still living stems" (113–14). The war of the worlds is exactly that, not just the struggle of a people to survive against the predatory Martians, but the struggle of an entire world that includes human beings against the new environment introduced by these outsiders. For many societies colonialism ushered in a similar state of ecological crisis, and entire worlds were lost or transformed.

In Wells's case the historical context that gave rise to this story of galactic imperial conflict is quite clear, for it emerged from a discussion of events much closer to home—the colonial destruction of the indigenous people of Tasmania. These events are briefly mentioned in the story. "The Tasmanians," he writes, "in spite of their human likeness, were entirely swept out of existence in a war of extermination waged by European immigrants, in the space of fifty years. Are we such apostles of mercy as to complain if the Martians warred in the same spirit?" (4). The "war of the worlds," in other words, is a fictional reflection of European colonial history. On one level these extraterrestrial invaders who display such indifference to the tragedies that accompany their expansionism are just displaced nineteenth-century imperialists. This dark doubling of the British and the Martians produces a complex range of feelings, from recognition and identification to revulsion and disavowal. The British attitude toward empire, however, was never that simple, for any reader would notice that the primary doubling is between the British and the Tasmanians. Wells seeks to gain insight into how imperialism looks through the eyes of those whose worlds have been irrevocably lost. What makes this narrative similar to the kind of writing I will be analyzing is that it applies the perception of the fragility of societies in the face of colonialism to Britain itself. Wells had no difficulty recognizing the tremendous technological advantages of Britain at the end of the nineteenth century. Nevertheless the novella postulates that this sword may be double-edged—always the dark side of imperial destruction. The Martians constitute an eerie double of British colonialism as the attitudes that shaped British actions in other social worlds come back to haunt the empire. The narrator learns what it is like to see one's entire world dismantled and destroyed by outsiders. *The War of the Worlds* might be seen, then, as an allegory of the nineteenth-century imperial unconscious—the recognition that despite its success in producing a global empire, Britain might suffer a similar fate. Like many of the works I will be discussing, this novella is a "double text" as the voice of the colonizer is disquieted by the voice and experience of the colonized.

In a profound irony, the Martian invasion of earth is foiled not through British military power, but through the action of "disease bacteria . . . the humblest things that God, in His wisdom, has put upon this earth" (133). Lacking biological resistance to common terrestrial microbes, the invading Martians (and the "red weed" they have brought with them) are destroyed by an epidemic of ordinary diseases. There can be little doubt that colonial history influenced Wells's decision to make disease a more important factor in the history of empire than military or technological power. In explaining why the colonizing Martians fall victim to the diseases of the colonized, the narrator suggests two possibilities: microbes "either never appeared upon Mars, or Martian sanitary science eliminated them ages ago. A hundred diseases, all the fevers and contagions of human life, consumption, cancers, tumours and such morbidities, never enter the scheme of their life" (101). In the first case the Martians succumb to what contemporary epidemiologists call a "virgin soil epidemic," the virulent outbreak of an infectious disease among a population previously isolated from it. Typical of the way the narrative undercuts stability by superimposing the experience of the colonized on that of the colonizer, the expansionist Martians suffer a fate similar to that of indigenous peoples facing the onslaught of new diseases brought from the Old World. In every part of the globe entire societies were decimated by wave after wave of diseases they had never experienced, bacteria and viruses against which they had built up no immunity. Yet Wells's focus is not the impact of disease on the colonized, but how it affects the invader. In the colonial context, the power of disease was not unidimensional: it could destroy a society or defend it from outsiders, a lesson Europeans painfully learned as they sought to extend their early success in colonizing temperate regions to the tropical environments of the West Indies, Africa, and Asia. The backdrop to these reflections, therefore, is not only the epidemiology of colonial peoples, a subject that has received extensive attention in recent years, but also the history—more rarely addressed—of the impact of disease on European colonists. As the narrator argues, through death and disease, "by the toll of a billion deaths," human beings have bought their "birthright of the earth," and it is theirs "against all comers" (134). The epidemic destruction of the Martians is thus not only a figure of colonial depopulation but also an anxious allegory of the fate of empire, one that probably had less to do with prophecy than with the actual experience of the British in the tropics over the previous two centuries.

Another reason the Martians are susceptible to terrestrial diseases, which adds another dimension to Wells's story, may be that they had previously eliminated these diseases from their world through advances in "sanitary science." With an irony that has become clearer in recent decades as Western nations face a panoply of emerging and reemerging diseases, the microbes did not disappear with the Martians' technological mastery over them, and these diseases, probably long forgotten, eventually prey on them. The victory of "civilization" over disease can never be permanent, especially when the pathogens continue to thrive elsewhere. "Sanitary science" was one of the great inventions of nineteenth-century European medicine, and "health" in its traditional meaning of *sanitas* was often seen as the distinctive contribution it offered a world that previously seemed unable to rise out of a pathogenic morass produced by a lack of knowledge, technology, and appropriate social institutions. Wells's nineteenth-century audience thus could hardly miss the significance of this allegory of vulnerability emerging out of a society's very success in eliminating disease from its borders. Perhaps the Western technological mastery over diseases—one of the great themes of imperial culture—was at best only temporary, and worse, perhaps a people's ability to isolate themselves from the diseases of the colonial world might eventually make them even more vulnerable. The narrative anxiously addresses the prospect that the very things that separate the "healthy" colonizer from the "sick" colonized might ultimately produce a tragic vulnerability. In a world where diseases were constantly being exchanged, where diseases traveled and any boundary could ultimately be breached, isolation was no longer possible, and the longer a society avoided contact with an infectious disease the more virulent would be the inevitable outbreak of infection. In *The War of the Worlds,* the pathogenic world of the colonized recoils on an empire whose very success in achieving perfect health through civilization makes it susceptible to epidemic. Through a circuit whose ironies can hardly be missed, the precolonial indigene and technologically advanced Martians meet in their inevitable encounter with diseases brought by colonial expansion.

Near the end of the story, as the narrator walks through a London that has now become a "dead city," he realizes that he might be "the last man." Here Wells pays tribute to Mary Shelley's novel *The Last Man,* written seventy-five years earlier. As a late Victorian text, Wells's novella stands outside the primary time frame of this book, which primarily treats the period from 1780 to 1848, when the first British Public Health Act was passed, but in concentrating on the impact of disease not only on the colonized but also on the colonist, Wells's narrative has much in common with the writers and colonial physicians I will be discussing in this study of the impact of colonial disease on British culture during the Romantic period. The novella crystallizes a range of epidemiological anxieties and uncertainties that came to dominate the British cultural understanding of colonialism. Colonial disease shaped British culture to a degree that has not been adequately recognized, as an entire range of writings reflected on this new epidemiological world and on its consequences for both colonizers and colonized. In a context in which the communication and exchange of new diseases between peoples proceeded at a pace never before seen, the framing of colonial disease was neither fixed nor secure. By "colonial disease," therefore, I do not mean "non-European" diseases but instead denote the new global expansion and exchange of diseases that took place at this time. Even as disease played a growing role in differentiating Europeans from others, it also established new forms of commonality. As the British grappled with understanding their place in this new world that colonial expansion had brought into being, a world in which threatening diseases surpassed their traditional boundaries, they anxiously looked to the colonial world. In an age of epidemiological crisis, they read colonial disease through others, sometimes projecting their fears onto colonial people, sometimes to assure themselves that the worst diseases would not reach Britain, and often to justify the introduction of Western technologies and political institutions in new regions of the world, but also as a mode of understanding. The colonial world was a dark mirror in which Europeans read their own destinies. From our current vantage point, in which disease is more than ever a global phenomenon, when every year seems to bring a new disease and the old ones, over which modern medicine thought it had gained control, are reappearing in new, drug-resistant forms, much can be learned from a study of how writers first responded to this new state of affairs. At a time of growing anxiety about the global movement of infectious diseases, we are more capable of understanding the anxieties that shaped British Romantic culture.

I am grateful to the Johns Hopkins University Press for permission to republish parts of an essay that appeared in the *Journal of English Literary History* 63 (1996): 773–808. I thank the Social Sciences and Humanities Research Council of Canada for the research support that was fundamental to my writing this book. I have benefited from the advice and assistance of many individuals, most notably David Arnold, Neil Fraistat, Hermione de Almeida, Anthony Harding, Heather Jackson, Robin Jackson, Elizabeth Jones, Michael Laplace-Sinatra, Nigel Leask, Jill Matus, and Timothy Morton. Philip D. Curtin generously allowed me to reproduce a map from his book *Death by Migration*. My thanks too for the invaluable assistance of fellow Romanticists on the NASSR-List. My research assistants, Nahoko Miyamoto, Julia Saric, and Jessica Wilson, helped keep this project under way, especially when administrative work put a premium on research time. I am greatly indebted to my editor Alice M. Bennett for her scrupulous attention to the manuscript and her judicious suggestions. Most of all I am grateful to my wife, Sharon, and my daughters, Carmen and Janet, who remain a continuing source of inspiration and support.

Romanticism and Colonial Disease

Colonialism and Disease

It is asserted, that on the arrival of a stranger (at St. Kilda)
all the inhabitants, in the common phraseology, catch a
cold.   —Charles Darwin, *The Voyage of the "Beagle"*

A legend among the Kiowas of the American Great Plains tells about an
encounter between Saynday, the mythic hero of the tribe, and a stranger
named Smallpox, dressed in a black suit and high hat. Smallpox speaks first:

"Who are you?" the stranger asked.

"I'm Saynday. I'm the Kiowas' Old Uncle Saynday. I'm the one who's always
coming along."

"I never heard of you," the stranger said, "and I never heard of the Kiowas. Who
are they?"

"The Kiowas are my people," Saynday said, and even in that hard time he stood up
proudly, like a man. "Who are you?"

"I'm Smallpox," the man answered.

"And I never heard of *you*," said Saynday. "Where do you come from and what do
you do and why are you here?"

"I come from far away, across the Eastern Ocean," Smallpox answered. "I am one
with the white men—they are my people as the Kiowas are yours. Sometimes I travel
ahead of them, and sometimes I lurk behind. But I am always their companion and
you will find me in their camps and in their houses."

"What do you do?" Saynday repeated.

"I bring death," Smallpox replied. "My breath causes children to wither like young
plants in the spring snow. I bring destruction. No matter how beautiful a woman is,
once she has looked at me she becomes as ugly as death. And to men I bring not death
alone, but the destruction of their children and the blighting of their wives. The

strongest warriors go down before me. No people who have looked on me will ever be the same." (Marriott and Rachlin 144–45)[1]

Saynday's encounter with Smallpox embodies an experience that was repeated in different places at different times throughout the colonial period. To a degree that historians and literary critics have not adequately recognized, colonial experience was profoundly structured by disease, both as metaphor and as reality. For different peoples at different times, it was an age of epidemiological crisis. In the legend one glimpses what it meant for a people to undergo total social collapse, the destruction of children, wives, and warriors. Smallpox's words powerfully articulate the depth of the changes wrought by colonial disease: "No people who have looked on me will ever be the same."

Like many other stories of the colonial period, the encounter between Saynday and Smallpox displays the complex ways a culture seeks to understand or "frame" a disease. In using this term I am drawing on Charles Rosenberg's analysis of the social and cultural processes by which ideas about diseases, about how they are transmitted and who is susceptible to them, are formed. There are substantial differences between having a disease, naming a disease, and having a named disease. Disease transmission requires its own kind of reception theory, for it is *communication* that really does change those who receive it both physically and culturally. Rosenberg has usefully suggested that we understand diseases as social and cultural "negotiations." The idea of a disease at a given time or place is thus not necessarily stable but has undergone arbitration between different social and cultural groups, classes, and institutions. As he remarks, "The negotiations surrounding the definition of and response to disease are complex and multilayered. They include cognitive and disciplinary elements, institutional and public policy responses, and the adjustments of particular individuals and their families. Involved at all levels is the doctor-patient relationship. . . . Disease can be seen as a dependent variable in such a negotiated situation; yet, once agreed upon, it becomes an actor in that social setting, legitimating and guiding social decision making" (Rosenberg and Golden, *Framing Disease* xxi). Rosenberg refers to such negotiations as "frames," a term that nicely captures the provisional character of conceptions of what a disease is, how it is transmitted, and who is likely to be sick from it. Although a frame might suggest consensus and stability, I employ the term in a more active sense, which recognizes that the framing of disease at any given time is not necessarily settled but is constantly open to negotiation, revision, and dispute. The framing of disease can also be seen as an attempt to cope with biological entities whose nature, causes, and behavior were frequently unknown or changing.

Framing diseases during the colonial period was particularly uncertain and unstable for a number of reasons. Of central importance was that different societies were grappling with *new* diseases. Colonialism may not have created new pathogens, but it did bring people who had previously been isolated into contact with each other and with diseases that were new to them. Precolonial peoples inhabited unique disease environments, ecologies that had been built up through the interaction of human beings and microbes over vast spans of time. They would have adapted themselves biologically and culturally to the pathogens around them, and in such circumstances the framing of diseases was largely stable. During the colonial period diseases began to *travel* as never before. Diseases that had previously been largely restricted in their geographical ranges, or had slowly made their way to Europe from the East (as had chicken pox, smallpox, and measles), began to travel at epidemic and pandemic speed. The boundaries that historically separated these disease environments were breached as new pathogens were exchanged on a scale far greater than ever before. Traditional physical environments and modes of behavior were also radically transformed, and these alterations provided opportunities for microbes to colonize new parts of the globe. For many indigenous populations, the first sign of this new world was not necessarily the appearance of white people, but the introduction of new diseases. The interaction of colonizer and colonized may be a history of failed communication and of increased social, political, and cultural differences, yet microbes were communicated regularly and tragically.

Mary Louise Pratt describes the "contact zone" as the "space of colonial encounters . . . [where] peoples geographically and historically separated come into contact with each other and establish ongoing relations, usually involving conditions of coercion, radical inequality, and intractable conflict" (6). We need to reconceptualize this notion to go beyond its explicit emphasis on cultural parameters and include biomedical contact, itself part of those larger new biomedical environments brought into being by colonialism. Contact zones were undoubtedly spaces of political, linguistic, and economic transformation, but they were also regions undergoing rapid biological transformation. Contact with new diseases also introduced new names and new metaphors into the disease vocabularies of different peoples, who then had to think about disease in new ways. The Saynday narrative describes the process of giving a strange disease a name. Yet in focusing on disease as an intrinsic part of colonial discourse, one must be careful not to disembody colonial contact, which was structured by bodies that exchanged pathogens, suffered from sickness, and frequently died. Disease was both a metaphor and a sad reality.

The global expansion of human travel also made possible the *globalization of disease,* the worldwide spread of viruses and bacteria that had previously occupied relatively local geographies. Viruses require contact and modes of transport, and the colonial period was adept at supplying both. At least Robert Southey thought so. "Pigs, Spanish dollars, and Norway rats are not the only commodities that have performed the circumnavigation, and are to be found wherever European ships have touched. Diseases also find their way from one part of the inhabited globe to another, where it is possible for them to exist" (*Thomas More* 1: 57–58). In an important essay on this topic, Emmanuel Le Roy Ladurie speaks of "the unification of the globe by disease," which he argues took place between the appearance of the bubonic plague in Europe in the fourteenth century and the massive depopulation of the New World from the fifteenth century to the seventeenth ("Concept" 29). In concentrating on the catastrophic epidemics of this period, Le Roy Ladurie's time frame is fairly arbitrary, especially since the peoples of Oceania had not even encountered white people yet. Also, he tends to minimize the importance of colonization in expediting this process. Edward Said has remarked that modern imperialism brought into being "a fully global world" (*Culture and Imperialism* 6). Nowadays, when microbes can travel almost anywhere by jet, one can appreciate what it means to be in a world that functions, in Le Roy Ladurie's terms, as "a common market of bacilli" ("Concept" 41). This new epidemiological reality is one of the legacies of colonialism.

Disease representations during the colonial period are triangulated, as expressions not only of the interaction between different groups of people (classes, societies, genders), but also of the interaction of human beings with a dynamic and changing world of microbes and parasites. The framing of colonial disease was particularly difficult, however, because there was no stability in these triangulated relationships. A striking feature of the new colonial disease ecologies is that there was no uniformity in the experiences of those who inhabited them. Because they comprised people coming from different parts of the world who had been exposed to different pathogens and had thus developed different degrees of resistance to different diseases, the same pathogen did not affect all people in the same way. One person might be sick, or an entire people might be dying from an epidemic, while another group inhabiting the same place, drinking the same water, and breathing the same air was unaffected. In *The Voyage of the "Beagle"* (1839), after observing that "the first intercourse between natives and Europeans, 'is invariably attended with the introduction of fever, dysentery, or some other disease, which carries off numbers of the people,'" Darwin goes on to remark the strange fact that "there might be no appearance of disease among the crew of the ship which conveyed this destructive importation" (376–77).[2] Although both groups now share the same diseases, one group is "healthy" while the other is in crisis. The colonial disease landscape was not uniform. Indeed, a fundamental register of geographical or social identity during this period lay in what diseases one was capable of dying from. The globalization of disease partly demolished, even as it vividly brought out, the differences between the immune systems of different people, deriving from their adaptation to different disease environments.

Major cultural myths—racial, cultural, technological, medical, theological—were built on these differences, often to the detriment of those most affected by disease. Not enough study has yet been given to the enormous role these differences played in Europeans' understanding of themselves and others, especially since they produced a tremendous confidence in the superiority of European culture, technology, biology, and morality. Even God seemed to be on the side of the healthy. For instance William Bradford, after observing that, in contact with smallpox, the natives of the Connecticut River "dye like rotten sheep," notes with some satisfaction that "by the marvelous goodnes and providens of God not one of the English was so much as sicke, or in the least measure tainted with this disease" (313). This lack of uniformity requires that we understand geographical and cultural representations of this period contextually. Whether a place or a people is described as healthy or sick substantially depends on who is doing the describing. A "healthy" physical and social environment for one people may be "unhealthy" for another, and cultural history, with all its moral evaluations, has largely been written by the "healthy."

Sander Gilman, in *Disease and Representation*, argues that Western representations of disease are dialectical structures: fearing our own collapse, we project this fear and thus gain control of it by locating disease in others, especially in those we believe are particularly prone to sickness (1–2). All disease representations can be said, then, to be both autobiographical, as expressions of an individual sense of pathogenic threat, and culturally specific, as they reflect the characteristic ways larger social groups see themselves and others. Gilman's model is valuable for understanding the dominant structures governing colonial representations, the way disease is frequently personified in terms of a diseased other. In the Kiowa myth, Saynday protects his tribe first by giving Smallpox a European face and then by tricking him into seeking instead the Pawnees, the traditional enemies of the Kiowas. " 'That's the Pawnees,' Saynday said jauntily. He began to feel better. The deathly smell was not so strong now. 'I think I'll go and visit the Pawnees first,' Smallpox remarked. 'Later on, perhaps, I can get back to the Kiowas' " (Marriott and Rachlin 146). The Kiowa myth is typical of many colonial representations of disease transmission in that it represents it as an *encounter* between two people, one of them a stranger or an outsider. Smallpox is personified as a European missionary dressed in black. Susan Sontag's observation that there is a "link between imagining disease and imagining foreignness" (*AIDS and Its Metaphors* 48) helps explain the role that different diseases played in the emergence of notions of cultural and racial identity. During the colonial period, susceptibility to specific diseases was one of the primary means by which differences between peoples were conceptualized. "Loathsome and dangerous diseases," Benjamin Rush remarks in *An Account of the Bilious Remitting Yellow Fever* (1794), "have been considered by all nations as of foreign extraction." Rush attacked this prejudice as a form of scapegoating and a way Philadelphians avoided recognizing their own responsibility for the yellow fever epidemic of 1793. "The venereal disease and the leprosy have no native country, if we believe all the authors who have written upon their origin," he writes. "Prosper Alpinus, derives the almost yearly plagues of Cairo from Syria, and Dr. Warren flattered the people of Barbadoes, by an attempt to persuade them that the yellow fever of the West Indies, was originally imported from Siam" (147). People like to blame others for the diseases that afflict them.

Ideas about disease are thus inseparably linked to the formation of social groups and their others. Politics also shapes disease representations during the colonial period. For instance, in the United Irishman satire *Billy Bluff and the Squire* (1796) the Squire's prejudices are obvious when he accuses a woman of being "a witch." "Who gave you that cut over the eye? How many nights in the week do you ride over the sea on a bendweed? Do you carry on treasonable correspondence with the French? Did you ever see Carnot? Was it you carried the Spanish fleet into the Mediterranean? Yes! you old yellow thief! the *Northern Star's* your guide. Did you ever raise the D——l? It is you who brought the yellow fever into our West India settlements—who promoted the Union of Irishmen" (Clifford 40).[3] Here the woman is accused of a series of crimes, from associating with revolutionary France and the devil to taking her directions on her night flights from the radical Irish newspaper the *Northern Star.* At once an outsider, a sorceress, and a "thief," her "yellow" skin leads to speculation that she not only promulgates the dangerous contagion of the "Union of Irishmen" but also brought the epidemic yellow fever to the West Indies.

Recent criticism, recognizing the proliferation of images of disease in colonial texts, has largely followed a psychological model in seeing them as expressions of European attitudes toward others. Without attending to the epidemiological context within which these representations were formed, historians and critics often view them as metaphoric projections of racial and cultural anxieties. Even as one recognizes that disease plays a primary role in representations of otherness, the social and political construction of disease during this period is complicated in that diseases usually *did* come from elsewhere. The most virulent ones are not those that a people have developed some biological or cultural immunity against, but those they are encountering for the first time. The most dangerous diseases during the colonial period therefore were indeed "foreign," either those that had traveled from somewhere else or those encountered through travel. Colonialism allowed "old" diseases to come into contact with populations as yet unacquainted with them, and because these populations had not yet developed biological defenses they were invariably more virulent. More than at any other time in history, people struggled to understand diseases that were new to them. They feared the "strange" maladies; they also feared "strangers" and travelers. Diseases and cultural contact were fundamentally entangled with each other. Smallpox *did* migrate to America with the Europeans and settled alongside them, becoming as much a part of the colonial landscape as the settlers and their livestock. Contact with others thus presented risks that were more than metaphoric. Epidemiological danger frequently resided in the encounter between peoples. The rise of a literature in which pathogenic images play a growing role in understanding colonial situations and the pervasive tendency of groups to personify disease, to portray it as an encounter with a stranger or to associate it with specific individuals or groups, are also expressive of a reality that should not be ignored. The proliferation of narratives, myths, images, and metaphors about sickness and death thus also speaks of realities that an exclusive focus on representations as cultural constructions is likely to minimize. We must remember that the framing of colonial disease largely took place in the context of epidemiological crisis, at a time when people were confronting unfamiliar sicknesses on a terrain that was unequal and constantly changing.

More than at any other time in history, disease was power, since the success of nations in expanding beyond their borders and occupying other lands frequently had less to do with military strength (as most histories of this period have imagined), than with the simple advantage that one people had already built up childhood immunity to diseases that another society was encountering for the first time. Philip D. Curtin has observed that "in the longer sweep of history over the past two or three millennia, increasing intercommunication has made disease environments more nearly alike, not more diverse; but each breach of previous isolation has brought higher death rates, as unfamiliar diseases attacked populations whose environment provided no source of immunity" ("Epidemiology and the Slave Trade" 195). In the New World, smallpox, diphtheria, influenza, measles, yellow fever, malaria, mumps, typhoid fever, whooping cough, chicken pox, dengue, and scarlet fever, among others, often silently preceded and largely made possible the colonization of the Americas. For Europeans, the emergence of these new disease environments often provided opportunities for expansion, as was the case in North and South America, the South Pacific, and South Africa. In many other areas, however, such as Asia and the East and West Indies, diseases represented a primary obstacle to empire. Colonialism was indeed a geopolitics of disease, because the outcome of the contest for land was frequently determined by pathogens. This contest was fought on unequal ground, since the disease environment, itself undergoing change, had different effects on the peoples involved. Thus one of primary distinctions between the loosely termed "settler" and "conquest" colonies was epidemiological; settler colonies were those in which the exchange of pathogens, and the power that lay within that exchange, favored Europeans. Frequently, as in the colonization of the Americas, Australia, and New Zealand, settlement followed in the wake of massive epidemiological destruction.

Where the exchange of diseases favored native populations, as in India and in sub-Saharan Africa, different colonial structures were required. The disease environments of Africa ensured its comparative isolation from Europe throughout the early colonial period. They were also a major factor behind the development of the slave plantation economies of the West Indies, a unique kind of settlement achieved by the forced relocation of an entire population to a new region of the globe, ostensibly because blacks could withstand diseases that regularly killed white people. The sad irony was that since the African slaves brought with them the same sicknesses and helminthic infections that the Europeans were seeking to avoid (yellow fever and African strains of malaria and dysentery; hookworm, onchocerciasis, and filariasis), the epidemiology of the West Indies ultimately became like that of

Africa, so Europeans were largely back where they started. The native populations of this region, however, lacking immunological and social practices to resist these microbes and parasites along with those first brought by Europeans, were decimated. When, after 1850, a ready supply of powdered quinine finally made it possible for Europeans to explore Africa and settle there—penetration that would be extended with the adoption of measures to control insects in the 1890s—the biological advantage that had protected Africans from extensive colonization was reversed, and they also suffered a major epidemiological crisis. "With the apparent partial exception of West Africa," argue Hartwig and Patterson, "the unhealthiest period in all African history was undoubtedly between 1890 and 1930" ("Disease Factor" 4). In a colonial context, medicine played an ambiguous role: it made possible colonial expansion and with it the increased exchange of pathogens even as it assisted in the scientific conquest of African diseases.

An adequate understanding of the literature and history of colonialism therefore requires attention to this world-making and world-shattering traffic in pathogens and to the massive epidemiological suffering produced by colonial commerce and expansion. In using the term "colonial disease" I am thus referring not to non-European disease (itself a European construction) but to this globalized expansion and exchange of diseases. Some work has been done on the political, historical, and economic dimensions of colonial medicine.[4] Valuable studies have also been done of the ecology and epidemiology of colonial disease.[5] More research is needed, however, to determine how these radically new disease environments were seen by those most affected by them, the people who occupied the "contact zones." For these people, colonialism was a time of extended crisis, when epidemics were the norm rather than the exception. This book seeks to contribute to a better understanding of how people during this time experienced this new disease reality. Although informed by the extensive work that has been done on the social, economic, demographic, and epidemiological consequences of colonialism, my primary attention is on the literature produced during this period of global epidemiological crisis.[6] Just as there is no uniformity of attitudes toward AIDS in our time, because AIDS means different things to different people, we should not expect uniformity in colonial responses to disease. The experience of disease cuts across a wide range of social, economic, and cultural contexts. The diseases themselves—how they were understood and controlled, who was sick and why—also differed among groups, classes, and cultures, so that to reconstruct what disease meant, we need to read it through the contextualized voicing of specific groups of people and societies. Here literature is an enormously valuable resource.

Recent studies of the epidemiology of colonial contact in the Americas have provided evidence that the Kiowa legend is not a fiction but a mythic distillation of history, as indigenous peoples struggled against wave after wave of epidemic diseases brought from Europe and Africa.[7] Some historians, such as Henry F. Dobyns, have estimated that New World populations underwent declines of 50 percent to 95 percent ("Outline of Andean Epidemic History"). Europeans encountered societies that were in a state of demographic crisis. The same process was at work elsewhere. Charles Darwin remarks: "Wherever the European has trod, death seems to pursue the aboriginal. We may look to the wide extent of the Americas, Polynesia, the Cape of Good Hope, and Australia, and we find the same result" (376). Despite the great suffering reflected by demographic studies of colonialism, the events themselves left little historical documentation. History, it seems, has been written by the healthy.

Although the impact of disease on indigenous and colonized peoples is receiving more attention from historians and demographers, it is ironic that there has been so little study of the enormous epidemiological cost of colonialism for Europeans, despite the greater number of written documents available. A general silence envelops European colonial disease and mortality. This situation can be partly explained by a general assumption of traditional and postcolonial critics alike that with few exceptions the dangers of colonial contact flowed in one direction, from the colonizers to the colonized. In most "temperate" regions, where the battery of diseases brought by Europeans far outnumbered those of indigenous populations, this was true. But in many other parts of the globe, notably in "tropical" regions, a different picture emerges. In India, Southeast Asia, the West Indies, and sub-Saharan Africa—areas that are the focus of this book and that were the primary arenas of European expansion during the eighteenth and nineteenth centuries—the mortality and morbidity rates for Europeans compete with those of indigenous peoples. Yet the European experience of colonial disease in these regions, like that of indigenes in other places, remains largely buried in history. When encountered in literary texts or historical documents, it is largely ignored or treated as a metaphoric projection of European insecurities or biases onto other parts of the globe.

Demographic and epidemiological statistics are available for the nineteenth century. As colonial administrators and physicians recognized that disease was a primary obstacle to establishing and maintaining colonial settlements, they began to keep health records, especially for military personnel. Philip D. Curtin, who is among those most influential in increasing our knowledge of the epidemiology of colonialism, has examined nineteenth-century military medical records in his important study *Death by Migration*. Its title power-fully encapsulates his major conclusion: that "every trading voyage, every military expedition beyond Europe, had its price in European lives lost" (xiii). Curtin makes statistically explicit the reality, rarely lost on eighteenth- and nineteenth-century colonists, that traveling, especially to the tropics, was dangerous to one's health. "Statistics have shown," writes Georges Pouchet, "the dangers of changing one's position on the globe" (92). Colonial history abounds in stories of adventure and the acquisition of wealth. Less obviously, but certainly more pervasively, it is structured in terms of the relation between travel and disease. Colonists talked a lot about how not to get sick in places that put one's health at risk. If one was lucky, a brief period of sickness on first arriving in the tropics ("seasoning") would yield an indeterminate period of relative health. Others, however, died within a couple of years or returned to Europe as invalids, their health permanently impaired. Epidemiological costs varied in different parts of the globe, but one thing was clear: with the exception of the Pacific Islands, where Europeans were healthier than at home, the cost in tropical regions was high. Curtin has produced a map for 1817–38 that provides a graphic description of European colonial mortality rates across the globe (see map 1).

The annual mortality rate of soldiers stationed in Great Britain was 15.30 per thousand, almost the same as that of soldiers stationed in the northern United States (15.00) and slightly lower than for France (20.17). Mortality rates in the West Indies were from six to more than eight times higher, from 85.00 in the Windward and Leeward Islands to 130.00 in Jamaica. In the British colonies in southern Asia mortality rates were slightly better, ranging from 17.70 in the Straits Settlements to 71.41 in Bengal. (The Dutch East Indies, notorious throughout the eighteenth century, had a rate of 170.00 per thousand.) Throughout the nineteenth century, Sierra Leone was known as "the white man's grave." Military records indicate that this association was no exaggeration, for the annual mortality rate for Europeans stationed there was 483.00 per thousand, more than thirty times that of England. Every year, in other words, *almost half* of the soldiers stationed there died. In one of the most influential texts on colonial medicine during the Romantic and Victorian periods, *The Influence of Tropical Climates on European Constitutions*, James Ranald Martin clarifies the meaning of these statistics when he remarks that a

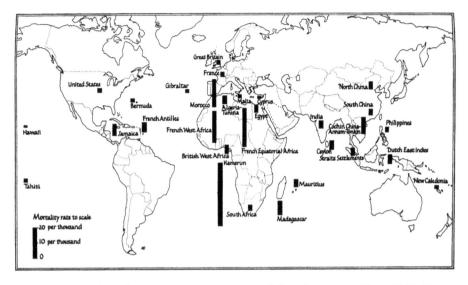

M A P 1. Mortality of European troops at home and abroad, 1817–38. From Philip D. Curtin, *Death by Migration: Europe's Encounter with the Tropical World in the Nineteenth Century* (Cambridge: Cambridge UP, 1989).

male over one hundred years old had a better statistical likelihood of living an entire year in England than a young soldier had in Sierra Leone (75).[8] Soldiers paid a much higher price than settlers or colonial administrators and servants, especially since most were males aged twenty to forty, a group that in normal circumstances would have had an annual mortality rate far below that of the general population.

Romanticism and Colonial Disease focuses on the British cultural response to colonial disease, how medical and literary writers from roughly the end of the eighteenth century to the middle of the nineteenth attempted to understand their own biomedical identities in relation to these new, more dangerous disease environments that colonial contact had brought into being.[9] Native cultures are not the only ones that developed myths about disease, and one objective of analyzing the British cultural response to colonial disease is to suggest why, indeed, the enormous loss of life associated with European colonialism remains an ever present yet rarely discussed aspect of colonial life, even within postcolonial criticism. The book charts a deepening British understanding of the scale and extent of colonial disease and mortality and the growing anxiety their insecurity aroused. The British experience of disease raised questions about where colonial contact begins and ends as the imperial metropole with its heterogeneous, impoverished, and anonymous populations seemed more and more to be a simulacrum of the periphery. Questions about the epidemiological cost, even the biological possibility, of a British empire are an increasingly important part of this writing.

Although there was a dramatic drop in the mortality rates of colonial servicemen over the course of the nineteenth century, through improvements in sanitation and hygiene combined with the increased use of quinine, military "invalidism" actually increased.[10] We lack adequate figures on how many people were "invalided" during the period. Nevertheless, by the early nineteenth century medical works were devoting considerable attention to the special requirements of this new kind of patient, people who returned home, as Charles Curtis remarked, with "a constitution, wasted and debilitated by the diseases of those climates; from which they recover with difficulty, or not at all" (171). For instance, Martin included a section of "practical observations on the nature and treatment of the diseases of Europeans on their return from tropical climates." Robert Dundas added to his *Sketches of Brazil* the ominous subtitle *Remarks on a Premature Decay of the System Incident to Europeans on Their Return from Hot Climates* (1852). By the end of the nineteenth century, far more servicemen were being discharged because of ill health than were dying overseas. This rising number suggests that the British did not learn about the risks of colonial activity solely from newspapers or correspondence. They discovered them at all levels of society: in the sick and indigent soldiers and sailors inhabiting their streets and hospitals; in colonial administrators, clerks, and officers seeking cures for chronic health complaints at the many resorts that were springing up everywhere; in the children of East Indian and African colonists who were being raised in England for fear that if they stayed in the colonies they would grow up sickly and degenerate; in the retired nabobs, such as Jos Sedley of Thackeray's *Vanity Fair*, who returned to England with wealth but not health; in women whose mental and reproductive capacities were feared to have been permanently damaged by the impact of tropical heat on their nerves and generative organs. "Tropical invalids" were figures of colonial return. In these people, the British saw not only the extent of their involvement in colonial activity but also its negative effect on their constitutions. Colonial disease was not therefore something that existed "over there." It was continually being registered in the bodies of sailors, soldiers, colonial clerks, missionaries, women, and administrators who had been to the tropics and returned. Encounters with tropical invalids in the literature of this period thus embody an entire range of attitudes toward colonialism and the world it produced.

I will say more about the impact of disease on colonists over the course of this book. Let me emphasize here that these high rates of mortality and invaliding were not simply statistics. Most people in Britain would have known someone who had died or been invalided through colonialism. Take, for instance, the range of personal and family connections that linked the writers of the Romantic period to colonialism and disease. Robert Southey's brother Tom was a sailor stationed in the Caribbean; Wordsworth's brother John was employed in the East India trade and drowned off the coast of England. Coleridge had two brothers who served in the military in India. Both died there in their twenties, John (1754–87) of consumption and Frank (1770–92) of a gunshot wound, self-inflicted in the confusion of fever. Coleridge writes: "He shot himself (having been left carelessly by his attendant) in a delirious fever brought on by his excessive exertions at the siege of Seringapatam" (*Collected Letters* 1: 311). After an abortive attempt at joining a company of dragoons and the failure of the Pantisocracy scheme, Coleridge considered emigrating to the West Indies. He looked to the patronage of John Pinney Senior, who not only had plantations on the sugar island of Nevis but owned Alfoxden, where Wordsworth was staying in 1798.[11] Sir Walter Scott had one brother who served in the navy under Rodney, another who was a major in the army, another who was paymaster to the Seventieth Regiment in Canada, and another who emigrated to Jamaica. De Quincey's father derived his income from trade in West Indian cotton, and he noted, referring to his uncle Thomas Penson, that "everybody has an Indian uncle" (*Collected Writings* 7: 22). Tracing his lineage on his father's side back to Barbados, Leigh Hunt emphasized in a number of works that he came from "a tropical race," suggesting that these origins explained certain aspects of his literary style: "What might have been affectation in a colder blood, was only enthusiasm in a warm one" (*Men, Women, and Books* iv).

Thomas Moore was a colonial administrator in Bermuda from 1803 to 1804. Charles Lamb and Thomas Love Peacock were both employed by the East India Company, the latter designing colonial gunboats. Before becoming Byron's private physician, Polidori considered taking a position in India, and in 1821 Shelley investigated working for an Indian prince. While a schoolboy at Eton, Shelley was greatly influenced by James Lind, who had served many years as a physician in India. Keats, like Thomas Chatterton before him, considered becoming a surgeon on an Indiaman. After the death of his brother Tom he resided in Wentworth Place, which his friend Charles Armitage Brown purchased with money he inherited on the sudden death of his brother James, an official of the East India Company. In Pisa Shelley renewed his friendship with his second cousin Thomas Medwin, now an invalid after serving six years as a lieutenant in the Twenty-fourth Light Dragoons stationed in Cawnpore, India, from 1813 to 1818. It was there, as part of the Grand Army of Lord Hastings, that Medwin met Edward Ellerker Williams, who was also an officer (in the Eighth Light Dragoons), and Jane Cleveland Johnson, who (unable to divorce her husband) lived with him as his wife. Williams drowned with Shelley in the Gulf of Spezia, and Edward Trelawny, who wrote a romantic account of his adventures in India, helped Byron cremate them. Charlotte Smith had four sons who survived to maturity. Two became civil servants in Bengal. Her third son, Charles, entered military service; shortly after losing a leg at Dunkirk in 1793, he died of yellow fever in Barbados. Her youngest son, George Augustus, became a lieutenant in the Sixteenth Foot and died of fever in Surinam in 1806. Jane Austen, whose father was a trustee of a plantation in Antigua, had two brothers who served in the British navy: Francis, who eventually became an admiral, served in India, the West Indies, and British North America. Charles Austen married the daughter of the attorney general of Bermuda, and after serving in the Mediterranean and the West Indies, he died of cholera in 1852 while serving on the Irrawaddy River in Burma.[12] Mary Shelley's half brother, William Godwin Jr., also died of cholera, and Coleridge may have contracted the disease in late 1831 and early 1832; Williams and Medwin were among the first Europeans to witness its pandemic outbreak in India in 1817.

Probably the best-known death from colonial disease is that of Byron, who died in the malaria-infested marshes of Missolonghi. But he was not the only writer to die prematurely. After inheriting two plantations in Jamaica when his father died in 1812, Matthew "Monk" Lewis, who wrote the *Journal of a West Indian Proprietor* (1733), visited the island twice, once in 1815 and again in 1818. Leaving England on his second voyage, Lewis left explicit instructions that if his mother's health were to decline, he was not to be informed: "It would affect me too heavily, and might kill me in such a climate" (Baron-Wilson 2: 191). Shortly after arriving in Jamaica early in February, Lewis wrote to his mother, "My health [is] still in perfection" (2: 207). By the end of March he seems to have developed an unbounded confidence about his prospects: "You see, I am still alive; and I am also still *well,* which is strange enough, for I have been doing everything that makes other people die outright here; However, it has done me no harm, and I begin to believe (like Macbeth) that so long as I stay in Jamaica, "*I bear a charmed life*" (2: 226). The style of assertion here is typical of colonial discourse, for in claiming a "charmed life" and identifying himself with Macbeth, Lewis admits the threat that he simultaneously denies. British colonial discourse on disease frequently functions in this ironic mode. Shortly after Lewis left Jamaica to return to England on 4 May 1818, yellow fever broke out on board the ship. On 14 May, after more than a week of agony, Lewis was dead. When his coffin, draped in canvas, was dropped overboard, it rose to the surface. A fellow passenger remarks that "the wind getting under the canvass acted as a sail, and the body was slowly borne down the current away from us, in the direction of Jamaica" (2: 235).

Sir William Jones died of liver inflammation brought on by malaria in 1794. John Leyden (1775–1811), who achieved recognition by assisting Sir Walter Scott in collecting materials for the early volumes of the *Border Minstrelsy*, was considering following the lead of Mungo Park in Africa when his friends, fearing for his health, arranged to have him appointed assistant surgeon at Madras in 1803. For eight years, as a surgeon, naturalist, linguist, and judge, he published work on the geology, diseases, and languages of the region, though he was rarely in good health. In 1805 he wrote that he had suffered under a "pestilent state of health. . . . I have . . . been given up by the physicians three or four times within these last eleven months, as any one might very well be, afflicted at once with the four most formidable diseases of India, *i.e.* liver, spleen, bloody flux, and fever of the jungles, which is reckoned much akin to the African yellow fever" (Constable 1: 205). He died of malaria in the 1811 expedition against Java. Maria Jane Jewsbury (1800–1833) came to notice with the 1825 publication of *Phantasmagoria, or Sketches of Life and Literature.* A friend of both Wordsworth and Felicia Hemans, she published poetry, essays, and narratives. In 1832 she married William Kew Fletcher, and in September of that year she left England for India, where he had taken up a chaplaincy with the East India Company, dreading "nothing but the mosquitoes" (qtd. in Gillett lxi). After a short stay in Colombo, Ceylon, where her host, the senior chaplain, was Keats's friend Benjamin Bailey, she arrived in Bombay—"alias biscuit-oven, alias brick-kiln, alias burning Babel, alias Pandemonium, alias everything hot, horrid, glaring, barren, dissonant, and detestable." In June 1833 she suffered a mild attack of "demi-semi-cholera, only demi-semi" (lxiii). By October she was dead and buried at Poona. Wordsworth's comment sums up a prevailing view of the frequent outcome of colonial migration: "From the first we had a fore-feeling that it would be so" (*Letters* 5: 719).

Jewsbury was not the only female British poet to die in India. Emma Roberts (1794–1840), a close friend of Letitia Landon, accompanied her newly married sister to India in 1828, living in the stations of Agra, Etawah, and Cawnpore, where she published a volume of poetry titled *Oriental Scenes.*[13]

With the early death of her sister in 1831 she moved to Calcutta, where she edited the newspaper *Oriental Observer* and became a noted contributor to the *Asiatic Journal* (many of these papers appearing in 1835 in the three-volume *Scenes and Characteristics of Hindoostan*). In 1832 Roberts was forced to return to England because of ill health. In 1839, however, having established herself as "the domestic historian of India" (Roberts xx), she went back there with a view to examining the social transformations taking place with the disappearance of the East India Company. Weakened by fever during the overland journey, she suffered a progressive gastrointestinal infection after her arrival in India. In April 1840 she writes: "My health is failing me, and I can scarcely bear any increased subject of anxiety" (xxiv). On 16 September she died at Poona, where she had gone for a "change of air," and was buried near the grave of Jewsbury.

As a study of the geographical dimensions of disease during the Romantic period, *Romanticism and Colonial Disease* examines the role played in the making and unmaking of national and cultural identities by ideas about the geographical distribution of diseases and what kind of people were susceptible to them. Geography framed diseases during the colonial period, and this pathologizing of the globe was instrumental both in describing the biomedical boundaries of the modern world and in bringing them into being. The period can thus be understood as an ongoing negotiation of this geographical frame, with its continually fluctuating and uncertain boundaries. Disease narratives provided a means of differentiating colonizers from the colonized, but these distinctions were often fragile and subject to change. European colonists had reason to be nervous about the new diseases they encountered in the contact zones. Diseases played a key role in producing difference as they provided an apparent racial or biological basis for asserting them, but their communicability also established a profound link with those being defined as other. This book adopts a form of ecological materialism inasmuch as it argues that the colonial world was radically shaped by the globalization of disease. My concentration, however, is on the cultural impact of this new disease reality. In this regard Smallpox's comment to Saynday—"No people who have looked on me will ever be the same"—applies as much to the British as to other groups, as they too struggled to understand these new disease environments and the people who inhabited them. The time roughly between the middle of the eighteenth and nineteenth centuries is crucial in the emergence of cultural constructions of disease. In this period, when substantially more colonists died from disease than by the late nineteenth century, the British became more and more anxious about the epidemiological implications of colonialism, not only for those who went abroad but for those who stayed home. These anxieties emerged most clearly after 1817, when pandemic cholera broke out in Bengal.

As I will argue throughout this book, medical geography played a primary role in the construction of "foreignness." During this period "the tropics" emerge as a unique biomedical construct. Originally the word was a mete-orological and astronomical term, referring to the climatic region lying be-tween the Tropic of Cancer and the Tropic of Capricorn, the two latitudes where the sun turns back or "tropes" the earth. Much of the early medical discourse on the tropics was about "climate" and its impact on European bodies or "constitutions." Yet, as Curtin notes, "People die from disease, not from climate, and the world contains many different disease environments, each with a range of viruses and bacteria that differ in varying degrees from those found elsewhere. Physical environment and climate obviously play a role, but epidemiological differences exist even where physical environment is the same" ("Epidemiology and the Slave Trade" 194–95). Over the course of the eighteenth century, though "climate" continued to be used to describe these environments, a much more sophisticated conception of the causes of illness in the tropics emerged, one that ascribed pathogenic qualities to a range of environmental, economic, and social factors. The "tropics" thus shifted from being a climatic term to being a social, biological, and medical construction. Central to this construction was the notion that the tropics were fundamentally sick and needed to be cured if they were ever to become fully habitable for human beings. Not only were they perceived as pathogenic spaces, but the kinds of diseases associated with them were also seen as more dangerous, more extreme, more loathsome. Whereas native peoples were being destroyed by a panoply of Old World diseases, the diseases that most frightened Europeans were the tropical ones—malaria, yellow fever, dysen-tery, cholera. Also, the malignity of common European diseases was felt to increase under the rays of a tropical sun. Perhaps malaria and yellow fever were simply more intense forms of the common agues and autumnal fevers of England. Perhaps yellow fever was typhus fever in a particularly intensified tropical form. Maybe leprosy was but an Eastern form of syphilis. Concepts of health and disease are relative matters. Europeans' representations of the trop-ics as a diseased space reflected their own experience there. Medical geogra-phy was a European invention, and as such it was a powerful expression of how Europeans saw the world and the distribution of diseases across it. One legacy of this endeavor, however, was that it pathologized large regions of the globe, dividing the world into those regions, like Europe, that were considered healthy and those that, for various reasons, needed to be cured if they were to become truly habitable.

The cultural consequences of the European biomedical construction of the tropics remain a central concern of this book. The world brought into being by colonial expansion, however, extended beyond the tropics. During the colonial period, disease environments were themselves undergoing radical changes, as new diseases under new conditions supplanted or settled alongside old ones. Here I examine how the British struggled to understand their place in this radically new world, where diseases no longer stayed put but traveled from place to place with the movement of peoples. Throughout I employ a *relational* or *differential* model of disease, arguing that British people's conceptions of their own biomedical identity were formulated within a global context, as part of their own response to the experience of colonial disease. In defining the healthiness of their part of the globe, they postulated other regions that were unhealthy or productive of other, nastier diseases. British "healthiness" was thus fundamentally structured in relation and often in opposition to colonial disease environments. My object is not to conflate diseases, but to suggest how tropical disease was instrumental in the construction of a British biomedical identity. Most diseases during this period cannot be understood without reference to colonial environments, and just as important, colonial environments cannot be understood without reference to the structurings of medical geography. The "tropics" were not, therefore, simply the dark edge bordering a Western biomedical identity; they were intrinsic to its formulation.[14] As time went on the boundaries between Europe and its pathological other seemed harder to maintain even as greater efforts were made to affirm them. Placing disease in the tropics—itself a comforting gesture, at least for those at home—became increasingly difficult to do.

Just as the transmission of disease was not a one-way street, neither was its cultural understanding. This book explores how the British learned to read themselves through colonial otherness.[15] This relational identity, I will stress, was constructed at a time of tremendous anxiety about England's inescapable immersion in the colonial marketplace of pathogens. In this regard the striking emergence of a British cultural emphasis on hygiene and discipline, on avoiding "unsafe" behavior, can itself be seen as an anxious response to colonial disease. Despite the attempts to control "tropical disease" by keeping the "tropics" at a geographical or climatic distance or by insisting that colonists maintain special moral and dietary discipline, the British grew worried about their susceptibility to sickness at home, an anxiety heightened by the succession of cholera pandemics that began in 1817. Having constructed "tropical" otherness, yet recognizing that the sources of tropical illness lay less in the climate than in a host of other factors, they deeply feared that being English was no guaranteed prophylactic. Perhaps England—or at least certain social groups within England—might also be tropicalized. Fear about the pathogenic conditions and character of the working class, initially refracted on poor Irish immigrants but then applied to the inhabitants of urban slums, drew much of its power from comparisons with colonial peoples. Maybe colonialism was making the English vulnerable to a "foreignness within" as it was producing spaces and peoples in England whose increasing cultural or social "foreignness" provided tropical diseases with a means of invading English society.[16] Maybe "foreign" diseases were not so foreign after all: perhaps, like malaria, they had always already been there, hidden, waiting for the right moment to reappear with increased virulence. Maybe all that was required was the heat of the factory or the overcrowding of an urban slum to transform a familiar endemic fever into its virulent tropical form.

In both the East and West Indies, tropical medicine already played a vital role in the colonies long before it was institutionalized during the 1890s in the medical schools of the metropolitan centers of empire. Since the contact zones were where the new reality of colonial disease was felt most immediately, and since these were the places where traditional disease ecologies were changing most rapidly, colonial physicians were among the first to understand this new reality and its implications for traditional ideas of the distribution and causes of diseases. In contexts where they saw the rapid emergence of new diseases and the disappearance of others, colonial physicians were the first to recognize the dynamic nature of modern disease ecologies. A central thesis of this book is that British people's understanding of their own place within this global disease exchange substantially derived from perspectives of colonial physicians on infectious disease, especially fevers. Although it took time, the British eventually grasped the fact, which modern epidemiologists have been rediscovering, that developed nations inherit the problems of emerging ones. During the early nineteenth century they learned to interpret their own susceptibility to epidemic disease through the experience of colonial physicians, military personnel, and settlers. In medical as well as cultural terms, they read themselves through their colonial others, even as they sought to reinforce boundaries.[17]

Anxiety about disease is rampant during the period. Percy Bysshe Shelley worried that English society was on the brink of being invaded by elephantiasis. Thomas De Quincey, as John Barrell observes, "was terrorised by the fear of an unending and interlinked chain of infections from the East, which threatened to enter his system and to overthrow it, leaving him visibly and permanently 'compromised' and orientalised" (15). He magnifies these anxieties as he describes his "Oriental dreams," in which "tropical heat" and "vertical sun-lights" provide the "connecting feeling" that brings together "all creatures, birds, beasts, reptiles, all trees and plants, usages and appearances, that are found in all tropical regions, and assembled them together in China or Indostan." In these nightmares all tropical regions share the same pathogenic identity. All are below "Cancer," and contact is contagious: "I was kissed, with cancerous kisses, by crocodiles; and laid, confounded with all unutterable slimy things, amongst reeds and Nilotic mud" (*Confessions* 109). In 1832 Samuel Taylor Coleridge wrote a poem advising the lower classes how to avoid the cholera shortly after he himself had recovered from it. Mary Shelley's *The Last Man* provides the most powerful articulation of the anxieties of the period, as she imagines a pandemic that destroys not only England but the entire human race. To the extent that this book recounts a general narrative, it describes the emergence among the British of global epidemiological anxieties, their increasing concern, even as they sought to keep the tropics at a safe geographical and cultural distance, that commercial and military expansion had left no place on earth safe from the diseases of others.

Common literary periodizations do not necessarily dovetail with those of medicine. Although with some exceptions the primary literary texts discussed here were written between 1780 and 1832, the medical context—focused on the emergence of the medical discourse on tropical environments—spans the broader period when topographical and environmental medicine was the dominant paradigm, from the rediscovery of Hippocrates in the late seventeenth century to the discovery of the bacterial transmission of disease in the 1870s. Definitions and periodizations of "colonialism" and "imperialism" are equally fraught with difficulties. The high point of British imperialism is normally understood as 1870 to 1914, when European nations scrambled to establish global empires. These years also roughly correspond to the rise of bacteriology as the dominant paradigm for medical practice. Yet as Martin Green suggests, the literature of imperialism has a much longer history, extending as far back as the late seventeenth century, with the union of England and Scotland (5). My attention therefore is on a very dynamic time in history, which in economic, political, and medical terms laid the foundations for the more actively pursued imperialism of the latter half of the nineteenth century. To distinguish the medical and literary culture produced during this earlier period from the more strident imperialism of late Victorian Britain, I use the word "colonialism" throughout. It refers not only to the physical undertaking of establishing settlements outside Britain but also to the cultural, ideological, and medical discourses that emerged with colonial expansion and contact. At the same time, I am cognizant that in some regions, particularly India, an imperial framework was largely established, culturally and politically, by the beginning of the nineteenth century.

Another reason I use "colonialism" more frequently than "imperialism" is to emphasize the fundamental fact that British expansion was made possible by real bodies entering and producing new disease environments. Whereas imperial relationships were of many kinds, some more explicitly forms of dominance than others, colonialism required bodies to travel from one place to another. The epidemiological consequences of this activity are the subject of this book. Early on, relatively little attention was given to the epidemiological costs of territorial expansion. By the nineteenth century these costs were an intrinsic part of colonial discourse, whether on moral, economic, or medical grounds. More abstract versions of colonialism that do not find it necessary to consider bodies that can get sick and die, therefore, are of less interest to me here. My own perspective is "postcolonial," not because I am engaged in a critique of European colonialism (Who nowadays is not?) but because I seek to place British culture within the globalized disease context that is one of its major legacies.

Sheila M. Rothman, in a groundbreaking study of the history of tuberculosis, has called for a new kind of history of disease that proceeds "from the perspective of the patient" rather than the doctor. "To move patients to the center of a history," she suggests, "requires breaking out of the language and constructs of medicine" (1). *Romanticism and Colonial Disease* is strongly influenced by this approach. It was originally conceived as a larger study of the nineteenth-century British colonial culture of disease, one that would seek to recover in detail, by analyzing letters, journals, diaries, and other biographical materials, how colonists thought about the new diseases and disease environments they were encountering. Material of this kind does appear here and will be the subject of future work. But early on it became apparent that some of the most important literature of the Romantic period offered an ideal opportunity for understanding the complex ways the British responded to colonial disease—in the West Indies, in Africa, and then in India.[18] Writers rather than patients are thus at the center of this book, but one should nevertheless recognize that many—among them Coleridge, Percy Bysshe Shelley, Keats, and De Quincey—were frequently sick, and that these anxieties shape both their writing about disease and their understanding of their place in a British colonial world. On the other hand, Wordsworth was, as is well known, intrepidly healthy, a fact not lost on contemporaries as they made him into an English cultural icon and read his health as a confirmation of the healthiness of his poetry. Even as this book contributes to the social history of disease by discussing the British framing of colonial disease, there-fore, its primary interest is in how writers during this period complicate this framing. Literary texts are primary cultural documents, which shape culture in profound ways and frequently offer a far more complex picture of cultural manifestations than many other written documents. Rather than seeking to show how writers *reflect* cultural assumptions and stereotypes about disease, therefore, I am interested in the complex ways they think through these ideas. At the same time, I hope this book will offer a new perspective on a wide range of Romantic literature whose struggle with colonial disease has not been adequately appreciated.

In many studies of the nineteenth century Romanticism appears in a rela-tively poor light, for it is frequently equated with the idealizing or mytholo-gizing of disease. This status, for better or worse, suggests that one cannot comprehend how Europeans in the nineteenth century understood disease without attending to the primary role this literature played in its representa-tion. However, I also suggest that Romantic attitudes toward colonialism and disease were far more complex and far less stable than has been thought. Many of the texts take no univocal position on colonialism, as readers are presented with alternative, often contradictory, views. In this regard I am very much indebted to recent work on Romanticism and colonialism, most nota-bly by Nigel Leask and John Barrell.[19] Literature cannot be understood apart from the historical contexts to which it contributes, so my readers will find the analysis of individual works of literature set alongside a wide range of historical materials that provide a context for examining the complex and often surprising ways they responded to the colonial disease world.

Colonial geography was, as much recent criticism has suggested, a gen-dered construction, in which race and sexuality were superimposed on each other. During the eighteenth and nineteenth centuries, colonial regions were frequently gendered as female spaces making themselves available to the ex-plorer, the settler, the adventurer. Especially in literary romances, colonialism is portrayed in terms of the male desire for adventure and for territorial and sexual conquest.[20] There is a danger, however, in representing colonial expe-rience as if it were an early advertisement for Club Med. Its complex sexuali-ties, as diverse then as now, should not be sensationalized and reduced to sim-plified patterns. The overlapping of discourses on sexuality, race, gender, and geography produced unstable and often contradictory relationships. More-

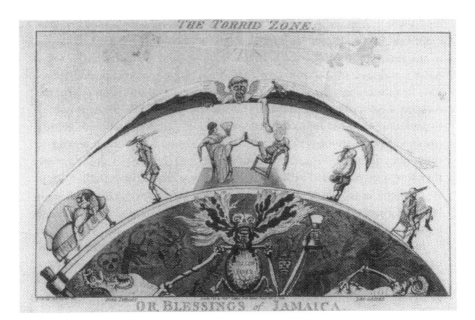

FIG. 1. A. J., *The Torrid Zone, or Blessings of Jamaica* (1800). The Wellcome Institute Library, London.

over, the gendering of the globe must also be read within the context of its pathologizing. Colonialism is indeed a discourse of desire, but the bodies that appear within it are less frequently healthy than anxious about their fragility either in the face of larger natural and social environments or in relation to other bodies (indigenous or foreign) that constitute an implicit threat. Fears about disease radically complicate colonial romance, as sexuality, disease, race, and tropical environments are mapped onto each other in extremely complex ways.

The colored aquatint *The Torrid Zone, or Blessings of Jamaica* (1800) (fig. 1) provides a graphic illustration of one version of these relationships. Patterned at once on traditional cosmographies and anatomical descriptions of the eye, the illustration is divided into three realms. In the upper, heavenly sphere, under the harsh light of a tropical sun, an angel/demon with a bottle of opium in hand hangs his leg over the horizon as he peers out. On one side is Leo, the astrological emblem of British power; on the other is the symbol of disease, Cancer. Below, colonists are engaged in their normal leisure occupations: one man reads a paper, a woman lies on a settee, and typical of the region's reputation for heavy drinking and sexual activity, a couple engage in sexual foreplay. Yet one cannot miss that these preoccupations take place on a scythe held by yellow fever, which divides the terrestrial realm from the pathogenic hell beneath them. Yellow fever with an hourglass in one skeletal hand is flanked by a man suffering from "sore throat" and another with "dry gripes." In the background a phantasmagoria of tribal images, demons, skulls, snakes, and lizards evokes the Torrid Zone as a "heart of darkness."

This illustration suggests that in considering European ideas of colonial race and sexuality we should not focus too exclusively on colonial hedonism—the middle ground—without considering the broader pathogenic contexts within which it was also understood. Rather than offering an easy fulfillment of masculine desire, the colonial world more frequently required a complex negotiation of disease and desire. Colonial narratives are filled with accounts of individuals who are said to have been excessively preoccupied with drinking, eating, and sex; yet one usually learns of these pursuits retroactively, as an explanation of why these people are now dead, invalided, or insane. Maria Falconbridge's offhand comment on the death of the captain of a cutter in Sierra Leone is typical of colonial discourse: "He drank too freely, and returning a little indisposed, signified a wish of going to the French factory for medical assistance" (84–85). Benjamin Moseley argued that "health is retainable by Europeans in hot climates," but it seemed that Europeans, when faced with "the rigid restrictions, and self-denials, which are still necessary to keep the body and soul in unison" in the tropics, proved "dissatisfied to exist in the insipid security of temperance" and seized "the present hour of pleasure, and dangerous enjoyment" (*A Treatise on Tropical Diseases* 2). In his *Narrative of a Five Years' Expedition against the Revolted Negroes of Surinam,* John G. Stedman noted the unusual physical debility of the planters. They were "as dry and sapless as a squeesed lemon—owing to their intemperate way of living such as late hours—hard drinking—and particularly their too frequent intercourse with the negro and mulatto female sex" (49). Although the colonial world offered increased sexual opportunities, Stedman's desire to maintain his health in this environment imposed a new set of constraints. In fact, in talking about the relationship of European bachelors and female slaves, he subordinated sexuality to nursing: "These Gentlemen all without Exception have a female Slave mostly a creole in their keeping who preserves their linnens clean and decent, dresses their Victuals with Skill, carefully attends them they being most excellent nurses during the frequent illnesses to which Europeans are exposed in this Country" (47). What has frequently been taken as a discourse on the fulfillment of desire, therefore, was more frequently about the necessity to regulate it. To the European, sexuality and the tropics were often linked as modes of disorder and sources of disease, an analogy that would be invoked again in descriptions of the tropicalized bodies of the urban working class. Faced with the dangerous climatic extremes that characterized tropical environments, British colonists increasingly sought to maintain a "temperate" climate within themselves, as a kind of prophylactic. By the later nineteenth century, notes Philippa Levine, the dangers of the tropics and of sex were powerfully fused: "Tropical sex, like tropical disease, was a cankerous entity unchecked by Western mores and *malignant*. Both—sex and disease—required the full power of medical, military, and judicial force to control the potential of contamination" (602). If diseases were products of disorder, either of places or of peoples, then colonists more than others needed to maintain regulation and discipline to ward off sickness. It is striking how far discipline shaped the lives of British, and especially Scottish, colonists. Read within the context of colonial epidemiology, the British emphasis on discipline may be less the expression of an intrinsic national moral outlook than a reflection of epidemiological anxiety—a fear that perhaps self-control was the only thing that might keep one alive.

ONE

Romantic Medical Geography

Empire, Disease, and the
Construction of Pathogenic Environments

Disease in India is not disease in England.
     —Charles Morehead, letter (1882)

In some countries foreigners and natives are as differently
affected by certain contagious disorders, as if they had
been different animals.
     —Charles Darwin, *The Voyage of the "Beagle"*

James Lind's description of the coastal regions of West Africa in his *Essay on Diseases Incidental to Europeans in Hot Climates* (1768) demonstrates that medical and aesthetic appreciations of landscape are not equivalent. "Upon examining the face of the country," he writes, "it is found clothed with a pleasant and perpetual verdure; but altogether uncultivated, excepting a few spots, which are generally surrounded with forests or thickets of trees, impenetrable to refreshing breezes, and fit only for the resort of wild beasts" (40–41). Lind's depiction of a land that is aesthetically pleasing, yet sick, can be usefully compared with another, Jane Eyre's description of the environs of the Lowood Orphan Asylum, which is also shaped as much by the language of medical geography as by aesthetics. It appears to be an idyllic scene. In spring "Lowood shook loose its tresses; it became all green, all flowery; its great elm, ash, and oak skeletons were restored to majestic life; woodland plants sprang up profusely in its recesses; unnumbered varieties of moss filled its hollows, and it made a strange ground-sunshine out of the wealth of its wild primrose plants"

(Brontë, *Jane Eyre* 76–77). Jane declares that "all this I enjoyed often and fully, freed, unwatched, and almost alone." The "unwonted liberty" that underlies what is almost a parody of Romantic naturalism, however, has been made possible by an outbreak of typhus at Lowood, which Jane blames on these very surroundings. An extraordinary dynamic thus underlies this landscape and its appreciation. Not only is it a diseased space, but disease has provided the conditions for its appreciation:

Have I not described a pleasant site for a dwelling, when I speak of it as bosomed in hill and wood, and rising from the verge of a stream? Assuredly, pleasant enough: but whether healthy or not is another question.

That forest-dell, where Lowood lay, was the cradle of fog and fog-bred pestilence; which, quickening with the quickening spring, crept into the Orphan Asylum, breathed typhus through its crowded school-room and dormitory, and, ere May arrived, transformed the seminary into an hospital. (77)

Recent work has shown that landscapes are social constructions and a primary medium for the representation of class and gender ideologies.[1] Brontë's description of Lowood suggests the important role that contemporary medical descriptions of "healthy" and "unhealthy" landscapes played in eighteenth- and nineteenth-century ideas of place. Brontë sets medicine against aesthetics, reading the physical environs of Lowood as a doctor would—as a "disease landscape." In the dense forest, with its profusion of "woodland plants," "unnumbered varieties of moss," and moisture-loving "primroses" and its many "recesses" and "hollows" where air is confined, she sees a strong indication of the presence of disease. Such landscapes may be "pleasant enough: but whether healthy or not is another question": as the "cradle" of "fog-bred pestilence," Lowood is uninhabitable.

This comparison of two "disease landscapes," spanning roughly a century, suggests that during this period medical ideas were not removed from the appreciation of landscapes but were instrumental in their differentiation and evaluation. Places, localities, and regions were thoroughly medicalized, as ideas drawn from medical geography (or medical topography, as it was frequently called) contributed fundamentally to how the British understood what George Levine has called "the geography of ordinary England" (204).[2] Whether in parts of England, in the nation as a whole, or in colonial regions, medicine shaped how space was perceived. Medical geography, with its focus on pathogenic places, provided a vocabulary, which has not been adequately recognized, for conceiving colonial spaces as places that were sick and needed to be cured.

Disease Landscapes

In 1792 Leonhard Ludwig Finke published the first two volumes of his three-volume *Versuch einer allgemeinen medicinisch-praktischen Geographie.* Often considered the first major text in medical geography, this publication marks the emergence of a medical discourse that was not only geographical in concern but global in scope, a science that sought to map the world's diseases, establishing correlations between the "places" where people lived and the diseases they suffered from.[3] "I have looked at the whole world from a medical point of view," Finke writes (qtd. in Barrett, "Medical Geographical Anniversary" 702). The idea that diseases have specific geographical ranges rather than being universally distributed across the globe was not new. Finke himself notes that it was a central tenet of Hippocratic medicine, forcefully articulated in *Of Airs, Waters, and Places,* an essay proposing that environments determine the diseases people suffer from.[4] The Bible also has served not only, in Northrop Frye's terms, as the "great code of art" but also as the great code of pathogenic geography. Through its depictions of the plagues of Egypt and the sufferings of Job, of blindness, leprosy, and plague, the Bible emphatically links disease with the Holy Land and establishes an equally pervasive link between disease and the transgression of moral codes.

European disease geographies can be seen as projecting Western fears onto other regions of the globe. But these representations were not simply the product of the ethnocentric inscription of pathologies onto blank spaces. They also constitute complex negotiations between biology and culture, articulated over a long history of colonial encounters. Europeans did not locate plague and leprosy in the "East" just because they had read the Bible: they had firsthand experience of the disastrous epidemiological consequences of their efforts to colonize the Middle East during the Crusades, and they knew that plague regularly traveled along the trade routes opened up to the East. The enormous population losses suffered by the indigenous peoples of the New World and the South Pacific made it quite clear that new diseases usually come from "somewhere else" and that colonial contact was structured by disease. Sir Thomas Browne provided a perceptive understanding of the dynamics of colonial disease when he declared that "the mercy of God hath scattered the great heap of diseases, and not loaded any one country with all: some may be new in one country which have been old in another. New discoveries of the earth discover new diseases; for besides the common swarm, there are endemial and local infirmities proper unto certain regions, which in the whole earth make no small number: and if Asia, Africa, and America should bring in their list, Pandora's Box would swell, and there must be a strange pathology" (4: 45). Browne recognizes both that different places frequently have different endemic and epidemic diseases and that no place is immune to disease. Geographical exploration is as much the discovery of new diseases as of new countries. Colonialism did indeed open up a biological Pandora's box, a world of unfamiliar diseases—"strange pathologies"—that constituted the anxiety-ridden horizon of colonialism.

Medical geography was thus not new, since human beings have always seen a connection between foreign diseases and foreign places, a link that colonial endeavors and narratives continually affirmed. What is distinctive about Finke's work, and that of others at this time, is the attempt to understand the geographic distribution of disease scientifically. As an undertaking that had enormous consequences for how nineteenth-century Europeans saw themselves and the world around them, medical geography constituted a radical medicalization of the globe. Not only were diseases considered *geographical* phenomena, but the entire world was mapped in terms of disease. Nations and societies were now compared and evaluated on a scientifically constructed axis according to the kinds of diseases that affected them and their success in dealing with them. The geography of nations was now largely rewritten in terms of the language of health, disease, and medical technology.

Such a mapping became possible because from the late seventeenth century until the emergence of modern germ theory in the 1870s, the dominant model of epidemic disease transmission was not contagion, but contamination. It was believed that people became sick, either directly or indirectly, from the noxious air or *miasmas* produced by the places where they lived. Since places rather than people produced disease, it was places more than people that were in need of curing. Especially in the nineteenth century, few physicians held a single, unitary model of the cause and transmission of disease, most believing that "the causes of epidemic diseases were multifactoral" (Cooter 90).[5] From the early eighteenth century onward, the focus of medical attention nevertheless shifted toward analysis of the disease-bearing aspects of physical environments. By the 1830s, with the emergence of the Sanitarian movement, the environmental cause of illness was raised almost to the level of dogma. In a period of major colonial expansion, geography and medicine were thus fundamentally linked. Medical theory, preeminently concerned with the description and analysis of "pathogenic environments," of "healthy" and "unhealthy" places, shaped how the colonial world was perceived.

The spread of disease was to be controlled in two ways. By locating and mapping the "unhealthy places" in a region, a country, or across the globe, physicians could ensure that everyday contact with them would be minimized or that proper safeguards could be taken when people moved through such areas. For the first time, Lloyd Stevenson observes, physicians were concerned with "putting disease on the map." Medical cartography emerged during the 1790s as American physicians attempted to understand the origins and spread of yellow fever epidemics, and it became increasingly important in England from the 1830s onward.[6] Once these "pathogenic places" had been identified, they could be modified and human beings might rid the earth of disease. By instituting proper methods of sanitation; by draining marshlands, which were believed to be the source of harmful miasmas; by improving the soil through agriculture and by avoiding its cultivation at certain times of the year; by cutting down forests or widening urban streets to improve ventilation; by ensuring that people lived at a distance from cemeteries, cesspools, marshes, tanneries, or slaughterhouses it was hoped that medicine might ultimately gain control over most human diseases. The health of people's bodies would be guaranteed by ensuring the health of their physical environments.

Without a knowledge of bacteria or of the role of vectors such as mosquitoes and lice in transmitting disease, many physicians, following Thomas Sydenham, believed the primary agent of transmission, especially for "fevers," was bad *air*, literally the "mal-aria." Although physicians differed on what caused the air to become noxious (putrid exhalations produced by decaying organic matter were the usual suspect), most agreed that disease would be controlled by improving its "salubrity." Since air itself was seen as the fundamental medium of fevers, meteorology became very much a concern of physicians. "Ventilation" takes on an almost mythical status in the medicine of the period, in accounts of "gaol fever," in naval doctors' recommendations about improving ventilation in ships, in an increasing emphasis on clearing forests and widening city streets, and in the burgeoning literature on the healthiness of sea air. Whether these diseased spots are narrow alleys, dockyards, lowlands, the depths of forests, or the confined spaces of jails, hospitals, ships, or small rooms, they can be cured by opening them up to the therapeutic power of breezes. Therapy, especially in regard to fevers, frequently amounted to a "change of air."

Since disease was perceived as a geographical phenomenon, physicians focused on constructing and interpreting landscapes, identifying those aspects of the environment that produced dangerous air. For the medical geographer, concerned with the global distribution of diseases, a key concern was "climate," a term derived from the traditional association of meteorology and medicine. Even more emphasis, however, was given to "medical topography," which sought to describe, Ludwig Finke notes, the disease-bearing features of "an individual locality" (qtd. in Barrett, "Medical Geographical Anniversary" 702). Concerned with mapping disease landscapes, medical topography thus worked alongside medical geography in the campaign against disease. In Johann Peter Frank's monumental treatise on public health titled *A System of Complete Medical Police* (1779–1817), a clear link is established between medical topography and state policy. "Humane physicians should be set to explore the nature, condition and constitution of the tiniest village," writes Frank. "They should investigate its diseases and their causes in the most precise detail" (qtd. in Rosen 187). He further notes that "correct topographies" are "an extremely important contribution for those who have to look after the health and well-being of a country. Every publicly employed physician or district physician, should supply the medical description of his region as accurately as possible, and compare every change in weather, every phenomenon concerning the healthiness of a place, with his site so that the science of the influence of human dwellings and the climate of each country becomes better known" (180).

Frank's emphasis on mapping disease landscapes in relation to climatic considerations should be set within the context of what Foucault has called "a politics of health, the consideration of disease as a political and economic problem for social collectivities which they must seek to resolve as a matter of overall policy" (166). England was more reluctant to support explicit state intervention in the area of public health. Nevertheless, by the late eighteenth century medical topographies had become integral to medical practice, not only through the identification of pathogenic places, but also through the commercial marketing of the increasingly popular "health spots." Thinking about disease and health had become inseparable from the medicalized representation of place.

Basing his observations on the belief that "the natural features and peculiarities of every locality affect materially the life and health of the inhabitants," James Martin provides a comprehensive model for how doctors are to interpret landscapes in medical terms. The "Medical Topographer," he writes,

should investigate all the circumstances which tend to deteriorate the human race, and to lower its vigour and vitality; all that relates to the external causes of diseases, their propagation, and their prevention; all plans for improving the physical, and, through it, the moral condition of the people. He should cultivate more extensively the medical topography of the empire. The natural features and peculiarities of every locality affect materially the life and health of the inhabitants. Any general system of sanitary inquiry should, therefore, embrace information respecting the surface and elevation of the ground, the stratification and composition of the soil, the supply and quality of the water, the extent of marshes and wet ground, the progress of drainage; the nature and amount of the products of the land; the condition, increase or decrease, and prevalent diseases of the animals maintained thereon; together with periodical reports of the temperature, pressure, humidity, motion, and electricity of the atmosphere. Without a knowledge of these facts it is impossible to draw satisfactory conclusions with respect to the occurrence of epidemic diseases, and variations in the rate of mortality and reproduction. (102)

Doctors must examine not only the physical "surface" of a locale (whether it is forested, under cultivation, marshland, and so on) but also soil composition, quality of water, and drainage; local animal species and the diseases they are subject to; and atmospheric factors such as pressure, temperature, winds, and electricity. The medicalization of space thus provided the theoretical grounds for the detailed study of local topographies and physical environments. Fundamental to this kind of medicine is the notion that the maladies of different global regions are unique. Nevertheless, these studies are subordinated to the larger theme of "improvement," since medical topography is concerned with "all plans for improving the physical, and, through it, the moral condition of the people."

Martin's assertion that the medical topographer should "cultivate more extensively the medical topography of the empire" reflects the close relation between medicine and colonialism. During the later eighteenth century and most of the nineteenth, a knowledge of the geography of disease was seen as fundamental to the successful expansion of empire. Since colonists in new regions of the world confronted pathogens against which they had not yet built up any immunity, and since medical geography was primarily a European enterprise, it is not surprising that colonial regions, especially those where Europeans' mortality rates were high, were largely viewed as "sick." (Here the exceptions provided by the "temperate" climates of Canada, the northern United States, Australia, South Africa, and especially New Zealand should be duly noted.) The importance of this global pathologizing of space to the politics and literature of empire has not been adequately recognized or understood, as critics frequently treat disease as a metaphor for something else. Among other effects, it "naturalized" disease, which was now believed to occupy space just as plants and animals did, with some "climates" breeding more of one kind of disease than another. For Robert Dundas, "diseases, not unlike plants and animals, have all their special climes and localities; and though their geographical distribution has not certainly been the object of that special consideration which it so justly deserves, it presents a field for investigation fraught with the highest interest to society, and which gives fair promise of an ample reward to those who would enter on its cultivation" (34). Nicolaas A. Rupke notes that in the medical geography of Alexander von Humboldt the analogy between the global distribution of infectious diseases and of plants is even more strongly emphasized. One of Humboldt's followers, Friedrich Schnurrer, remarks, "It is impossible to found a science of plants on the flora of a single region, but one must compare types of plants from across the earth; equally, an understanding of diseases is not possible when these are taken in isolation, but they must be considered in their totality, and nosological systems can only be constructed when the most important types of diseases and their causes have been compared" (qtd. in Rupke 298). These ideas influenced even the placement of military settlements in colonial regions. Since "the diseases of the tropics seem[ed], like the vegetable productions of the same regions, to be restricted to certain altitudes and particular degrees of temperature," garrisons were increasingly established at altitudes of more than 2,500 feet (Tulloch and Marshall 103).

By seeing disease as essentially geographical, a problem of places more than of peoples, colonial medicine provided a powerful ideological underpinning for European expansion. Since colonial regions were largely seen as "sick" environments that needed curing, medical geography provided a scientific rationale for making colonial ecologies more like those of Europe and thus introducing European methods of land use, social organization, and resource management. The colonization of bodies thus proceeded from, and was largely supported by, the medical colonization of physical space. If colonial peoples were sick, they could be cured by changing their environments. In this way medical geography was instrumental in shaping how Europeans looked at landscapes and the people who inhabited them. The appreciation of the aesthetic qualities of both national and foreign landscapes—embodied in fiction, travel literature, and anthropological narratives—was thus underwritten by powerful ideas about the role such spaces played in promoting health or disease. And these constructions of space often fundamentally influenced colonial settlement practices and attitudes. The "quest for beauty" is certainly a central feature of nineteenth-century colonial landscapes, which were increasingly made to conform to European ideas of the beautiful, the sublime, and the picturesque. But we misunderstand these landscapes if we ignore the colonists' "quest for health" and the ways environmental medicine supplied a template for distinguishing "sick" spaces from "healthy" ones and justified a pattern of land-use changes that promised to cure the former.

Tropical Medicine and the Framing of "Tropical Climates"

The diversity of environments analyzed and evaluated by medical geographers and topographers during this period is too extensive to address here. Instead I want to examine the biomedical framing of "tropical climates," otherwise known as hot, warm, torrid, or intemperate climates, for it was here that European colonization confronted its greatest epidemiological challenges. Tropical regions had long been portrayed as places of tremendous fertility and excessive growth. Yet just as important, they were spaces of disease (Sir Walter Raleigh called them "*Terrae Vitiosae*" [28]), and this idea lasted long after Europeans were disabused of their belief in the spontaneous richness of tropical soils.

In his magisterial study of the history of tropical medicine, Henry Harold Scott points out how little sense this field makes theoretically. "We have no definition of the term 'Tropical Medicine,'" he writes.

If we take its narrow interpretation as "disease restricted to the tropics," *i.e.* to 23° 27′ of latitude on either side of the equator, we could with a close approximation to the truth say that it is non-existent. If we extend our limits to "diseases met with in warm climates," this apparently small extension in reality comes to include nearly all the ills that flesh is heir to, except, perhaps, frost-bite, and even that might occur on the mountain heights of a country generally regarded as among warm climates— Fujiyama, Kilima-Njaro, Mount Kenya, for example. (1: vi)

An added problem is that the geographical distribution of diseases has not remained constant throughout history. Especially in the past five hundred years, largely as a result of colonialism, they have traveled, so that even if one could establish the "prevailing" tropical diseases, one would still need to specify a time span. Tuberculosis, for instance, was largely seen as a Western disease throughout the nineteenth century, yet by the middle of the twentieth it had become primarily a disease of tropical and underdeveloped regions. Given a context in which the subject of study seems to evade theoretical description, no wonder Andrew Balfour would remark that "there is in one sense no such thing as tropical medicine" (191). The emergence of tropical medicine during the eighteenth century (primarily in the East and West Indies), its growing importance throughout the nineteenth century, and its ultimate institutionalization as a medical field at the end of that century express the increasing sophistication with which European imperial nations grappled with the realities of colonial environments: the field both responded to and reinforced the European experience of these regions.[7] John Farley notes the fundamental relation between tropical medicine and imperialism: "The discipline arose as part of Western imperialism when explorers, military personnel, colonial administrators, businessmen, and finally settlers came face to face with a new set of diseases—tropical diseases, for which they had no answer and which were, at times, particularly virulent" (1).

The consequences of this pathologizing of large areas of the globe should not be minimized. "Tropical medicine," as a field that inherited the geographical assumptions of colonial medicine, played (and continues to play) a key role in this development. Of the relatively large number of eighteenth-century texts dealing with the specific diseases affecting Europeans in tropical regions, especially those by doctors who had stayed for some time in the West Indies, the best known and most influential was undoubtedly James Lind's *Essay on the Diseases Incidental to Europeans in Hot Climates,* which went through six editions between 1768 and its first American edition in 1811.[8] As its title indicates, Lind views tropical environments strictly from the perspective of their impact on the health of white Europeans. Although some doctors, especially those serving the slave plantations of the West Indies, dealt with the diseases of black slaves, it would take more than a century before European physicians began to study in detail the relation between tropical climates and indigenous populations. Biogeography—the field of natural history concerned with the geographical origin and distribution of plants and animals across the globe—shaped Lind's ideas of how climate influenced human health. Some climates, he observes, "are healthy and favourable to European constitutions, as some soils are favourable to the production of European plants. But most of the Countries beyond the limits of Europe, which are frequented by Europeans, unfortunately prove unhealthy to them" (2). In his introduction, Lind strikes a familiar note as he argues that the central factor in successful colonizing is not military power, but the control of disease. As proof, he cites "the unhappy fate" of "the Portuguese who, in the 15th and 16th centuries, spread their settlements over the coast of Guinea, and a great part of India. They *suffered* more by *sickness,* than by shipwreck, . . . [or] by their wars with the natives, and every other accident. In many places on the coast of Guinea, where they were formerly settled, we can now hardly trace any vestige of their posterity" (3). Lind suggests that they failed because of incorrect medical beliefs. Having observed that if settlers could avoid dying shortly after their arrival in the tropics they frequently remained in good health, the Portuguese concluded that during this period of "seasoning" their blood was changed by their diet. Hoping to speed up this process, they bled newly arrived Europeans, making them more vulnerable to fevers. Lind's

Essay aims to ensure the successful British colonization of tropical regions. In fact he speaks of it as a "sequel" to his *A Treatise on the Scurvy* (1753) and *An Essay on the most Effectual Means of Preserving the Health of Seamen* (1757). Having extended the capacity of the British navy to reach foreign lands, he now stresses the need to "preserve unimpaired their health and constitutions during their residence in a foreign climate" (xvii).[9]

Lind is typical in believing that fevers are caused primarily by the noxious vapors released from marshes or moist soil. Among the signs of an unhealthy country, he writes, is the appearance of "thick noisome fogs, rising chiefly after sun-set, from the vallies, and particularly from the mud, slime, or other impurities" (134). Such a view, with its emphasis on the role of heat, humidity, and rich soils in engendering pathogenic atmospheres, made the "tropics" places where disease was thought to be rampant. Thus Lind concludes that "on the whole face of the earth, there is scarce to be found a more unhealthy country" than tropical Guinea "during the rainy season" (66). He quotes from Robert Robertson's journal manuscript, later published as *A Physical Journal Kept on Board His Majesty's Ship "Rainbow," during Three Voyages to the Coast of Africa, and West Indies, in Years 1772, 1773, and 1774* (1777):

It seemed more wonderful to me, that any white people ever recover, while they continue to breathe so pestiferous an air. . . . We were, as I have already observed, thirty miles distant from the sea, in a country altogether uncultivated, overflowed with water, surrounded with thick, impenetrable woods, and over-run with slime. The air was vitiated, noisome, and thick, insomuch that lighted torches or candles burnt dim, and seemed ready to be extinguished; even the human voice lost its natural tone. The smell of the ground and of the houses was raw and offensive; the vapour arising from the putrid water in the ditches which surround the town, was much worse. All this however seemed tolerable, when compared with the infinite numbers of insects swarming every where, both on the ground and in the air, which as they seemed to be produced and cherished by the putrefaction of the atmosphere, so they contributed greatly to increase its impurity. (67–68)

West Africa is portrayed as a country "over-run with slime." Contaminated by the stink thrown up by rotting earth, marshy ooze, and putrid ditches, the air is so "vitiated, noisome, and thick," so "pestiferous," that even "candles burn dim." Robertson sees the "infinite numbers" of insects as another sign of a pathogenic environment, for in feeding off the "putrefaction of the atmosphere" they increase its impurity. What surprises Lind is that despite these dangers, European settlers appear to have done little to improve their situation. "It is not uncommon," he declares, "in many trading factories, to meet with a few Europeans, pent up in a small spot of low, damp ground, so entirely surrounded with thick woods, that they can scarcely have the benefit of walking a few hundred yards, and where there is not so much as an avenue cut through any part of the woods for the admission of wholesome and refreshing breezes" (49–50). Such environments, however, can be cured. "If any tract of land in Guinea was as well improved as the island of Barbadoes, and as perfectly freed from trees, underwood, marshes, etc.," Lind writes, "the air would be rendered equally healthful there, as in that pleasant West Indian island" (50).

The East Indies and the West Indies in general fare little better than West Africa, both being described as rampant with fever. The "number of English sacrificed to the climate" of Jamaica, Lind argues, "is hardly credible, and only to be guessed at from common computation, that this island formerly buried to the amount of the whole number of its white inhabitants once in five years; however, it has of late become more healthy" (8–9). Similarly, he notes that "in all parts of the East Indies, situated near large swamps, on the muddy banks of rivers, or the foul shores of the sea, the vapours exhaling from the putrid stagnated water, whether fresh or salt, from the corrupted vegetable and other impurities, produce mortal diseases, especially during the rainy season" (78–79). Most of Africa, large parts of Asia, and many islands in the West Indies are thus seen as essentially diseased environments. These pathogenic landscapes have much in common: invariably, the water in marshes, ditches, or standing pools has become putrid as animal and vegetable matter decays under the heat of a tropical sun, producing poisons that are absorbed into the air, which reaches a high level of toxicity when these spaces lack ventilating winds. Yet the pathogenic nature of these environments is not fixed. As in Lind's contention that even tropical Guinea might be transformed into another Barbados and that Jamaica "has of late become more healthy," they can be "improved." "In the East Indies," he writes, "and in the southern parts of Asia in general, we find, that the countries which are well improved by human industry and culture, such as China, and several other places in that part of the world, are blessed with a temperate and pure air, favourable to the European constitution. On the other hand, the woody and uncultivated parts, such as the islands Java, Borneo, and Sumatra, the coasts of Arakan and Pegu, the islands of Negrais . . . have proved fatal to a multitude of Europeans and others, who have been accustomed to breath a purer air" (77–78). By claiming that "countries that are well improved by human industry and culture" are "blessed with a temperate and pure air," Lind suggests that "tropical climates" are susceptible to transformation. People must endure tropical climates, it seems, not because of their distance from the equator, but because they have not yet "improved" them. Colonialism was indeed structured by the notion of improving minds and cultures, but we should not forget that, under the banner of health, it also set out to improve colonial ecologies and the bodies (both foreign and indigenous) that inhabited them.

Lind's medical writings were enormously influential during the latter half of the eighteenth century as they shaped the colonial diagnosis of pathogenic spaces. The medical text that succeeded Lind's as the primary reference on tropical climates, *The Influence of Tropical Climates on European Constitutions,* written first by James Johnson, then by James Martin, also sees colonial medicine as being essentially concerned with the health of Europeans in the tropics rather than with that of indigenous or slave populations, and Martin emphasizes its importance in furthering the establishment of a British empire. He also believes that tropical climates and landscapes are sick, and like Lind he believes they can be cured. "When . . . we look back to our native country, and boast of its pure and bracing air," he writes, quoting the French geographer Conrad Malte-Brun, "let us not forget the important fact, 'that it is man himself who has in a great measure created these salubrious climates. France, Germany, and England, not more than twenty ages ago, resembled Canada and Chinese Tartary, countries situated, as well as our Europe, at a mean distance between the equator and the pole' " (4).

As Richard Grove has persuasively demonstrated, it was in colonial regions, which underwent rapid transformation as a consequence of the introduction of capitalist plantation agriculture, that ideas about humans' power to transform natural environments and climates were first articulated.[10] Since medical geography produced a map of the world that was basically critical of non-European ecologies, it seemed obvious to most physicians that the easiest way to improve these places would be to make them more like Europe, especially by bringing them under cultivation. "Agriculture," Martin writes, "is everywhere the most powerful improver of climate, and . . . its advancement ministers not only to the support of man in the production of his food, but in a greater degree to his health and vigour, by purifying the air he breathes" (102). The same medicine that was transforming the English landscape, justifying the enclosure of uncultivated land and the draining of marshes and fens (thus ridding England of endemic malaria), also saw agriculture as the answer to the prevalence of diseases elsewhere in the world. With his eye on the region that was believed to be the cradle of cholera, Martin asserts: "That the clearing of the extensive surface of the Sunderbunds, or of any considerable portion of it, leaving belts and clumps of forest trees, would tend greatly to improve the local climate, in and around Calcutta, there can be no doubt.

Such a measure would open out the city to the more free influence of the sea-breezes, diminish the moisture of its atmosphere, and purify it. These are no speculative results" (30–31).

European environmental medicine thus justified introducing European methods of land cultivation into other regions of the world. The settler who opened a clearing in the woods or a tropical rain forest or the immigrant who put the land under the plow, drained a marsh, or enclosed a piece of land, was not simply working for his own economic benefit; he was also the agent by which a sick, unimproved land would be cured of its endemic diseases. Thus Ira Allen speaks of the American settler engaged in forest clearance as one who "sees the effect of his own powers, aided by the goodness of Providence; he sees that man can embellish the most rude spot, the stagnant air vanishes with the woods, the rank vegetation feels the purifying influence of the sun; he drains the swamp, putrid exhalations flit off on lazy wing, and fevers and agues accompany them" (qtd. in E. Martin 175). Similarly, the physician Charles Caldwell responds to "the super-abundance of *marsh miasma* in the United States, compared with most parts of Europe" by stressing the value of draining swamps. "A neglect of this rational, salutary, and lucrative practice, subjects thousands in the United States to the malignant action of marsh miasma, who would otherwise escape this deleterious poison" (14, 21). Caldwell's appeal to reason, health, and economic gain suggests the fusion of concepts of order, medicine, and economics in the transforming of colonial environments. In Jamaica, Edward Long writes that the healthiest places are those "where the ground is cleared from wood and bushes; has no stagnating water upon or near its surface; where the soil is fertile, and favours the cultivation of European plants, and the health of European animals." Such places, he argues, "by industry and cultivation, might be converted into the most healthy and delightful rural retirements" (2: 512).

The benefits that were to accrue from introducing European agricultural methods to new regions of the globe were not, however, all that obvious to contemporary observers, since in many cases the immediate result was not a decline but an increase in epidemics. Benjamin Rush gives a classic exposition of this irony when he notes, in a paper originally delivered to the American Philosophical Society in 1785, that "Pennsylvania for some years past, has become more sickly than formerly. Fevers, which a few years ago appeared chiefly on the banks of creeks and rivers, and in the neighbourhood of mill-ponds, now appear in parts remote from them all, and in the highest situations." A rising number of millponds contributed to the problem, but a more significant factor was the clearing of forests: "Intermittents [in distinction from continued fevers] on the shores of the Susquehannah, have kept an exact pace with the passages which have been opened for the propagation of marsh effluvia, by cutting down the wood which formerly grew in its neighbourhood" ("Inquiry" 267–68). Having admitted that European land use was a primary cause of an increase in epidemics, Rush nevertheless goes on to argue that cultivating land *makes it healthy.* "While clearing a country makes it sickly," he writes, "*cultivating* a country, that is, draining swamps, destroying weeds, burning brush, and exhaling the unwholesome and superfluous moisture of the earth, by means of frequent crops of grain, grasses, and vegetables of all kinds, render it healthy" (268). Colonial soils, in their unimproved state, were considered dangerous, and the first effect of colonial contact was to open them to the heat of the sun, releasing the pestilential vapors that had been building up since the beginning of time. Laying in crops helped the earth recover its proper balance, ridding it of dangerous superfluous moisture.[11]

James Annesley's *Researches into the Causes, Nature, and Treatment of the More Prevalent Diseases of India* (1828) also deserves mention. After citing Rush and noting that the clearing of forests in Bengal has produced "the most malignant and most pestilential diseases," Annesley, who served as a physician in India for thirty-seven years, also speaks of the medical powers of agriculture: "It was not until the soil has been subjected to cultivation for a long series of years, that a tolerable degree of healthiness was restored." Annesley is hopeful, but less certain, however, that "the same industry will be followed by so happy an effect within the tropics" (22). Faced with contradiction and diseases at every stage, colonial physicians developed complex theories to justify their faith in the healthiness of European modes of land use when they seemed to be producing the opposite results. The increase of epidemic disease in many regions could thus be seen as a temporary negative stage in curing the soil, like bringing a patient to the crisis point in a fever so that a cure might be achieved by the epidemic release of endemic poisons.[12]

Especially after the outbreak of cholera in 1817, the emphasis on the curative powers of agriculture came to be replaced by an emphasis on hygiene, sanitation engineering, and urban planning as a means of curing colonial spaces. Unhealthy places are seen increasingly as "dirty" spaces. "Go into the native town and around you will see on all sides filth immeasurable and indescribable, and at places almost unfathomable," writes a commission on the condition of Bombay in 1861; "filthy animals, filthy habits, filthy streets, and with filthy courtyards around the dwelling of the poor; foul and loathsome trades, crowded houses, foul markets, foul meat and food, foul wells, tanks and swamps, foul smells at every turn, drains unventilated and sewers choked, and the garbage of an Oriental city. Men, women and children, the rich and the poor, living with animals of all kinds and vermin, seeing all this and inhaling the deadly atmosphere and dying by the thousand" (qtd. in Scott 1: 98). Eight years later, another report speaks of the "marvellous revolution" wrought by the establishment of health officers in 1864: "Except in a few obscure lanes, the city is almost devoid of bad odours. Its area is nearly thrice that of municipal Calcutta and yet every street and house and every road is daily swept as well as watered and the dust is carefully removed. The natural effect has been seen, not merely in the comfort of all classes of the inhabitants, but in the fact that cholera, which used to be endemic in the city . . . has not been known for some time" (qtd. in Scott 1: 98).

This approach was not restricted to the East Indies but can be seen in all areas of the colonial world. These geographies produced a map of the world in which colonial spaces were largely perceived as dirty or unclean and European civilization was expected to cleanse or sanitize peoples and places. The 1889 World Exhibition in Paris provides a striking example of the way such ideas influenced the representation of non-European societies. Muhammad Amin Fikri, who saw the Egyptian exhibit on his way to the Eighth International Congress of Orientalists, writes that "it was intended to resemble the old aspect of Cairo," so much so that "even the paint on the buildings was made dirty" (qtd. in T. Mitchell 1).[13] Although climate continued to be the central term in the vocabulary of colonial medicine, dirt becomes an increasingly prominent aspect of the nineteenth-century mapping of pathogenic environments. Seeing colonial spaces as dirty and disordered, however, was part of the way Europeans marked themselves off from what they feared.

Colonialism was profoundly underwritten by medical discourse in defining itself as the means by which unimproved peoples, living in unimproved lands, could gain control over their diseased environments. In the following passage, Martin articulates the fundamental link between notions of improvement and ideas of empire:

Let us contemplate a desert country, the rivers, abandoned to themselves, become choked and overflow, and their waters serve only to form pestilential marshes. A labyrinth of thickets and of brambles overspread the most fertile hills. In the meadows the unsightly wild mushroom, and the useless moss choke the nutritious herbs; forests become impenetrable to the rays of the sun; no wind disperses the putrid exhalations of the trees which have fallen under the pressure of age; the soil, excluded from [the] genial and purifying warmth of the air, exhales nothing but poison; and an atmosphere of death gathers over all the country. But what do not industry and perseverance accomplish? The marshes are drained; the rivers flow in their disencum-bered channels; the axe and the fire clear away the forests; the earth furrowed by the plough is opened to the rays of the sun, and the influence of the wind; the air, the soil, and the waters acquire by degrees a character of salubrity; and vanquished nature yields its empire to man, who thus creates a country for himself.

Agriculture must be much improved in Bengal before the European . . . can be said to have created a country for himself. (21).

Martin is here describing and justifying a radical transformation of physical space, as European land-use technologies are called on to rid India of the pestilential air, the "atmosphere of death," that hangs over it. His imperialist perspective is quite obvious in that he sees Bengal as a "country" that Euro-peans are creating. The diseased environments that are the signs of nature's "empire" over mankind must give way to those new environments, "opened to the rays of the sun, and the influence of the wind," whose salubrious air signifies the wisdom of a man-made, British empire.

Colonial comparisons of the merits of geographical regions were also comparisons of the cultural and physical merits of the people who inhabited them. To a degree that colonial historians have not adequately recognized, the health of a people was considered to be a verdict on the merits of the society. This was especially true of early British imperial medicine, which sought to remake people by remaking their environments. Colonial physi-cians insisted on attaching more than ordinary importance to moral restraint. Asked "What has the medical topographer to do with the morals of the natives of a country?" Martin responds that the morality and discipline of a people contribute to the health of a region:

Place [a sober and industrious race of people] . . . in a district overrun with noxious weeds and timber, and fast degenerating into a morass, and can there exist any rational doubt that they will clear it sooner, and preserve it longer in that improved state than men of a different disposition? Place in a similar situation, or even in a district thus improved, a body of men who are idle and intemperate, and the immediate result will be that the soil will deteriorate for want of proper care, the weeds will reappear, the drains will become obstructed, the edible products of the earth will lessen in quantity, and diminish in their nutritive quality; the inhabitants will become unhealthy from the bad state of their grounds; and the diminution of their physical powers thus produced will disable them progressively more and more from remedying the causes of the evil. Many of these effects will doubtless first be felt in their own persons, but it is undeniable that they must ultimately operate on their visitors. On this obvious principle is founded the axiom in Medical Topography—"that a slothful, squalid-looking population invariably characterizes an unhealthy country" (138).

We have thus come full circle: not only do the physical characteristics of the world's environments express the capacities of the people who inhabit them, but the observation of the physical and moral characteristics of indigenous people is itself a fundamental aspect of "medical topography," as a primary index of the healthiness of their lands. People are read through the landscapes they inhabit, while landscapes are seen as the physical expression—the topographical indexes—of the moral discipline and technological power of those who inhabit them. The sickness of a people is therefore intricately bound up with the sickness of their surroundings. Curing one cures the other. Thus the American Alexander Wilson claims that "the European inhabitants who were transplanted to that continent, seemed for a time to degenerate; but the face of the country, being by degrees changed from woods and morasses to a clear surface and cultivated fields . . . the natural effects have begun to flow from these changes. . . . [T]he more quickly it is deprived of its woody covering, the more rapid will its improvements be in every thing that hath distinguished the European nations in equal latitudes" (275–76).

Baron Antoine-Jean Gros's *Napoleon Visiting the Pesthouse at Jaffa* (*Napoléon visitant les pestiférés de Jaffa*) (fig. 2), first displayed in the Louvre in 1804, provides a powerful artistic representation of the ideological link between Western medicine and the curing of colonial spaces. During Napoleon's military expedition into Palestine in 1799, the bubonic plague broke out among his troops at Jaffa. To boost their morale while demonstrating that they need not fear the plague because it was *not* contagious, Napoleon made an official visit to the wards of a makeshift hospital and is said to have lifted one of the sick men in his arms. Touching a bubo, the French commander supposedly declared, "You see, it is nothing." The leading physician of the expedition, René Desgenettes, went further, lancing a bubo and then pricking himself in the groin and armpit. He was lucky not to die.

The painting celebrates the power of Western medical knowledge over Eastern superstition, yet it achieves its power by drawing on and displacing biblical geography, with its evocation of Christ walking among the sick and curing them. As Walter Friedlander observed, "Bonaparte imitates the behaviour of Christian saints . . . , who in Italian paintings of the sixteenth and seventeenth centuries . . . are seen walking in the midst of the plague-stricken people, bringing them comfort and spiritual relief, but also healing miraculously by touching" (140). Having reduced disease to an irrational fear, a product of superstition, Napoleon shows that he is not afraid of the darkness of the plague. The blind man pictured at the right of the painting groping his way toward the French commander is thus not only a biblical type but also a

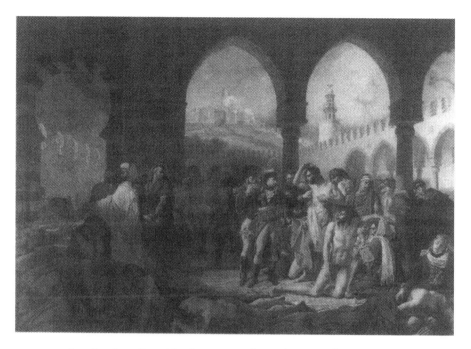

FIG. 2. Antoine-Jean Gros, *Napoleon Visiting the Pesthouse at Jaffa* (*Napoléon visitant les pestiférés de Jaffa*) (1804). La Réunion des Musées Nationaux de France.

figure of the darkness and blindness that is being dispersed by French enlightenment. Napoleon by his very presence seems to have literally opened up a space of light in the darkness of this Oriental setting. And through the two main windows we see the French flag and the Christian cross, bathed in light, rising above the buildings of Jaffa.

In Gros's painting the conquest of territory is portrayed as a conquest of disease, as a curing of place. The West's relation to the East was thus not simply that of free man to enslaved, or of male lover to female object of desire, but also that of doctor to patient. Freedom had a medical dimension: Napoleon is portrayed as a liberator who frees peoples by curing their environments. He is a *roi thaumaturge,* a king whose touch heals. Yet his power extends beyond the individual to include the healing of an entire region. Nevertheless, a few comments are perhaps in order. First, the medical knowledge that is being celebrated in the painting, that the bubonic plague is transmitted by places, not people, is incorrect, for the bacillus *Yersinia pestis,* when not transmitted by the bite of an infected flea, is highly contagious in its pulmonary form. Although Eastern medicine is shown as having turned its back on enlightenment (notably in the Middle Eastern physician on the left), traditional practices, most commonly quarantine, were not unjustified. Second, what is represented in the painting is imperial ideology rather than historical reality, especially when seen in the context of what actually took place in the hospital at Jaffa. Louis-Antoine Bourrienne, Napoleon's secretary, claimed not only that the story of Napoleon's touching the sick was fictitious, but also that Napoleon, concerned that these sick soldiers might impede his retreat, decided to have them poisoned.

Hybrid Landscapes

It would be misleading to argue that Romantic literature simply reflects an imperialist "geography of disease." Too frequently nineteenth-century literature is seen as a direct reflection of a homogeneous imperial culture, and British writers, just because they wrote at this time, are considered promoters of empire or of the values that make it possible. My object here is less overtly polemical, for I wish to show that geographical constructions of the relative health of England and other parts of the globe were a primary discursive medium through which positions, both supportive and critical, were taken with regard to nationalism and imperialism. Colonialism was very much a geographical discourse on health and disease and on the relative merits of social environments. Stands on nationalist and imperialist ideologies, not necessarily supporting them, shape the very ways these writers talk about the healthiness or unhealthiness of domestic, national, and foreign environments.

Disease geographies are complex symbolic and biomedical structures. Their increasing importance during the nineteenth century is one sign of the significance the West was ascribing to the negotiation of disease on a world scale, itself a consequence of its globalization. The emergence of a global conception of the distribution of diseases suggests that even the most local ones were intrinsically understood in terms of their place within a larger geography. All diseases were thus constructed in *relational* or *differential* terms: to inhabit one disease environment was to not inhabit another. Knowing one's epidemiological place, in other words, was increasingly based on global comparisons. Insofar as these European medical geographies provided a method for placing diseases somewhere else, a symbolic means of localizing them within specific regions or climatic zones, they could alleviate anxieties about the global transmission of disease. Just as maps intrinsically produce an impression of stability for the elements they analyze, colonial disease geographies tended to produce a relatively stable picture of the global distribution of diseases, even as ecologies were rapidly changing. This goal is explicit, for instance, in one of the earliest attempts to collect this kind of material, Friedrich Hoffmann's *A Dissertation on Endemial Diseases* (1746), which claims that endemic diseases, "drawing their Origin from a fixed and static Cause essential to the Country, remain without Change or Variation for many Years" (2). Since diseases were also bound up with cultural and biological identities, they provided a means by which Europeans could distinguish themselves and their environments from other regions where disease was believed to be rampant. J. B. Harley has noted that Mercator's projection affirmed European notions of cultural superiority by placing Europe at the center of the world and making the temperate regions seem much larger than they were (290). Disease geographies functioned in a similar manner. Notions of health, like those of climate, were differentially constructed: the healthiness of one place always assessed in contrast to another place that was sicker or produced more loathsome diseases. Disease geographies tended to affirm the wholesomeness of temperate climates because these were the regions where Europeans were normally the healthiest. As the epidemiologist William Farr would remark in 1852, basing his claim on this newly emerging science, "England, according to the latest observations, is the healthiest country in the world" (*Report* vii).

Although disease geographies can be said to be hierarchical, then—stabilizing mechanisms that spatially separated Europe and differentiated it from the global context of microbial exchange opened up by colonial contact—these biomedical structurings were constantly being undercut. Medical geography simultaneously produced a picture of the world in which the disease environments of the West, despite their apparent superiority, were close to other regions where frightening diseases thrived. Sontag has observed that "part of the self-definition of Europe and the neo-European countries" is that in the former "major calamities are history-making, transformative, while in poor, African or Asian countries they are part of a cycle, and therefore something like an aspect of nature" (*AIDS and Its Metaphors* 83–84). Epidemics were thus perceived as a "natural" part of colonial landscapes and thus hardly merited the status of news. Yet they did become history when they moved—as did the epidemics of plague, yellow fever, malaria, and cholera. The possibility of epidemic invasion was always there, so the stability of disease geographies was always uncertain. The dynamics of colonial landscape transformation further contributed to and emphasized this instability. Given the assumption that colonial landscapes were not *essentially* sick but could be radically improved, their topographies were seen not as unchangeable, but instead as being in transition from one state to another. Colonialism continually affirmed that the map would change.

Colonial landscapes can be seen as intrinsically *hybrid* structures. "Hybridity" conveys a complex range of meanings within contemporary postcolonial studies, so I should explain how I am using it. Originally derived from a biological context, to refer to plants or animals of mixed origins, over the nineteenth century the term developed a racial meaning, applied to people of mixed backgrounds. Although I insist on the relevance of this biological dimension to the colonial framing of hybridity, my emphasis is on the geographical and environmental understanding of human biomedical identities. In this context hybridity describes the change in physiology—in the physical "constitution"—produced by a change of climate or environment. Colonial landscapes are hybrid because they exhibit in diverse and often contradictory ways the complex biomedical impacts and negotiations that emerged from Europeans' attempts to transpose their own biosocial ecologies to other regions of the globe. In postcolonial studies, notably through the influence of Homi Bhabha, "hybridity" has been given a more specialized, linguistic meaning, related to the way colonial representation "reverses the effects of the colonialist disavowal, so that other 'denied' knowledges enter upon the dominant discourse and estrange the basis of its authority" (114). Hybrid disease landscapes, in this sense, upset the stability of colonial disease geography by questioning and displacing European epidemiological certainties and securities. Take, for instance, the problems raised by the epidemic increase of yellow fever in Pennsylvania through the clearing of forests and building of millponds. Rush argued that this rise in disease was only temporary. Just as settlers had to undergo a period of sickness or "seasoning" to adapt to new climates, so the hybrid landscapes of the New World seemed to require a similar period of greater sickness to become like their European counterparts. Epidemics thus have an unstable meaning, both as a symptom of the pathogenic spaces that the colonial settler is seeking to transform and as a promise of the utopian health regime being initiated by European culture.

"Hybridity" has largely been reserved for describing colonial cultures and the relation between colonizers and colonized. Yet it should be stressed that the exchange of pathogens was far more a two-way street than has been imagined. The "contact zone" expanded over the eighteenth and nineteenth centuries to include Europe as much as any colonial region. Whatever confidence might be gained by placing the world's "worst" diseases somewhere else was negated in that these geographies blurred the differences between European and colonial diseases. All over England, pathogenic spaces were

being recognized that seemed to have less in common with an idealized understanding of England's temperate environment than with disease-bearing
foreign spaces. This was especially so for "fevers," a topic that dominated
medicine during the early nineteenth century.[14] The emergence of fever as a
primary concern of Europeans, itself reflective of the increase of this class of
diseases through the growth of towns and cities, cannot be understood without reference to its importance within a colonial context, where it dominated
medical practice. Many physicians did not understand that fever could be a
symptom of many diseases but instead considered it the *same* malady taking
on various forms in different climates or circumstances. Margaret Pelling
writes: "Reports were . . . increasingly received of the behaviour of epidemic
diseases in other countries or in their countries of origin. Some writers were
prepared to merge the intermittent and continued fevers into a single class
whose members owed their peculiarities to factors in the different climates in
which they arose" (19). Fever was notorious for its protean powers of imitation. For physicians seeking to describe the etiology and characteristics of a
wide range of fevers across the globe, fever was itself hybrid: there frequently
was controversy over whether outbreaks were endemic or imported. With
the growing prominence given to "tropical medicine" in medical journals
during the early nineteenth century, "fever" itself takes on a colonial inflection, as the "tropical disease" par excellence.[15]

Reading English fevers through the lens of tropical medicine, physicians
could not help but notice the similarities between the conditions of many
people in England and those of their colonial counterparts. For instance, in
his *Treatise on Fever* (1830) Thomas Southwood Smith writes that "the room
of a fever-patient, in a small and heated apartment in London, with no
perflation of fresh air, is perfectly analogous to a stagnant pool in Ethiopia, full
of the bodies of dead locusts. The poison generated in both cases is the same;
the difference is merely in the degree of its potency." Reflecting on this
similarity, Smith comes to the extraordinary conclusion that the miasmatic
environments produced by London poverty are equivalent to those of the
tropics: "Nature, with her burning sun, her stilled and pent-up wind, her
stagnant and teeming marsh, manufactures plague on a large and fearful scale:
poverty in her hut, covered with her rags, surrounded with her filth, striving
with all her might, to keep out the pure air, and to increase the heat, imitates
nature but too successfully; the process and the product are the same, the only
difference is in the magnitude of the result. Penury and ignorance can thus at
any time, and in any place, create a mortal plague" (364). Smith was discovering that in "process and product" the "fever-nests" of urban England were

not fundamentally different from the pathogenic "nature" of the tropics. Yet here the assumed relation between European and colonial environments is reversed, as the English "fever-nest"—socially produced by "poverty" and "ignorance"—is now seen as a mimic double of colonial nature. The importance given to responding to these "fever-nests," especially since they were seen as the seedbeds of epidemics that spread outward to threaten the entire urban social order, is one sign of a growing anxiety about the mirroring incursion of the tropical within temperate spaces.

Throughout the nineteenth century, colonial spaces retain their status as paradigms of pathogenic space, whose magnitude makes them ideal models for understanding the dynamics of disease in less obvious places. Yet they appeared more and more frequently in medical texts dealing with English illness as English physicians came to see English fever in terms of colonial medicine. Doctors found to their surprise that the disease experience of the urban poor did not appear to be fundamentally different from that of people in the tropics, since "fever" seemed as much a product of socioeconomic conditions as of climate. The primary difference seemed to be that the presence of endemic fever in the large manufacturing cities had largely gone unnoticed. James Currie, for instance, remarks that though many believed typhus was "seldom to be met with" in Liverpool, "among the inhabitants of the cellars, and of . . . back houses, the typhus is constantly present; and the number of persons under this disease that apply for medical assistance to the charitable institutions the public will be astonished to hear, exceeds three thousand annually" (221–24). Urban doctors were discovering the silent mortality that was taking place among the working classes. The pathogenic spaces of colonialism were progressively found not in the heart of Africa, but in British manufacturing cities.

In the doubling of landscapes, contemporary England emerges as another space of hybrid darkness, perhaps no less frightening than the tropical world constructed by colonial physicians. Undoubtedly, the primary function of colonial medical geography was to assert the health of Europe compared with other regions of the globe. Yet the instability and uncertainty that shape this view of the world should not be ignored. As Hermione de Almeida observes, the reports of colonial physicians "expanded the classifications of current European nosologies, rendered far more complex notions on the multiplicity of disease, and undermined all functioning theories of disease in contemporary use" (184). One goal of this book is to describe how colonial experience radically changed the ways English writers looked on the health of their own environments, with attendant fears that perhaps they were not removed from the problems produced by colonial contact. Colonial disease darkly mirrored English social space. The "foreign" diseases that the British were encountering outside their island seemed to reflect a foreignness within. In a world where the boundaries of colonial contact had become fluid and in which commerce, travel, and pathogenic exchange were global, the destabilizing power of "hybridity" erupted within their representations of themselves.

"The Ruined Cottage"

"The Ruined Cottage" has long been viewed as a classic example of Wordsworth's extraordinary ability to use landscape to convey the complexity of human psychology and feeling. Many critics have noted, as do Kenneth Johnston and Jonathan Barron, that "most of the signs of Margaret's decline and decay are in fact deduced from her garden" (67). For earlier critics the garden was read symbolically, as a poetic means of establishing continuity and eliciting aesthetic harmony where the bare circumstances of the tale would produce unalleviated pain. New historicist critics have reached a similar conclusion, only the imagery is now understood as a strategy for naturalizing history and thus distancing readers from the social context of Margaret's suffering.[16] Both approaches to the poem are weakened by an inability to see "nature" as itself historically inflected. Natural landscapes were hardly ahistorical or politically neutral during the Romantic period, because the comparison of the relative merits of physical environments was the basis of colonial understanding. Although Wordsworth's description of the cottage does function symbolically (no description of a garden or an English cottage can avoid doing that), it is more useful to recognize the poet's employment of the aims and techniques of contemporary "medical topography": it consistently reads Margaret's moral and psychological well-being through the social landscape she inhabits (and inhabited), while simultaneously reading the landscape through her. The poem refuses to separate the consideration of human health from a consideration of social and physical environments. Strikingly, it describes the emergence of a pathogenic space in what was believed to be the ideological heart of Englishness—the life of rural cottagers. Wordsworth clearly blames colonial military action—the "plague of war" (*"Ruined Cottage,"* MS B 188)—for the poverty, the unemployment, and ultimately the fever that incapacitates and impoverishes Robert and his family. "In disease / He lingered long" (lines 201–2), and this disease, this "plague," spreads to the rest of his family, not by contagion, but because the social environment itself—England—has become sick. By detailing how this pathogenic space has come into being, Wordsworth engages in a critique of the social consequences of English colonialism in the West Indies. (I will return to this topic in a fuller analysis of this poem in the next chapter.)

Wordsworth's focus on landscape is less an escape from history than a critique of the ecology and pathology of English colonialism. It is worth recognizing how the narrative is inflected across a colonial register, as readers are shown the progressive deterioration of the cottage into a sick wilderness:

> It was a plot
> Of garden-ground, now wild
>
> .   .   .   .
>
>   Within that cheerless spot,
> Where two tall hedgerows of thick willow boughs
> Joined in a damp cold nook, I found a well
> Half choked [with willow flowers and weeds].
>
> (116–25)

It is not by accident that Wordsworth's depiction of this uninhabitable space has much in common with James Martin's description of the deleterious impact of an idle people on the environment: "Let us contemplate a desert country, the rivers, abandoned to themselves, become choked and overflow, and their waters serve only to form pestilential marshes. A labyrinth of thickets and of brambles overspread the most fertile hills. In the meadows the unsightly wild mushroom, and the useless moss choke the nutritious herbs." Just as Martin argues that physical landscapes reflect the moral character—the "sobriety" and "industry"—of the people who inhabit them, Wordsworth maps Margaret's despondency onto her cottage and garden. An obvious conclusion to be drawn from her story is that for the rural poor England was itself becoming a colonial space. Margaret struggles with a wilderness outside and a wildness within, both ultimately the result of England's expansionary policies.

Take the framing of the poem. A puzzling feature is Wordsworth's early emphasis on the difficulty the wanderer has in traveling through this harsh physical environment:

> Across a bare wide Common I had toiled
> With languid feet which by the slippery ground
> Were baffled still; and when I sought repose
> On the brown earth my limbs from very heat
> Could find no rest nor my weak arm disperse

The insect host which gathered round my face
And joined their murmurs to the tedious noise
Of seeds of bursting gorse which crackled round.
(18–25)

Where is this landscape coming from? The common gorse (*Ulex europaeus*) is
not a New World plant, but Wordsworth's description of the vast extent of
land covered with its excessive growth suggests descriptions of colonial wildernesses, now transposed to a British setting.[17] The "insect host" is also
reminiscent of tropical environments: Lind notes that when the air in a place
"swarms with numberless insects and animalcules, [it is] a sure sign of its malignant disposition" (*Essay on the Most Effectual Means* 52). Set in this wilderness, the wanderer comes upon the ruins of a cottage, "a spot" so pathogenic
that even a "wandering gypsey in a stormy night / Would pass it . . . to
house / On the open plain" (32–34). The Pedlar tells his tale of Margaret
from within this space, as he sits on a bench "studded o'er with fungus
flowers" (38), a place where "you see the toadstool's lazy head" (488).

Wordsworth's history of the emergence of this pathogenic space is a mas-
terpiece of topographical detail. Throughout, disease is understood as a product of disorder. In her grief, Margaret allows her cottage and garden to fall
into neglect; under "a sleepy hand of negligence; / The floor was neither dry
nor neat, the hearth / Was comfortless" (440–42). Just as Martin equates the
healthfulness of a landscape with the moral discipline of its inhabitants, the
Pedlar reads the signs of disease and moral disorder into the landscape. Margaret's negligence and sleepy idleness, linked to somnambulism, are not so
much expressions of an individualized character as refractions of an entire
corpus of travelers' descriptions in which aboriginal populations are described as having these specific moral traits. In many parts of the world, where
chronic infections and helminthic diseases frequently sapped the energy of
entire populations, when climate was not seen as the cause of a people's
general physical lassitude it was blamed on their "laziness" or "backwardness."
Much of the negative image of the American South as a culture suffering
from indolence and poverty, for instance, originated in the impact of chronic
malaria, hookworm, and pellagra, what George Brown Tindall calls the
"Southern trilogy of 'lazy diseases' " (227).[18]

The Pedlar's description of Margaret also emphasizes her inability to raise
herself from the torpor of grief. On the cottage wall "knots of worthless
stone-crop started out . . . and grew like weeds / Against the lower panes"
(368–70), while in the garden "the unprofitable bindweed spread his bells /

From side to side" (372–73). The Pedlar discriminates among the various kinds of plants. The "unprofitability" of some makes them "weeds," the telltale signs of wilderness and, with it, disease. He also associates disease with dirt. One of the most powerful disease images in the poem is the encroachment of the sheep to the very foundation of the cottage:

> looking round I saw the corner stones,
> Till then unmarked, on either side the door
> With dull red stains discoloured and stuck o'er
> With tufts of hairs of wool, as if the sheep
> That feed upon the commons thither came
> As to a couching-place and rubbed their sides
> Even at her threshold.   (388–94)

Although Wordsworth is explicitly referring to the traces of paint left by the sheep, this passage also draws on the symbolism of blood, sexuality, and dirt in an image of a wilderness that is "rubbing" itself up against the order once maintained (though under economic stress) within the cottage. Throughout, the Pedlar consistently recognizes that the wilderness he is describing is a hybrid one; it is not "natural" but a product of economic factors linked to war. At one point this connection is clearly asserted:

> poverty and grief
> Were now come nearer to her: all was hard,
> With weeds defaced and knots of withered grass.
>   (452–54)

Poverty and war are the plague. They are seen in the ecology of the place and in Margaret's ultimate incapacity to resist the progressive decay of her world. By the end of the poem the cottage no longer affords any shelter from her environment—"when she slept the nightly damps / Did chill her breast, and in the stormy day / Her tattered clothes were ruffled by the wind" (519–21). "The Ruined Cottage" is a psychological study of grief, but it is more than that. Manuscript B ends by reaffirming the poem's status as a disease narrative: "In sickness she remained, and here she died, / Last human tenant of these ruined walls" (527–28). The phrase "in sickness she remained" may be an awkward way of saying Margaret was ill, yet in many ways it captures the environmental sense that she dwelled "in" sickness, that it is the place itself that no longer supports human life. The Pedlar uses the same phrasing to describe Robert's fever: "In disease / He lingered long" (201–2). The sickness of one cannot be seen in isolation from the sickness of the other.

To watch somebody die from sickness while being unable to do anything was common during the colonial period. Although indeed most recent attention has focused on how Wordsworth seeks some means of continuing in the face of this loss, the poem is hardly an apology for colonialism. The Pedlar's anger and his sense of impotence are clearly registered throughout the poem, as in the following passage:

> She is dead,
> And nettles rot and adders sun themselves
> Where we have sat together while she nursed
> Her infant at her bosom.   (162–65)

The Pedlar feels he must apologize to his listener for losing control over the narrative: "You will forgive me, Sir, / I feel I play the truant with my tale" (170–71). In addition to the nettles and the adders, which provoke him because they have supplanted Margaret and her infant, the Pedlar also includes the "weeds" and "rank spear-grass" (162) that now thrive on top of the cottage walls, *rank* meaning both excessive and disgusting. By the end of the tale the same weeds and spear-grass will be seen in aesthetic terms, providing some consolation for the Pedlar through "an image of tranquillity" that allows him to deal with "the uneasy thoughts which filled my mind" (MS D 517–19). Contemporary readers have frequently been critical of this effort; they have perhaps been too willing to accept the Pedlar as the only voice of Wordsworth in the poem. But this response tends to minimize the anxieties of the tale and the enormous sense of loss it evokes.

"The Brothers"

Wordsworth's "The Brothers" provides another example of the complex ways the interpretation of landscapes during the Romantic period provided a material medium for thinking through the fracturings and mimetic structurings of identity that emerged in England with colonialism. The poem is about a failed homecoming. After spending twenty years as a sailor in the West Indies and building up "some small wealth / Acquir'd by traffic" (63–64) there, Leonard Ewbank returns to his birthplace, his "determin'd purpose to resume / The life which he liv'd there" (66–67) and be reunited with his brother James. Although the word "traffic" might be read simply as meaning Leonard engaged in maritime commerce, when used in relation to the West Indies it suggests that he has also been involved in the "traffic in slaves," an interpretation reinforced by his being at one point "in slavery among the

Moors / Upon the Barbary Coast" (312–13).[19] Leonard hopes to return to his native home, as if it could remain unaffected by these dealings. He asks the local priest whether his brother James is still living. The resulting dialogue is a brilliant play of misunderstandings and misidentifications, as it unsettles the stable categories that once operated in this world, between those who are "natives" and those who are "strangers." The priest, mistaking Leonard for a "tourist," an outsider, recounts the tragic history of the Ewbanks, little knowing that he is speaking to one of the principals in his story. Dramatic irony shapes the dialogue, undercutting and redefining the claims of each speaker at each moment. Leonard never reveals himself to the priest. He claims that "it was from the weakness of his heart / He had not dared to tell him [the priest], who he was" (427–28). Yet this reticence may reflect his no longer really knowing who he is. The poem is thus an extraordinary study in the ambiguity and instability of colonial identities. By its end Leonard relinquishes his claim to a "native" identity; he returns "shipboard, and is now / A Seaman, a grey headed Mariner" (429–30). The dialogue takes place in a graveyard—a suitable setting, for one learns not only that James has been dead for twelve years, but also that Leonard is dead to this community. The returning sailor discovers there is no return.

"The Brothers" is a radical rewriting of Coleridge's "Rime of the Ancient Mariner." A critique of colonialism without the supernatural machinery Coleridge employed, it too seeks to convey through a dialogue of a sailor with a "native son" that "being at home," isolated from the outside world, is no longer possible. Whereas Coleridge's poem tends toward monologue, "The Brothers" is structured as dramatic and ironic interaction. Everything the priest says must be "put in quotation marks" because he is speaking to Leonard, who is a hybrid identity, since he is both a "native son" and an "outsider." Yet this mixing, registered in the poem as confusion, is not restricted to him alone: it also shapes the world he is seeking to recover. The landscape Leonard enters has become oddly foreign to him. Although during his childhood "every corner / Among these rocks and every hollow place / Where foot could come . . . was known" (268–71), he no longer recognizes them:

> looking round he thought that he perceived
> Strange alteration wrought on every side
> Among the woods and fields, and that the rocks,
> And the eternal hills, themselves were changed.
>
> (93–96)

Earlier in the afternoon Leonard lost his way on the path "through fields which once had been well known to him" (90), and as he stands in the graveyard, looking at the burial place of his brother, he cannot remember whether he has seen this grave before: "as he gazed, there grew / Such a confusion in his memory" (83–84). One might explain away this confusion by arguing that Leonard has changed, not Ennerdale, and that this change in the look of things serves his psychological need to deny the death of his brother; however, this confusion also suggests a deeper instability within the landscape itself, as if it were indeed a mirror of Leonard's own estrangement.

This estranged doubling of landscape—the foreign landscape that seems to occupy the space formerly occupied by Leonard's birthplace—mirrors the fracturing of identity that is symbolically expressed in the two brothers. Mark Schoenfield notes that "the poem continually uses paired images, the 'two Springs which bubbled side by side' [141], the 'two bells' which would ring if Leonard returned [320], the two brothers 'like two young ravens on the crags' [283], and the 'pair of diaries' [164]" (156). The parallel mirroring of the two brothers, both in themselves and in the landscape, is fractured by Leonard's decision to go to sea. Now each brother represents a different choice within the colonial context—the brother who went to sea, ironically "chiefly for his brother's sake" (300), and the one who stayed home—yet they remain linked in their division. In the landscape this division is mirrored by the "brother fountains" (141) that produce two different streams, two different histories: "One is dead and gone, / The other, left behind, is flowing still" (142–43). Throughout the poem, changes in social identity, the doubling and division that constitute the identity of the two brothers, are clearly registered in the doubling and division within the social landscape.

"The Brothers" is a study in colonial psychology: it explores the psychological dimensions of the new world brought into being by global commercial expansion—the "profitable life" (2)—intimating that it is one in which there is a destabilized fracturing of identities, a world of mirrors that produce unfamiliar and confusing reflections, as the familiar presents itself as foreign and vice versa. In exploring this new kind of space, Wordsworth drew on Coleridge's "Rime" ("Is this mine own countree?" [467]), but even more important, on one of the oldest texts in the Western tradition, *The Odyssey.* Awakening on the island of Ithaca, in book 13, Odysseus experiences a similar disorientation, not being able to "tell what land it was / after so many years away" (235). Ithaca initially appears foreign as it takes on a semioneiric quality strongly similar to what greets Leonard's eyes: "The landscape then looked strange, unearthly strange / to the Lord Odysseus" (236). In an extraordinary moment in the poem, Odysseus responds to Ithaca, his home, as if it were just another strange island in the middle of nowhere:

> And then he wept,
> despairing, for his own land, trudging down
> beside the endless wash of the wide, wide sea,
> weary and desolate as the sea.   (236–37)

In *The Odyssey* one can see the beginning of a concept of colonial hybridity, not surprisingly since it is the first major poem in Western literature to deal with the catastrophic consequences of colonial conflict. Odysseus's *nostos* or "homecoming" is ostensibly portrayed as successful (depending on how one reads its conclusion), yet it is set within the context of failed homecomings, as the narrative shifts away from the fall of Troy to the negative impact this war has had on the supposedly victorious Akhaians. Written at a time when Troy and the world of the Akhaians were only faded memories, the *Odyssey* is critical of this earlier colonial struggle, suggesting that these events have caused the disappearance of an entire way of life.

Where Homer presents Odysseus's defamiliarization as temporary, rectified by his heroic remaking of his home, Wordsworth presents a more pessimistic view in which colonialism is read as pathogenic. Note the strange, yet complementary, illnesses that afflict the two brothers. While in the tropics, Leonard suffered from "calenture." Throughout the eighteenth century, calenture was generally accepted as another name for tropical fever, since it derived from Spanish *calentura,* meaning heat. Robinson Crusoe thus speaks of "being thrown into a violent Calenture by the excessive Heat of the Climate" (Defoe 16) while slave trading on the Guinea coast, and Gulliver mentions "I had several Men died in my Ship of Calentures, so that I was forced to get Recruits out of *Barbadoes,* and the *Leeward Islands*" (Swift, *Prose Works* 11: 221). Samuel Johnson uses the word similarly when he argues that is it not military power but disease and hurricanes that protect the Spanish colonies in the West Indies; they "are defended," he remarks, "not by walls mounted with cannon which by cannon may be battered, but by the storms of the deep and the vapours of the land, by the flames of calenture and blasts of pestilence" (*Works* 10: 373–74). In the *Dictionary,* however, Johnson defines "calenture" in a narrower sense as "a distemper peculiar to sailors, in hot climates; wherein they imagine the sea to be green fields, and will throw themselves into it, if not restrained." In *Zoönomia,* which Wordsworth read early in 1798, Erasmus Darwin considers calenture a form of "nostalgia" that produces "an unconquerable desire of returning to one's native country, frequent in long voyages, in which the patients become so insane as to throw themselves into the sea, mistaking it for green fields or meadows" (2: 367). We are likely nowadays to treat "nostalgia" as a vague sentimental idealization of the past. During the eighteenth century, however, it still had a clear geographical meaning as homesickness. It was believed to be an extremely dangerous illness that primarily affected soldiers and sailors. "By the end of the eighteenth century," Jean Starobinski remarks, "throughout all the countries of Europe, all doctors recognized nostalgia as a frequently fatal disease" (95). Whether fever was the cause of the homesickness or vice versa, the notion of calenture helped to explain why English sailors so frequently threw themselves overboard in the tropics.[20] By transforming tropical fever into a form of nostalgia, English doctors made calenture into a dangerous psychological disorder that afflicted colonial servicemen, a state of delusion in which the victim perished in the effort to reenter a native landscape primarily of his own making. Wordsworth's description of Leonard's illness conforms to this narrower interpretation as it makes calenture into a disease of the imagination:

> he, in those hours
> Of tiresome indolence would often hang
> Over the vessel's side, and gaze and gaze,
> And, while the broad green wave and sparkling foam
> Flashed round him images and hues, that wrought
> In union with the employment of his heart,
> He, thus by feverish passion overcome,
> Even with the organs of his bodily eye,
> Below him, in the bosom of the deep,
> Saw mountains, saw the forms of sheep that grazed
> On verdant hills, with dwellings among trees,
> And Shepherds clad in the same country grey
> Which he himself had worn. (50–62)

Subtitled "A Pastoral Poem," "The Brothers" was originally intended, Wordsworth notes, "to be the concluding poem of a series of pastorals" (*"Lyrical Ballads"* 142). James Butler argues that as such it is "literally and figuratively the last poem of an expiring century" (10). Without diminishing the importance of "pastoral" as a central, positive term within Wordsworth's poetry, one should also recognize the contradictory way in which, as it emerges within a tropical context, English pastoral verges on psychopathology. In *The Country and the City* Raymond Williams notes how late nineteenth-century colonists entertained the fantasy of "rural England . . . its green peace contrasted with the tropical or arid places of actual work." They hoped that through colonialism they could eventually afford to live in rural society: "The country, now, was a place to retire in" (281–82). Where many have seen Wordsworth as a naive promoter of cultural imperialism, Leonard's nostalgia indicates his willingness to address the dangers implicit in such fictions, providing new insight into the role that pastoral played for those engaged in colonial commerce. Here it is obviously a product of fever—it *is* calenture—and Leonard is shown to have been in danger of falling victim to a fiction, of drowning in a landscape of his own making. As Keats remarks: "on the shores of darkness there is light, / And precipices show untrodden green" ("To Homer" 9–10).

An interesting aspect of Wordsworth's portrayal of calenture is that he understands it as a waking dream, a mistaken superimposition of a "native" landscape onto a "foreign" one. Death lies in the confusion of the two. This problematic fusion of landscapes finds its complement in the somnambulism that afflicts Leonard's brother James. His illness is not that different from Leonard's. In *Zoönomia*, Darwin distinguishes somnambulism from sleepwalking. Rather than equating it with sleep, he asserts that it is a form of *reverie*, "a hallucination of the senses" (2: 361). Citing the case of a woman who suffered from the illness, Darwin insists that her mind was "so strenuously employed in pursuing its own trains of voluntary and sensitive ideas, that no common stimuli could so far excite her attention as to disunite them; that is, the quantity of volition or sensation already existing was greater than any, which could be produced in consequence of common degrees of stimulation" (1: 224). The somnambulist is thus so preoccupied with a specific train of thought that he does not attend to the outside world; sensory impressions from outside cannot break the chains of reverie. The priest of Ennerdale understands James's illness as an expression of his psychological *displacement*, his search for his absent brother:

> 'tis my belief
> His absent Brother still was at his heart.
> And, when he lived beneath our roof, we found
> (A practice till this time unknown to him)
> That often, rising from his bed at night,
> He in his sleep would walk about, and sleeping
> He sought his Brother Leonard.   (342–48)

Where Leonard risked being drowned in the fevered recreation of his native home, James appears to have suffered from the opposite problem: in his somnambulistic state, he no longer attended to the native world around him, and he wandered through foreign landscapes of his own making in search of his brother. Where Leonard escaped a precipitous fall into nostalgia, James is not so lucky. The parish conjectures that, after falling asleep on Pillar Mountain, James "to the margin of the precipice / Had walked, and from the summit had fallen head-long" (395–96).[21] The irony of this accident cannot be missed: though physically at home in the Ennerdale countryside, James dies while wandering through an imagined colonial landscape. Within the unstable geographies produced in the poem, he dies away from home.

To a great extent James's condition mirrors Margaret's in "The Ruined Cottage," for her madness is also caused by a loved one's sacrifice to colonial service. Both wander through semioneiric landscapes. We hear of the "*sleepy hand of negligence*" (*"Ruined Cottage,"* MS B 440) that characterizes Margaret's cottage, that "evermore / Her eye-lids droop'd" (415–16), and that she spent most of her time sitting on an old bench engaged in reverie: "evermore her eye / Was busy in the distance, shaping things / Which made her heart beat quick" (491–93). Margaret is portrayed as a nostalgic somnambulist, pacing "to and fro" on the same path, "from a belt of flax / That girt her waist spinning the long-drawn thread / With backward steps" (496–98). Wordsworth does provide some clue to how the world must have appeared to James. Leonard's dreamlike experience of a native landscape that becomes foreign and unrecognizable probably acts out James's own alienation. Within the fractured mirroring of "The Brothers," where James is an othered twin of Leonard, where the "native" mimes the "foreign," where Ennerdale is seen in the waters of the West Indies and the latter is seen from the heights of Pillar Mountain, landscape no longer supports a stable, *placed* identity, for either subjects or localities. Bhabha describes how the colonial mimicry of British identity is a doubling that is both resemblance and menace, because the colonized other is "a subject of a difference that is almost the same, but not quite" (86). "The Brothers" describes a similar mimicry that also undercuts any stable authority: in the brothers' doubling of each other, and in James's intrinsic mimicking of the story being told to him by the very fact that he disavows his connection to it, knowing more than the teller of the tale, the poem explores the division registered within colonial society and the "disinherited" families that were one of its primary motors.

In seeking to understand the impact of colonialism on English rural society, Wordsworth was influenced by the work of William Gilbert, best known for his poem *The Hurricane: A Theosophical and Western Eclogue* (1796).[22] In a note to "The Brothers," Wordsworth declared that his "description of the Calenture is sketch'd from an imperfect recollection of an admirable one in prose by Mr. Gilbert, author of the Hurricane" (*William Wordsworth* 695). This source is not known, but if it developed out of the same theosophical context as *The Hurricane* one can see its relevance to "The Brothers." In a poem whose closest similarities are to the epic geographical contests of Blake's minor prophecies, Gilbert, originally a lawyer from Antigua, argues that the European colonization of America will ultimately lead to England's historical supersession. In his preface he argues: "The European subjugation of AMERICA, the AMERICAN MIND or LIFE only suffered a powerful affusion of the European; and, that as the solution proceeds it acquires a stronger and stronger tincture of the Subject, till at length that, which was first subdued, assumes an absolute, inexpungable predominancey, and a FINAL" (v).[23] Gilbert's metaphor for the forces that will destroy European empire is the hurricane that devastates it at the end of the poem. Wordsworth does not portray the destruction of English rural life in such sweeping terms, yet both "The Ruined Cottage" and "The Brothers" are poems about depopulation, which deal with the collapse of families as expressive of a larger historical condition. As such they share with Gilbert the thesis that Europe "depopulated America, and now AMERICA MUST depopulate her" (vii).

"The Brothers" is a contradictory reflection on rural English society in an age of travel and colonial commerce. It is also shaped, however, by Wordsworth's experience in a family that had been divided since the death of his father. Butler notes that the poem was written at "a time pivotal in developing his mature artistic temperament," as Wordsworth, seeking to establish a permanent "home at Grasmere," sought to define his own poetic identity "by weighing the tourist against the native son" (2). Just as important, the poem was written while his brother John, who had gone to sea in 1788, was enjoying a brief visit to Grasmere. During the twelve-year period when he had served first in the West Indies and then on the *Earl of Abergavenny,* an East Indiaman, John had been in England for only a few months. As Stephen Gill notes, the visit was welcome, since it seemed to knit "together [their] fragmented lives" (183). In 1798 John had offered to purchase a house in Grasmere for Wordsworth. Like Leonard, he appears to have been willing to sacrifice his own happiness for his brother's benefit. As Wordsworth declared, "He encouraged me to persist in the plan of life which I had adopted; I will work for you was his language and you shall attempt to do something for the world" (*Letters* 563). Wordsworth felt himself dependent on an economic endeavor that he considered as much a primary threat and source of fragmentation to English rural lives as it was for people in faraway places.

Late in 1800, shortly before John, now captain of the *Abergavenny,* left

Grasmere on a commercial venture to India, Wordsworth began work on "When first I journey'd hither, to a home," a poem that was largely complete by March 1804. Here he sought to establish some sense of kinship with his brother, whom he says "from all the life / And beauty of his native hills . . . went / To be a Sea-boy on the barren seas" (*William Wordsworth* 45–47). Shortly after John's arrival, he began daily visits to a fir grove near the cottage. Wordsworth describes his delight at discovering that his brother had, quite literally, inscribed his being into the grove by continually pacing along a self-made path. Colonialism functions in reverse, as John takes possession of a wilderness found in England and makes it his own:

> more loth to part
> From place so lovely he had worn the track,
> One of his own deep paths! by pacing here
> With that habitual restlessness of foot
> Wherewith the Sailor measures o'er and o'er
> His short domain upon the Vessel's deck
> While she is travelling through the dreary seas.
>
> (68–74)

Walking is here portrayed as a primary means of marking one's identity in space, a point Anne D. Wallace makes in proposing that Wordsworth used walking as a substitute for agricultural labor. In Wordsworth's poetry, she argues, spaces are given their social dimension—as "places"—through walking rather than through labor. "Against the background of a disappearing or subordinated georgic and the simultaneous economic decline of freeholders and rural laborers, his replacement of farmer with walker extends georgic's literary function into an era in which the culturally stabilizing capacity of agriculture seemed to have faded or failed" (149).[24] Wallace's insights are particularly appropriate for understanding the poem, because in it Wordsworth explicitly draws a comparison between pacing the grove and pacing "the Vessel's deck," an analogy that works in both directions. He describes how he discovered this grove after John had "Back to the joyless ocean . . . gone" (92), and tells how pleased he was that John had inscribed this pathway or social space, where the poet had seen none: "hither he had brought a finer eye, / A heart more wakeful" (67–68). Wordsworth named "the path-way" after John, so that "John's walk," both on the deck of the *Abergavenny* and in the grove doubles upon itself.

As if matters were not complicated enough, Wordsworth repeats John's actions: he literally walks John's walk, in both senses. Wordsworth custom-

arily composed while walking, so the creation of the poem is in many ways a
voiced doubling of John's silent pacing on both the deck and the pathway of
the grove. John is portrayed as "a silent Poet" (88), whose bond to Wordsworth seems less that of a brother than a kindred lover of nature: "thou a
School-boy to the Sea hadst carried / Undying recollections" (84–85). In
Wordsworth's world being a lover of nature was not enough. Memory either
fails or becomes pathological when one is in the tropics. Nature needed to be
supplemented by poetry. In the final lines of the poem, Wordsworth describes
how he frequently returns to John's grove, and he imagines that possibly,
despite the vast space separating him from his brother, the two men are
sharing the same poem at the same moment:

> Nor seldom, if I rightly guess, when Thou,
> Muttering the verses which I mutter'd first
> Among the mountains, through the midnight watch
> Art pacing to and fro' the Vessel's deck
> In some far region, here, while o'er my head
> At every impulse of the moving breeze
> The fir-grove murmurs with a sea-like sound,
> Alone I tread this path, for aught I know
> Timing my steps to thine, and with a store
> Of indistinguishable sympathies
> Mingling most earnest wishes for the day
> When We, and others whom we love shall meet
> A second time in Grasmere's happy Vale.
>
> (105–17)

Where is Wordsworth when in the grove he (like Margaret) walks, listening
to the "sea-like" sounds of the fir grove and timing his feet (both metrical and
physical) to those of his brother pacing the deck of his East Indiaman? And
what kind of space does John walk as he "mutters" and times his pace to "the
verses which I mutter'd first / Among the mountains"? Each brother carried
his own "store": John of the goods he hoped to use in trade; Wordsworth, a
"store" of "sympathies" and "wishes" for his safe return. The venture that
John hoped would profit himself, his brother, and his sister Dorothy proved
catastrophic. On 5 February the *Abergavenny* struck the shambles off Portland
Bill and, along with 231 other passengers and crew (among whom was Sir
Walter Scott's cousin John Rutherford, a new ensign of the East India Company), John was drowned.

Critics have long recognized that "Elegiac Stanzas Suggested by a Picture
of Peele Castle" expresses Wordsworth's response to nature in the light of his

brother's death. One idea of nature, in which the poet "could have fancied that the mighty Deep / Was even the gentlest of all gentle Things" (*William Wordsworth* 11–12), in which the castle, like England, was but "a treasure-house, a mine / Of peaceful years" (21–22), gives way to another, in which the castle opposes itself to a darker nature, "a pageantry of fear" (48). The poem is more than a statement of personal loss, for it reflects Wordsworth's changing understanding of England's place in the colonial world. In the "glassy sea" (4), which once mirrored a "Poet's dream" (16) of financial prosperity, he now sees betrayal and ruin. Instead of participating in the fiction of an England that confidently rides the waves, he now feels he must submit to a new economy, "a new controul," figured in a castle that "braves, / Cased in the unfeeling armour of old time, / The light'ning, the fierce wind, and trampling waves" (34, 50–52). Colonial labor and commerce now find their appropriate figure in a "Hulk which labours in the deadly swell" (47).

"Voices of Dead Complaint"

Colonial Military Disease Narratives

"you were left, as if
You were not born to live."
—William Wordsworth,
"The Ruined Cottage"

In a well-known essay written many years ago Robert Mayo argued that the poetry of Wordsworth's *Lyrical Ballads,* instead of being new, was typical of the sentimental magazine poetry of the 1790s. With obvious relish, Mayo noted that the subjects of these poems—bereaved mothers, forsaken and mad women; beggars, convicts, and prisoners; the old, sick, and indigent—were to be found everywhere in the popular literature of the day. They were conventional figures in the literary landscape of the decade, "stereotypes" "perfectly in line with contemporary taste" (495–96). Although Mayo leaves little doubt that the Romantic period saw an extraordinary rise in the literary appearance of such figures, his explanation is less satisfactory. For him they are a "literary fashion" (502), an excessive stage in the development of sentimental literature and social protest poetry. Wordsworth's beggars thus take their place in a "long procession of mendicants who infested the poetry departments of the *Lady's Magazine,* the *Edinburgh Magazine,* and other popular miscellanies in the last years of the eighteenth century" (500). No doubt these poems frequently do offer "stereotyped pathos and generalized poverty, hardship, and old age" (505). Nevertheless, it is worth asking whether this literature, despite its sentimentalism, is responding to a historical reality that has been largely ignored. Theodor Adorno once asked whether after Auschwitz the literary representation of suffering was any longer possible. Can it be that Romantic poets struggled with similar problems in attempting to portray suffering that existed on a scale that is hardly imaginable?

One group of "pariahs" that Mayo singles out is "soldiers and sailors who have fallen on evil times" (501). These people have rarely received much sympathy, yet in the literature of the 1790s they are everywhere, as are their bereaved mothers, their orphaned children, and their poverty-stricken and often abandoned wives, who Mayo tells us "were almost a rage in the poetry departments of the 1790s" (496). Even the Ancient Mariner, he notes, "is not completely unrelated to the anguished and homeless old sailors of the poetry departments," and "some of the difficulties readers had with this poem resulted from their trying to view it in terms of this stereotype" (502). The antiwar literature of the Romantic period, from Joseph Fawcett's *The Art of War* (1795) and Burns's "Soldier's Joy" to Byron's description of the attack on Ismail in *Don Juan,* has its share of poems that speak of servicemen who have been maimed or killed. The soldier bleeding in the sanguinary field is a common image, and not surprisingly so, since England was at war with France from 1793 to 1815.[1] One of the more popular genres, employed by both critics and supporters of war, is the "serviceman's return." Whereas in the patriotic press these events are happy ones, most of this literature uses the homecoming for critical purposes. The anonymous Irish street ballad of the 1760s, "Johnny, I Hardly Knew Ye," for instance, parodies such happy homecomings as a young woman resorts to black humor to deal with the shocking, maimed body of her lover:

> You haven't an arm and you haven't a leg,
> You're an eyeless, noseless, chickenless egg;
> You'll have to be put with a bowl to beg:
>   Och, Johnny, I hardly knew ye!
> With drums and guns, and guns and drums,
> The enemy nearly slew ye;
> My darling dear, you look so queer,
>   Och, Johnny, I hardly knew ye!
>   (Tillotson 1525)

Like many returned servicemen, her lover has been reduced to beggary. Similar representations of maimed and invalided soldiers and sailors can be found in contemporary engravings, notably by Gillray and Cruickshank. In

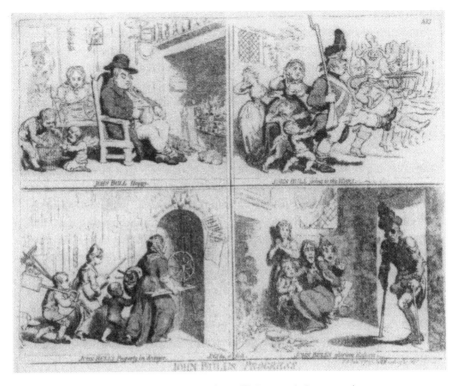

FIG. 3. James Gillray, *John Bull's Progress* (3 June 1793).

John Bull's Progress (3 June 1793) (fig. 3), for instance, the fat and dozing Bull of the first tableau finally returns to his now impoverished family as a gaunt, lame beggar.

Literary accounts of these individuals are significant not only from the standpoint of antiwar protest. Since soldiers and sailors played a key role in the military and commercial efforts of European nation-states to build and maintain their empires, their stories are very much bound up with colonialism. They were the primary workers in the massive expansion of sea trade and naval power that occurred over the seventeenth and eighteenth centuries. Living on board ships that drew their crews from several nations, or inhabiting the seaport towns that were springing up everywhere as the hubs in a complex network of commercial exchange and maritime transport, soldiers and sailors were part of a culture that was increasingly characterized by mobility, anonymity, and internationalism.[2] Charles White, searching for "skulls" for his racial science, did not have to travel far, for he found them "amongst the omnigenous seafaring population of Liverpool, illustrating all the races of men" (De Quincey, *Collected Writings* 1: 383). By situation and probably by attitude, sailors and soldiers were perceived as a people set apart, with their own separate culture. As the magistrate John Fielding suggests, "When one goes into Rotherhite and Wapping, which places are chiefly inhabited by sailors, but that somewhat of the same language is spoken, a man would be apt to suspect himself in another country. Their manner of living, speaking, acting, dressing, and behaving are so peculiar to themselves" (28–29). Although much of the literature of the Romantic period focuses on homecomings, for many there was no return. Because these were the people most likely to occupy the epidemiological contact zones opened up by colonial expansion, they were the ones most affected by colonial disease. Their stories thus raise a range of issues about how the epidemiological suffering produced by colonialism was understood. In representing colonial servicemen, the British reflected on colonialism as it was seen at home.

The number of people who died or lost their health in European colonial ventures is appalling, yet perhaps even more disturbing is the general silence that, with few exceptions, blankets these deaths. Drawn largely from the lowest rungs of society, either from the unskilled laborers who increasingly inhabited towns and seaports or from the merchant navy, common soldiers and sailors did not leave much of a documentary history. Gary Nash, speaking of the free unskilled laborers who manned the merchant navies and worked in American seaports, notes that they "are perhaps the most elusive social group in early American history because they moved from port to port with far greater frequency than other urban dwellers, shifted occupations, died young, and, as the poorest members of the free white community, least often left behind traces of their lives on the tax lists or in land and probate records" (16). Since conditions in the army and navy were usually even worse than in the merchant marine, eighteenth-century servicemen represent an even more elusive subcategory of this group, those who by circumstances and education were at the bottom of the social hierarchy. John Gabriel Stedman, in his *Narrative of a Five Years' Expedition against the Revolted Negroes of Surinam,* labels "private Men" as "being a Composition of Scum—Composed of all nations—ages shapes—and sizes by chance & by chance wafted together from all the different Corners of the Globe." He nevertheless notes that this *international* population "fight like little Devils, and have on many different Occasions been of infinite Service to this Settlement" (82). Rev. Henry Zouch of Wakefield speaks of the new "recruits from Sheffield, Leeds, Halifax, etc. [as] . . . the very sweepings of the street" (qtd. in Wells 80). E. P. Thompson calls them "casualties" or "casual laborers." "Distinct from the labourers (stablemen, streetsweepers, waterside-workers, unskilled builders, carters, and so on), were those for whom 'casualty' had become a way of life: street-sellers, beggars and cadgers, paupers, casual and professional criminals, the Army" (264). Given their low social status, it is perhaps not surprising that even as this social group is frequently seen in eighteenth- and early nineteenth-century literary and historical texts (How could they not be, given their primary importance to colonial expansion?), they rarely speak in them, and their disease experience is usually ignored. Complete records of deaths by sickness in naval hospitals were not kept until 1779, and deaths on board ships were not systematically recorded until 1811, when the Naval Office, responding to increasing concerns about mortality rates, instructed all commanders to provide them annually. Before this time, sailors were quite literally of no account. Most frequently their experience of disease appears in passing references, such as Gulliver's declaration, "I was Commander of the ship and had about fifty *Yahoos* under me, many of which died at Sea, and I was forced to supply them by others picked out from several Nations" (Swift, *Prose Works* 11: 227).

Even in death, other military ranks speak of their experience. For instance, the following inscription can be found on the funerary monument of Major Thomas Drinkwater, in Trinity Church, Salford:

> Thrice had his foot Domingo's island prest,
> Midst horrid wars and fierce barbarian wiles;
> Thrice had his blood repell'd the yellow pest
> That stalks, gigantic, through the Western isles!
>
> (Qtd. in Scott 1: 334)

Stedman, fearing he was not going to survive a fever in Suriname, had the foresight to compose a poetic epitaph:

> Under this Stone,
> Lays the Skin and the Bone,
> While the Flesh was Long gone of *poor Stedman*
>
> Who Still took up his Pen,
> And Exousted his Brain,
> In the Hopes these Last Lines Might be red Man,
>
> Of his Life he was tir'd,
> At no more he Aspir'd,
> D——nd the rogues, Shut his Eyes & Went Quietly to bed man.
>
> (375)

For common soldiers or sailors, who frequently ended up being thrown overboard or buried either in shallow graves on the beaches of the New World or in fields outside colonial settlements, we have no such epitaphs, and even their final resting places have been forgotten. In Robert Merry's "The Wounded Soldier," this subaltern population remains the "unnam'd dead" (B. Bennett 244).

Death in the West Indies

A few words must be said about how greatly disease affected this group. My focus will be on British operations in the West Indies, because it was here that the link between colonialism and disease was most obvious; however, mortality and morbidity rates were comparable in other tropical regions. One point must be stressed at the outset. As John R. McNeill observes, "European soldiers assigned to the West Indies could not expect to come home" (35). Normally, mortality among soldiers and sailors ran about twice that of civilian populations, as typhus, scurvy, venereal disease, and dysentery combined with crowded living conditions, poor hygiene, and inadequate nutrition in ships and camps to undermine their health. James Martin remarks, "The worst enemy to the soldier has, everywhere and at all times, been disease" (81). He goes on to speculate that over the course of the eighteenth and nineteenth centuries more men had been lost to disease *every twenty* years than had "fallen in our battles from the landing of Julius Caesar to the present time" (414). James Lind observes that "the number of seamen in time of war, who died by shipwreck, capture, famine, fire, or sword, are but inconsiderable, in respect of such as are destroyed by the ship diseases, and by the usual maladies of intemperate climates" (*Essay on the Most Effectual Means* 27). From such a perspective, the popular representation of the maimed or wounded soldier was itself a substantial distortion of their actual experience, a point noted by Samuel Johnson:

The life of a modern soldier is ill represented by heroick fiction. War has means of destruction more formidable than the cannon and the sword. Of the thousands and ten thousands that perished in our late contests with France and Spain, a very small part ever felt the stroke of an enemy; the rest languished in tents and ships, amidst damps and putrefaction; pale, torpid, spiritless, and helpless; gasping and groaning, unpitied among men made obdurate by long continuance of hopeless misery; and were at last whelmed in pits, or heaved into the ocean, without notice and without remembrance. By incommodious encampments and unwholesome stations, where courage is useless, and enterprise impracticable, fleets are silently dispeopled, and armies sluggishly melted away. (*Works* 10: 370–71)

In tropical regions, death rates were higher than elsewhere. There the traditional military assumption that power lay in amassing large numbers of troops
was contradicted by the fact that such large groupings favored the outbreak of
epidemics of malaria and yellow fever. J. W. Fortescue, the renowned historian of the British army, notes that "to assemble any great number of white
men together in the West Indies was the certain way to bring about an
epidemic of yellow fever" (4: part 1, 385). If full-scale military operations
were the worst of times for European servicemen, the best times were not
much better. Fortescue notes that in the normal course of operations "each
British battalion in the West Indies required to be renewed in its entirety
every two years" because of death and sickness (4: pt. 1, 141). Even as I
emphasize situations where mortality rates were particularly high, one should
recognize that the colonial norm for military personnel was not much better.
In the East Indies, prospects for survival were slightly better; on the West
Coast of Africa they were much, much worse. F. H. Lamb is somewhat surprised, on discovering a manuscript of the daily orders from the headquarters
of the Royal Marines in Fort Amsterdam, Curaçao, for a four-month period
in 1807, by the "somewhat macabre aspect of this chronicle" since "funeral
parties were detailed almost daily" (92). A modern reader needs to realize that
such a chronicle might have been written in almost any tropical region during
this period. Until the end of the eighteenth century, scurvy continued to
plague sailors on long voyages at sea. On shore or on short voyages, an array of
other infectious diseases were constantly at work.

As early as 1585, with Sir Francis Drake's attack on Spanish-held towns
in the West Indies, the British began losing large numbers of sailors there
to disease (among them Drake himself), and losses increased throughout
the seventeenth century, especially among the Spanish and French, as yellow fever and malaria took hold in the New World. Sailing from the Windward Islands in 1693–94, Francis Wheeler was forced to call off an attack
on Quebec when he lost 1,300 out of 1,800 sailors and 1,800 out of 2,100
soldiers to fever (Creighton 2: 103). In the journal of Captain Thomas Phillips, who commanded a merchantman in the West Indies, we learn how
difficult it was for him to keep his crew as His Majesty's ships kept pressing
his sailors into service to meet their declining complements. Captain Sher-
man of the *Tiger* told Phillips he had buried 600 men in two years, though
his ship's complement was only 220, "still pressing new [men] out of the
merchant ships that came in, to recruit his number in the room of those that
died daily" (237). The first major loss of men in the eighteenth century
occurred when Rear Admiral Hosier was sent in 1726 to Porto Bello, on the

coast of Panama, to blockade the Spanish galleons there. For six months Hosier sat in the harbor, blocking ships that were in fact empty, while his sailors died of yellow fever. By December 1726 he had lost so many that he was forced to return to Jamaica, where he obtained fresh crews. From there he spent the next six months blockading the ports of Vera Cruz and Havana. His ships' complement never exceeded 3,300 men, but out of a squadron of 4,750 he lost over 4,000 through disease—without a shot's being fired. In Jamaica he himself fell ill and died on 27 August 1728, as did his successors Commodore St. Lo and Rear Admiral Hopsonn (Lloyd and Coulter 98). John Campbell, in *Lives of the Admirals,* first published in 1744, was appalled: "I cannot prevail upon myself to enter into the particulars of a disaster which I heartily wish could be blotted out of the annals of this nation" (qtd. in Lloyd and Coulter 97). Colonial disease was very much a scandal, dealt with through silence.

When Admiral Vernon succeeded in capturing Porto Bello in 1740, Richard Glover penned "Admiral Hosier's Ghost," a poem that might initially seem to counter this silence and to criticize colonial activities in the tropics. In the midst of the on-board celebrations, "a sad troop of ghosts" appears— three thousand men in all—each shrouded in the "dreary hammocks" in which they died. Among them appears the shade of Hosier, who hails victorious Vernon to tell his "fatal story" (Masefield 131). "When you think on our undoing," Hosier's ghost declares, "You will mix your joy with tears" (131). Writing during the War of Jenkins' Ear, however, Glover has no intention of questioning England's expansionary efforts in the West Indies. The cause of the tragedy, Hosier claims, is ineptitude among naval authorities— that is, he was given orders "*not to fight*" (132, emphasis added). Too late, he realizes that he should have ignored his orders and "quelled the pride of Spain" (132). Even though he might have been condemned as a traitor, he would have "obey'd my heart's warm motion" and "play'd an English part" rather than suffering the pain and guilt of seeing his men die for nothing:

> "Unrepining at thy glory,
> 　Thy successful arms we hail;
> But remember our sad story,
> 　And let Hosier's wrongs prevail.
> Sent in this foul clime to languish,
> 　Think what thousands fell in vain,
> Wasted with disease and anguish,
> 　Not in glorious battle slain."
> 　　　　　　　　　(Masefield 132)

For Glover, colonial disease is a form of shame that can be erased only through military vengeance upon the Spanish:

> "O'er these waves for ever mourning
>   Shall we roam depriv'd of rest,
> If to Britain's shores returning
>   You neglect my just request;
> After this proud foe subduing,
>   When your patriot friends you see,
> Think on vengeance for my ruin,
>   And for England sham'd in me."
>
> (133)

Glover's poem expresses a typical British response to colonial disease in arguing that military "glory" and colonial gain can make up for the shame and indignity of tropical sickness. There is nothing heroic about dying from yellow fever, so Glover gives it a Spanish face; three thousand unburied dead will rest only when military vengeance has been exacted upon a recognizable enemy, when Vernon has "play'd an English part."[3] Glover thus uses the scandal of disease to further colonialism and to reassert military and patriotic values. Nevertheless, despite its propagandizing, the poem powerfully evokes, in ways that will be repeated by later writers, the image of colonial space as a region haunted by European ghosts. In its evocation of the specters of the colonizing dead—"these mournful spectres sweeping / Ghastly o'er this hated wave" (131)—Glover's poem captures what every eighteenth-century sailor knew about the West Indies, that it was the watery burial ground of innumerable servicemen.

The events that followed place Glover's poem in an ironic light. Jubilant over Vernon's success, the British decided to stage a massive deployment of soldiers and marines in the West Indies. Under the direction of Lord Cathcart, 8,000 British soldiers were enlisted. After numerous delays, Cathcart left England in October 1740, but by this time an epidemic of dysentery had struck the fleet, leaving 1,500 men sick and 600 dead (among them Lord Cathcart) by the time it reached Jamaica. There, having joined four battalions of men enlisted from the New England colonies, the soldiers embarked with Vernon for Cartagena, Colombia, in a fleet of fifty-eight ships and 18,760 men. The soldiers, now under the command of Lieutenant General Wentworth, landed in March 1741, and by 9 April they had taken possession of one of the major forts protecting Cartagena, losing 43 officers and 600 men in the assault. A week later the land forces were reduced from 8,000 to 3,500 by disease. They were forced to abandon the attack, but rather than leaving the area, the navy transports, now converted into hospital ships, remained anchored off Cartagena. J. W. Fortescue describes what happened:

> while the commanders [of the army and the navy] quarrelled the soldiers perished. Officers died as fast as the men, all discipline on the transports came to an end, and the men gave themselves up to that abandoned listlessness which was seen in Schomberg's camp in Ireland, when the bodies of dead comrades were used to stop the draughts in the tents. Day after day the sailors rowed ashore to bury their boats' loads of corpses, for there was always order and discipline in the ships of war; but the raw soldiers simply dragged their dead comrades up on deck and dropped them overboard, without so much as a shroud to their bodies or a shot to their heels. . . . So after a few hours the bodies that had sunk beneath the water came up again to the surface and floated, hideous and ghastly beyond description, about the transports, while schools of sharks jostled each other in the scramble to tear them limb from limb. . . . Thus the air was still further poisoned, sickness increased, and the harbour became as a charnel-house. At length, on the 5th of May, it was resolved to return to Jamaica and two days later the fleet sailed away from the horrors of Carthagena. (2: 73)

Of the combined forces, over 8,400 men died of fever. Of the approximately 12,000 soldiers who embarked on the expedition, only 3,569 remained when they left Cartagena, and of these, not above 1,000 were healthy (2: 70). Having returned to Jamaica, while the commanders deliberated what to do next 1,400 more died. Finally, like gamblers unable to quit the game, they decided to redeem their fortunes by attacking Santiago de Cuba. There, in three weeks, 2,260 more soldiers died of fever, leaving "less than three hundred privates fit for duty" (2: 75). One might have thought that matters would finally end here. However, 3,000 healthy reinforcements had just arrived from Britain, and Wentworth and Vernon decided to attack Porto Bello, which was once again under Spanish control (having brought England full circle). One thousand more men were thus lost to sickness and disease. By this time nine out of ten of the men who had originally sailed with Lord Cathcart had perished (2: 76).

Another large force was sent to attack Havana in 1763, during the Seven Years' War. After a two months' siege, the British army return indicates that 290 had been killed and 626 wounded. However, 694 men had died from disease. Two weeks later the losses of the combined forces were 636 killed, while nearly ten times that number, 5,508, were dead from dysentery and fever (Lloyd and Coulter 120). A letter written on 24 October 1762 by a major in the army stationed in Havana gives a more concrete picture of the impact of disease on the soldiers:

I think myself extremely happy in being among the number of the living, considering the deplorable condition we are now in. You will hardly believe me, when I tell you, that I have only 33 men of my company now alive, out of 100 when I landed. Our regiment has lost 8 officers, and 500 men. They mostly died of fluxes and intermitting fevers, the general diseases here. The other regiments have lost in proportion. We are now very sickly, as you may imagine, when out of 17 battalions here, we cannot muster 600 men fit for duty. The appearance of this country is most beautiful, and its natural advantages are many; yet a man's life in it is extremely uncertain, as many are in health one morning, and dead before the next. (Qtd. in Lind, *Essay on Diseases* 130–31)

The *Annual Register* for 1763 provides some idea of the human cost of the Seven Years' War, in which England gained control over Canada, India, many of the islands of the West Indies, and the Philippines: of 184,899 men enlisted during the period, 1,512 died in action, and 133,708 servicemen were lost to the navy either through disease or through desertion, the one recourse available to servicemen (qtd. in Blane, "Comparative Health" 205).[4] During the American War, 175,990 seamen and marines were raised; 1,243 of these died in action, while 18,545 died by sickness (losses through invaliding and desertion are not listed) (206).

Whatever benefits in general might have derived from eighteenth-century advances in living conditions and the medical knowledge of disease, and whatever particularly accrued to sailors from the Royal Navy's new understanding of antiscorbutic diets, for military personnel serving in the West Indies the century was not one of progress, for the worst was yet to come. Between 1793 and 1798, in an attempt to seize the Sugar Islands and to put down the black rebellion in St. Domingue (now Haiti), the British annually buried about 12,000 men (Fortescue 4: pt. 1, 496; 4: pt. 1, 565).[5] Fortescue concludes that "the West Indian campaigns, both to windward and to leeward, which were the essence of Pitt's military policy, cost England in Army and Navy little fewer than one hundred thousand men, about one-half of them dead, the remainder permanently unfitted for service" (Fortescue 4: pt. 1, 565). In his journal, Lieutenant Bartholomew James provides a personal view of the suffering behind these numbers:

The dreadful sickness that now prevailed in the West Indies is beyond the power of tongue or pen to describe. In a few days after I arrived at St. Pierre [Martinique] I buried every man belonging to my boat twice, and nearly all of the third boat's crew, in fevers; and, shocking and serious to relate, the master, mate, and every man and boy belonging to the Acorn transport, that I came from England in . . . the constant affecting scenes of sudden death was in fact dreadful to behold, and nothing was scarcely to be met but funeral processions in this town, of both officers and soldiers; and the ships of war was so extremely distressed that many of them had buried almost all their officers and seamen. (241–42)

He goes on to note that "out of about ten thousand soldiers and sailors which left Europe in the fleet from Spithead on November 27, 1793, I was one of about five hundred that ever lived to see [England] again" (269). Lieutenant Thomas Phipps Howard draws a similar picture of the misery of St. Domingue: "It is impossible for words to express the horror that presented itself at this time to those who were still able to crawl about. 30 Negroes were constantly employed in digging Graves & burying the unhappy wretches that perished; & scarcely could they working the whole of the Day, from sun rise to sun set, again dig Holes enough for the Dead, tho' three, four & five were tumbled into the same Grave together" (49). Howard cannot conceive that if the government were "perfectly informed of the work of Death that is so rapidly going on here, that they would any longer permit a Soldier of theirs to stay in such an Accursed Country" (118). If they did so knowingly, he concludes, "the great Characteristic of the Nation no longer exists & a System of the most unheard of cruelty & Inhumanity has arisen in its place" (118).

In January 1802 Napoleon sent his brother-in-law General Charles-Victor-Emmanuel Leclerc to St. Domingue in command of over 25,000 troops to put down the slave rebellion. The French had superior military force, and Toussaint-l'Ouverture was captured in April 1802. Seven months later, however, despite the monthly addition of new troops, 40,000 men were dead from fever. In May of the next year only 8,000 were left to surrender to the British, and the blacks took control of the island. The emergence of the first black state in the New World chiefly owed its existence to the decimating power of disease.[6]

Epidemics, the Military, and British Social Policy

This cursory examination of the disease history of eighteenth-century soldiers and sailors serving in the West Indies suggests that, at least for one segment of European society—mostly white lower-class males aged twenty to forty—the expansion of military power and trade into this region was catastrophic. During the nineteenth century, colonial military activity shifted to the East Indies and to Africa with similar high mortality rates. What is clear is that for marines, soldiers, and sailors serving in this region, *epidemics were the rule rather than the exception.* Why, then, does the tremendous suffering indicated by these numbers so rarely enter into either the literature of the period or our contemporary understanding of it?[7]

One factor is that high disease rates were seen to be *endemic* to military operations, so that the distinction between epidemic and endemic diseases became blurred; in a context where there was little expectation of health, at a time when an appalling number of sailors were dying of scurvy, epidemics were more easily ignored by authorities. James Martin notes, "We have lost an army in every quarter of the globe, and precedent has consoled us: it has always been so in our campaigns, and in our colonies" (413). Furthermore, these diseases did not affect all Europeans equally; they were largely restricted to a specific class that was generally seen as both a danger and a burden to society. Given our contemporary experience of the politics of AIDS, we are perhaps in a better position to understand how an epidemic that had a massive impact on a marginalized group within English society could be largely ignored. In many ways the silence that surrounds the disease experience of colonial servicemen can be seen as a paradigm of colonial disease in general: distributed differently across populations, it might appear to some to hardly exist or barely deserve mention. Those most affected by it, from indigenes to European subalterns, were rarely in a position to make their suffering known; frequently they did not survive to tell their stories, even if anyone cared to listen. Kai Erikson observes that "traumatic experiences work their way so thoroughly into the grain of the affected community that they come to supply its prevailing mood and temper, dominating its imagery and its sense of self, govern the ways its members relate to one another" (190). Colonial military subalterns powerfully exemplify the dynamics of social trauma: viewed as pariahs even as they were exploited to do the dirty work of empire, their culture—conveniently seen as a society unto itself—reflects the impact of a continuing epidemiological crisis that was ignored by others.

Servicemen were also seen to be especially predisposed to the sicknesses that ravaged their frames, brought on them by their animality, intemperance, moral laxity, poor hygiene, general ill health, and lack of prudence and discipline. In a remark that powerfully captures this general view, Gilbert Blane recommends that a general muster inspection be regularly used to instill proper hygiene, since otherwise "there will be men who will escape notice, and skulk below, indulging in filth and laziness" (*Short Account* 15).[8] The pathogenic living conditions on board ships were thus seen as a reflection of the disordered character of this population. "How necessary subordination and discipline are to health," Blane later remarks, as he goes on to claim that a major increase in morbidity in 1797 was "owing to the irregularities connected with the alarming mutiny which broke out in the beginning of that year, and was not suppressed for several months" ("Comparative Health" 177). The powerful association between moral discipline and colonial British culture has often been noted, but one of its origins, in the medical treatment of colonial servicemen, has not been recognized. Colonial medicine, with its concern for improving the health of populations that were considered sick because of inadequate hygiene or disorderly behavior, can be traced back to the medical management techniques of military physicians, who saw their role as one of reforming a population whose conduct made them fundamentally prone to disease. Not only did many colonial physicians draw their experience from military service, but their success in bettering the health of seamen and soldiers by improving hygiene, diet, and discipline was repeatedly remarked throughout the nineteenth century. These methods were extended to other populations—from prisons, to colonial settlements, to British society in general. The British obsession with discipline was thus not separate from anxieties about disease. The figure of the diseased sailor or the invalid soldier served as a moral exemplum to others of the need for discipline in the face of a tropical environment. By the Victorian period, colonial disease was almost exclusively seen as a moral problem. As the Victorian physician R. S. Mair writes, the appeal to climate as the cause of disease was "the bugbear always convenient to cover a multitude of personal sins." People "whose constitutions have been so impaired, as to necessitate a return to their native country, should assign the cause to their own imprudence, and want of self-restraint, rather than to any direct influence of the climate" (213). Sickness testified to a failure of moral character.

Critics are divided on to what extent British military authorities should be blamed for the epidemic conditions common sailors and soldiers lived under. The Admiralty was aware of these appalling conditions, and it did take some steps to rectify them. Military physicians, among them Lind, John Pringle, Thomas Trotter, Robert Jackson, Henry Marshall, Sir George Ballingall, William Fergusson, and Blane, played a key role in publicizing these conditions, especially from the 1780s onward. The naval surgeon Charles Fletcher is not unusual in drawing a parallel between cities and ships, and thus between the disease experience of the maritime and urban proletariat: "Shall we say that great Ships, like great cities, are the graves of the human species?" (41). Improvements were also made in diet and hygiene during the final decades of the eighteenth century. Yet for many navy doctors, epidemics were not necessarily exclusively caused by ships: they also were closely bound up with the populations from which the navy drew its recruits. Military physicians frequently argued that disease did not derive from the regular servicemen's ranks but instead came from the *outside,* through the practice of impressment. Two populations of servicemen were thus produced: the good sailor or soldier, shaped by military discipline, and the dangerous outsider, introduced by impressment. Blane argues: "It is . . . one of the principal means both of generating and spreading the seeds of disease, in consequence of that indiscriminate seizure of men for the public service, and the confinement that is necessary to secure them" ("Observations on the Diseases of Seamen" 154). "Ships newly commissioned, by receiving raw landmen, and drafts of seamen from crowded guard-ships, tenders, and hospitals," remarks Thomas Trotter, "are the most liable to suffer from infection" (1: 1). Lind divides these "outsiders" into "two sorts of men . . . viz. Sailors imprest after a long voyage from the East or West-Indies, or the Coast of Guinea; and such idle fellows as are picked from the streets or the prisons" (*Essay on the Most Effectual Means* 28). Lind was undoubtedly correct in recognizing that criminals were frequently infected with typhus or "jail fever" and that sailors recently come from the tropics would be carriers of malaria and yellow fever. Nevertheless, the division of sailors into these two groups was an artificial one that was difficult to maintain in the context of the colonial employment and frequent unemployment of servicemen.

Significantly, even though naval doctors argued *against* impressment, the practice continued despite its high mortality rates. A major reason for its continuance, beyond the simplistic view that sailors and marines were in short supply, is that the English government had long accepted the notion, at least tacitly, that these death rates were not a problem. It had learned how to use military service, with its high mortality, as a form of social control. The period does provide evidence of "managed" epidemics. In 1763, for instance, Sir Jeffrey Amherst, commander of the British forces in North America, is said to have distributed blankets inoculated with smallpox in order to control the Pontiac Indians of the Western Territories. The tribe was destroyed.[9] In the case of soldiers and sailors a less obvious mode of social control was employed. Although war was a threat to business for many merchants working within an increasingly international commercial context, for others in the propertied class, from at least the sixteenth century onward, war and disease frequently served a *productive* purpose, as they rid English society of the most dangerous segment of the working class—young, unemployed males: "Fellows of desperate Fortunes, forced to fly from the Places of their Birth, on Account of their Poverty or their Crimes" (Swift, *Prose Works* 11: 243–44).[10] A. L. Beier notes that "governments consciously recruited paupers and miscreants. Vagrants had been drafted since Edward I's reign, but under Elizabeth they became the mainstays of foreign expeditions, the Privy Council considering them 'such men as are fittest'" (94). For instance, in a letter written to Hampshire magistrates in 1624, Whitehall argued that pressing such individuals to serve in Holland would be for "the ease and benefit of the country, [which] will find it[self] being disburdened of many unnecessary persons that now want employment and live lewdly and unprofitably" (qtd. in Beier 94). This policy, which became even more pronounced during the eighteenth century, is given its most vivid illustration in Hogarth's portrayal *The Idle 'Prentice Turn'd Away, and Sent to Sea,* from the *Industry and Idleness* series. As with many sailors, Tom Idle's last appearance is on his way to the gallows at Tyburn.[11] As Douglas Hay has observed, "War was an invaluable device for the removal of the idle, and hence dangerous, poor" (141).[12] He further notes that "the Marine Society[,] founded by Jonas Hanway in 1756, clothed and equipped ten thousand impoverished men and boys from London and put them into the navy; as early as 1759, Hanway observed that after four years of war there were comparatively few ragged and vagabond men left in London for the society to send to the Admiralty" (141). Press gangs served a similar purpose, since individuals who had no visible means of support or who were unemployed were liable to conscription. Impressment was thus, Leon Radzinowicz notes, "one of the major expedients of British penal policy" (4: 79–104). Also, during periods of war criminals were often given the alternative of conscription in lieu of punishment or transportation. The "prison or the ship" is indeed the choice offered the young sailor in Southey's "The Sailor's Mother" when he is convicted of poaching (*Poetical Works* 153). We learn that his choice has cost him his sight, and probably also his life.

In focusing on "crime" and "poverty" as the primary factors influencing the recruitment of this broad population exported from Britain through colonial activity, one should not forget that this population also included those most likely to be engaged in *political* resistance to British domestic and imperial policy. Linebaugh and Rediker note: "Seamen in particular and wage workers in general were foremost among the most radical parts of the colonial population" (235), and they were active in the sporadic rebellions that marked the eighteenth century. They conclude:

The circulation of working-class experience, especially certain forms of struggle, emerges as another theme, linking urban mobs, slave revolts, shipboard mutinies, agrarian risings, strikes, and prison riots, and the many different kinds of workers who made them—sailors, slaves, spalpeens, coalheavers, dockworkers, and others, many of whom occupied positions of strategic importance in the international division of labor. That much of this working-class experience circulated *to the eastward*, from American slave plantations, Irish commons, and Atlantic vessels, back to the streets of the metropolis, London, cannot be overemphasized. (244)

The management of colonial disease therefore cannot be separated from the management of the politics of the international working-class population that they refer to as "the Atlantic Working-Class."

One of the more popular punishments for servicemen who had broken the law was to require them to serve in colonial regiments for life, as was the case of many involved in the 1797 naval mutiny (Wells 89).[13] On the West African coast, where slightly less than half of the soldiers stationed there died each year, the Royal Africa Corps was staffed with "Commuted Punishment men from England, composed of deserters and persons confined on board the Hulks who desire on being pardoned to serve His Majesty abroad" (Crooks 2). As Philip D. Curtin notes, "Out of 350 men sent to the Gold Coast in 1782, only seven were alive and on duty in 1785. The rest had either gone over to the Dutch, escaped and turned pirate, or died of disease—mostly the latter" (*Image of Africa* 91). Even though military officials were frequently opposed to impressment, especially of criminals, recruitment through the law courts remained popular. Even James Lind falls into this kind of thinking: observing the epidemiological dangers of clearing tropical regions of trees and shrubs, especially during the rainy season, he suggests that it should be undertaken only as "a proper punishment for such convicts as were saved from the gallows for this purpose" (*Essay on Diseases* 143).

Given the high mortality of enlisted men in the tropics, colonialism might be said to have served the purposes of the English propertied class in at least two ways: even as it contributed to the expansion of empire, it maintained the security of property at home by allowing the authorities to be rid of people they considered politically or socially dangerous. There were advantages to an administrative policy that ensured that a specific segment of British society would be most affected by colonial disease. For the propertied class, colonialism was a form of social or population control, as "it swept out of England thousands of men and boys from the class and age group most likely to face unemployment and destitution, those thought to be most likely to commit crimes, and a considerable although indeterminate number who had" (Hay 142). Joseph Townsend, in his *Dissertation on the Poor Laws* (1786), makes poverty a key element in a divinely authorized social system. "It seems to be a law of nature," he writes, that the poor should be to a certain degree improvident, that there may always be some to fulfil the most servile, the most sordid, and the most ignoble offices in the community. . . . The fleets and armies of a state would soon be in want of soldiers and of sailors, if sobriety and diligence universally prevailed: for what is it but distress and poverty which can prevail upon the lower classes of the people to encounter all the horrors which await them on the tempestuous ocean, or in the field of battle? Men who are easy in their circumstances are not among the foremost to engage in a seafaring or military life. There must be a degree of pressure, and that which is attended with the least violence will be the best. (35–36)

Parish relief, he argues, "tends to destroy the harmony and beauty, the symmetry and order of that system, which God and nature have established in the world" (35).

The silence about the epidemiological cost of colonization can thus be seen as an aspect of domestic administrative policy. The link between law and indentured labor in the colonies was another example of a policy that produced the following comment from the Jamaican Edward Long: "America has long been made the very common sewer and dungyard to Britain" (2: 270). This policy was directed toward what A. L. Beier calls "masterless men," that is, England's subaltern populations. Implicitly, the English landed gentry used colonial disease as a two-edged sword, augmenting their power both domestically and abroad. Empires were built using an expendable labor force. It was also, as Blane said, a population "no one takes cognizance of." He would later remark that sailors "in former times . . . had not the attention paid to them, which would have been due even to inanimate machines of equal utility; for there seemed to be much more anxiety about preserving arms from rusting, and cordage from rotting, than about maintaining men in an effective state of health" ("Comparative Health" 187).

Roderick Random *and "The Private Centinel"*

To understand the literary context within which Romantics took up the question of colonial sickness among common soldiers and sailors, a brief discussion of the important contribution of Smollett and Goldsmith will be of value. Thomas Carlyle had no difficulty recognizing Smollett's importance when he declared that this Scottish writer's "mission [was] to take Portraiture of english Seamanhood with due grimness, due fidelity; and convey the same to remote generations before it vanish" (qtd. in Boucé 17). A primary text in this delineation is *Roderick Random,* Smollett's semiautobiographical indictment of the Royal Navy. One of the most powerful passages in the novel is his description of the inadequate medical treatment of sick sailors on board *The Thunder:*

> But when I followed him [Thomson] with the medicines into the sick birth or hospital, and observed the situation of the patients, I was much less surprised to find people die on board, than astonished to find any body recover.—Here I saw about fifty miserable distempered wretches suspended in rows, so huddled one upon another, that not more than fourteen inches of space was allotted for each with his bed and bedding; and deprived of the light of the day, as well as of fresh air; breathing nothing but a noisome atmosphere of the morbid steams exhaling from their own excrements and diseased bodies, devoured with vermin hatched in the filth that surrounded them, and destitute of every convenience necessary for people in that helpless condition. (149)

For the medically trained Smollett, the naval vessel is a floating plague house where filth and putrefaction combine with stagnant air to produce the dreadful miasmas that cause epidemic fever.

In drawing attention to the pathetic conditions of military personnel, Smollett shared the outlook of many surgeons and physicians of the period, most of them also trained in Edinburgh. But Smollett also recognized that disease cannot be understood apart from the politics of national differences, as is clear in his account of the scandalous review of the sick sailors on the quarterdeck of *The Thunder.* Captain Oakhum (his name a pun on both oak and oakum, the tarred hemp used to seal wooden ships) "brought along with him a surgeon *of his own country*" (156, emphasis added). When the first mate, Morgan, known throughout as "the Welchman," brings the list of the sick to his attention, the captain insists that "I'll have no sick in my ship, by G—d." Angered by Oakhum's unwillingess to recognize disease as a reality, Morgan is about to risk insubordination when the captain's steward, "who *being Morgan's countryman,*" hurries him "out of the cabbin before he had time to exasperate his master to a greater degree" (157, emphasis added). Below deck, Morgan finds the Scots—"Thomson and me"—"at work preparing medicines" (157). The only way Morgan can deal with his indignation over Oakhum's assumption that "by his sole word and power and command, [he has] driven sickness a pegging to the tevil, and there was no more malady on poard" is to reaffirm his colonial identity, as he sings "a Welch song with great earnestness of visage, voice and gesture" (157). Thus readers are prepared to recognize that the horrors of the quarterdeck review, in which the English surgeon supports Oakhum's contention that there are no sick sailors on board, originate as much in English attitudes toward their newly subordinated "British" countrymen as in class affiliations. "It would be tedious and disagreeable," writes Roderick, "to describe the fate of every miserable object that suffered by the inhumanity and ignorance of the captain and surgeon, who so wantonly sacrificed the lives of their fellow-creatures. Many were brought up in the height of fevers, and rendered delirious by the injuries they suffered in the way.—Some gave up the ghost in the presence of their inspectors; and others, who were ordered to their duty, languished a few days at work, among their fellows, and then departed without any ceremony" (159). Smollett's experience as a Scot allowed him to recognize how far the framing of disease was informed by national prejudices and class. The unwillingness of the Admiralty to accept the reality of disease was thus mediated by its attitudes toward the subaltern and colonial populations it employed.

Roderick—like Smollett and the many other middle-class Scots who found advancement in colonial medical service—sees colonialism as an evil, but it offers him an otherwise denied opportunity for advancement. (For the Irish, who were largely common servicemen in the British navy and land forces, colonial service was hardly a career opportunity.) Early in the novel Smollett details how difficult it is for Roderick, as a Scot, to find work in England; thus one sees what Joseph Townsend meant by that "degree of pressure" that plays the crucial role in forcing individuals "to engage in seafaring or military life." When Roderick is given the choice between returning to England or staying in the West Indies, he chooses the latter. "When I recalled to my remembrance the miseries I had undergone in England," he writes, "where I had not one friend to promote my interest, or favour my advancement in the navy, and at the same time, reflected on the present dearth of surgeons in the West-Indies, and the unhealthiness of the climate, which every day, almost, reduced the number, I could not help thinking my success would be much more certain and expeditious, by staying where I was, than by returning to Europe" (199). Having pointed to the obstacles that stand in the way of a Scottish surgeon's establishing a career either in England or in the English navy, he concludes that the very unhealthiness of the West Indies is an *opportunity:* not only are surgeons in short supply with so many servicemen becoming sick, but also, "every day, almost," disease was producing new professional openings as the surgeons themselves fell ill. Advancement is "more certain and expeditious" in the West Indies—if one survives.[14] Having achieved some success, Roderick leaves Jamaica, as did Smollett: "I felt excessive pleasure in finding myself out of sight of that fatal island, which has been the grave of so many Europeans" (207). Colonialism is a gamble: you win only because someone else loses. (John Stedman makes the same observation in regard to military advancement: the death of high-ranking officers, though "regretted by every one," did have its consolations "to the Inferior gentry who were preferr'd in their places" [111–12].) Yet where Townsend celebrates "the harmony and beauty, the symmetry and order of [a] system" that leaves people with little choice, Smollett is critical of it. He points out that many of those engaged in colonial ventures are themselves products of earlier colonialism and choose to face disease rather than starvation.

The later venture of Roderick and his uncle Bowling in slave trading is not unconnected with the reflection on colonial disease introduced by Roderick's participation in Vernon's Cartagena expedition. Slavery was, of course, the basis of West Indian plantation economies, so any consideration of this region ultimately had to address it. As in many slaving ventures, Roderick (like the sailors) is denied knowledge of the destination of the voyage until the ship was "about 200 leagues from the Land's end" (407). Also, the merchants have made no provisions "for those [sailors] who are maimed in their service" (408). Roderick is initially quite pleased with his success as a surgeon; he succeeded in losing only one sailor to "those dangerous fevers to which northern constitutions are subject in hot climates" (407). He describes how, with four hundred slaves on board, they left "Cape Negro, and arrived in the Rio de la Plata in six weeks, having met with nothing remarkable in our voyage, except an epidemic fever, not unlike the jail distemper, which broke out among our slaves, and carried off a good many of the ship's company; among whom I lost one of my mates, and poor Strap had well nigh given up the ghost" (410). Roderick's callous lack of concern about fever among the slaves makes him at this point little different from Captain Oakhum, who also responds to sickness by ignoring it. Roderick is thus shown to be deeply involved in the economic relations and moral duplicities that victimize him. Throughout, Smollett portrays colonialism as a pervasive sickness, which feeds on masters and slaves alike. Roderick's identification with the situation of the slaves is not simply an overstated means of self-justification; it also expresses a profound sense of the constraints colonialism imposes on individuals. "Our ship being freed from the disagreeable lading of Negroes, to whom indeed I had been a miserable slave, since our leaving the coast of Guinea, I began to enjoy myself, and breathe with pleasure the pure air of Paraguay, this part of which is reckoned the Montpelier of South America, and has obtained, on account of its climate, the name of Buenos Ayres" (410). For Roderick, colonial space is a dangerous disease environment where freedom is denied; unlike the slaves, however, he sees it as a temporary situation that can ultimately be replaced by a "salubrious air" ("buenos ayres"), the "healthy" environment that colonialism has made possible. Smollett seeks to escape the oppressive aspects of colonial control by making it work to his advantage. Like the illnesses that were so much a part of it, tropical colonialism, for a middle-class Scot, is a stepping-stone to better things, if one can survive.

Although Oliver Goldsmith is best known for the *Deserted Village,* which remains one of the most important anticolonialist poems of the eighteenth century, an essay he wrote for the June 1760 issue of the *British Magazine* and later included as letter 119 of *The Citizen of the World* provides a valuable analysis of the life of a common soldier during the latter part of the century. Titled "On the Distresses of the Poor, Exemplified in the Life of a Private Centinel," it describes the encounter between the Chinese philosopher-naïf Lien Chi Altangi and a disabled soldier reduced to begging. The essay is laced with irony, for despite his miserable life the soldier continues to celebrate the ideal of English liberty and to thank providence that he is not worse off. "Except for the loss of my limb, and my being obliged to beg, I don't know any reason, thank heaven, that I have to complain; there are some who have lost both legs, and an eye; but, thank heaven, it is not quite so bad with me" (*Collected Works* 2: 460). (Southey employs the same kind of irony when in "The Sailor's Mother" the traveler remarks: "Old England's gratitude / Makes the maimed sailor happy" [152].) Altangi, on his part, is just as uncritical: "Every day is to him a day of misery, and yet he bears his hard fate without repining" (459). The narrative thus exposes the contradiction between British nationalistic ideology and the reality faced by the poor. The soldier recounts how, as an orphan, he was passed from one parish to another, each disclaiming responsibility for him: "At last it was thought I belonged to no parish at all" (460). After five years in a workhouse and a brief stint working for a farmer, he joins the ranks of casual laborers, "working when I could get employment, and starving when I could get none" (461). One day, passing through a field owned by a magistrate, he kills a hare and is sentenced under the vagrancy laws to transportation to the American plantations. Confined with two hundred others in the ship's hold, the soldier remarks that though others "died very fast, for want of sweet air and provisions," providence was "kind" to him because a continuous fever "took away my desire of eating" (462). "Sold to the planters" as an indentured laborer, he serves seven years, "obliged to work among the negroes." Finally he succeeds in making his way back to England, but without a parish to return to, lest he be "indicted for a vagabond once more" he stays in town, working as a casual laborer, doing "little jobbs when I could get them." As might be expected, this situation leads to his impressment as a soldier on the Continent, where he receives a chest wound. Discharged when peace comes and unable to work, he finds employment as a mercenary for the East India Company. After fighting in India and raising himself to the rank of corporal, he "fell sick, and when I became good for nothing, got leave to return home with forty pounds in my pocket (468)." In England he is once more pressed into the navy (it is now the beginning of the Seven Years' War). On board, he is accused of feigning "sickness to be idle" and is beaten. A series of mishaps follows, during the last of which he loses four fingers and a leg. Had he been maimed on a king's ship rather than a privateer, he claims, "I should have been entitled to cloathing and maintenance during the rest of my life, but that was not my chance; one man is born with a silver spoon in his mouth, and another with a wooden ladle" (465).

Goldsmith's portrayal of the miserable life of the private centinel is a powerful indictment of English parish and vagrancy laws, which conspire to produce a large group of people who, being denied a "place" in English society and common social rights, are made available for employment in the colonial military forces. Christopher Brooks has noted that in both a legal and an economic sense, the centinel is of "no account" ("Guilty of Being Poor").[15] Unable to establish an affiliation with a specific parish, he has no social identity. When he is being prosecuted as a vagrant, the centinel attempts "to give a full account of all that I knew of my breed, seed, and generation; but though I gave a very true account, the justice said, I could give no account; so I was indicted" (461). Later, when he seeks to avoid being pressed into service, the same thing happens: "As I could give no account of myself, (that was the thing that always hobbled me,) I had my choice left, whether to go on board a man of war, or list for a soldier" (462). Victimized by English society and legally denied a "place" within it, the centinel nevertheless "limps off" still proudly mouthing the clichés of British imperialism. "Blessed be God, I enjoy good health, and will for ever love liberty and Old England. Liberty, property, and Old England, for ever, huzza!" (465). Earlier, without apparent recognition that he himself is little better than a slave, he expresses a detestation of the French, "because they are all slaves, and wear wooden shoes" (464). As Brooks has observed, "The centinel possesses no property, no liberty to be an economic being, and apparently nothing possesses him except Newgate, the press-gang, and misfortune" ("Guilty of Being Poor").

Stedman's "Heart of Darkness"

Although "The Private Centinel" provides a valuable portrait of the life of an English servicemen during the eighteenth century, a more concrete view of what it meant to be a soldier stationed in the tropics is provided by John Gabriel Stedman in his *Narrative of a Five Years' Expedition against the Revolted Negroes of Surinam*. Based on the journal Stedman kept between 1773 and 1778 while serving as a captain in a regiment of volunteers sent to Dutch Suriname to put down a slave rebellion, the narrative was published by Joseph Johnson in 1796. Stedman's reasons for joining this expedition confirm Smollett's views. "I should never have engaged" in this war, he writes, "had I known any other way to push my fortune" (86). In debt, Stedman had originally resigned himself to "the desperate ressourse of going as a common sailor to North America or the Mediterranean, or even up the Baltick incognito for a voyage not longer than 9 months" (xxi); but when he heard of the expedition he concluded that participation in "so Hazardous a Service" (29) would be rewarded with military advancement. At the time a lieutenant in Holland's Scots Brigade, he was immediately made a captain. Although Stedman is not a Conrad, his journal is very much a "heart of darkness" narrative, which shows his progressively deeper understanding of the scale of the losses sustained by European troops in their attempt to put down an organized slave rebellion.

The early part of the book, covering the five months when Stedman was stationed in Paramaribo, provides a general description of the geography and history of the Dutch settlements in Suriname, an account of the luxury and violence of the plantations, interspersed with studies of the region's flora and fauna. Late in February, three weeks after their arrival, sickness breaks out among the officers, and Stedman attributes it to the effects of dissipation in a tropical climate: "In a Climate where an European is so much debilitated by perpetual perspiration even when he does nothing but sit still . . . the Smallest Exercise and particularly excesses must be to him of the most pernicious Consequence" (49). Stedman resolves to avoid such activities "as the only means of preserving my health." By early May, however, he too comes down with a fever, with little expectation of recovery. Little is said about sickness among the common servicemen until late April, when out of a company of eight hundred men "Five or Six sailors now were buried every day" (97). One sailor, he says, castrated himself in a fit of fever. Whereas Stedman sees luxury and dissipation as having sent "Thousands to the Grave" (49) among the landowning class, he argues that common servicemen are dying through abusive overwork and neglect by their commanding officers. "How often have I heard the Groans of the helpless and agonising young Man—allowed to die for mere neglect and want where both the proper attendants and necessary comforts in plenty might be had, and with but Little trouble while his naked trembling and half Starved Companions exausted with navy and military hardships and fatigue had Scarsely strength sufficient left to carry him to the Grave. . . . [S]uch Numbers of Stout able and blooming young Men are now dayly swept to the Grave—whole crews and Companys of whom if properly look'd after might have lived for Years to the Good and Glory of theyr Country—" (78). On 23 May "Lieutenant Collonel *Lantman* [died] while a number of our Officers lay Seek—amongst whom at last in place of Joy and discipation pale Mortality began to take Place, & which from Day to Day encreased amongst the private Men at a most Lamentable rate—" (102). By late June only about four hundred able-bodied men are left of the original company of eight hundred, "the Hospital being crowded by invalids of every kind" (113). "Officers and Soldiers were indeed riding post haste on the highway to eternity," Stedman writes, "and all hitherto to no purpose" (111).

Early in July Stedman is finally ordered to set out with forty-two men and two river barges, which he named the *Charon* and the *Cerberus,* to establish defense outposts on the Cottica River, in eastern Suriname—"after having been kept fidling, dancing, and dying for 5 months at Paramaribo the Manoeuvres were fairly begun" (116). Death within the context of military action makes sense; dying through inaction does not. These ten weeks constitute the psychological heart of the narrative, as Stedman describes his feelings of frustration, isolation, and powerlessness while waiting, in the depths of "the most horrid and inpenetrable woods" (118), for a sign of the rebel slaves. As Stedman is setting out, a plantation owner warns him of the futility of the enterprise. "As for the Enemy . . . you may depend on not seeing one single Soul of them. . . . But the Climate, the Climate will murder you all" (122). As in the West Indies, blacks had learned that success lay less in fighting than in delaying European troops long enough for yellow fever and malaria to take their toll. On 18 July Stedman receives news that fever has broken out on the *Cerberus.* On the twenty-second a sergeant and private are sent downstream to the hospital established at the military post called Devils Harwar. On 28 July he learns that the commanding officer on the *Cerberus,* Lieutenant Stromer, has a fever and that a man has died at Devils Harwar. The next day he delivers Stromer and five other sick men to the hospital. On 4 August, however, Stromer is dead, and burial efforts prove horrific: "Having contrived to make a Coffin of old boards, the Corps[e] drop'd through it before it reach'd to the Grave and afforded absolutely a shocking Spectacle" (135). On 8 August another officer named Macdonald falls sick (he lived long enough to die on the return trip to Holland in 1777), followed by Second Lieutenant

Baron Ower on the twelfth and Second Lieutenant Cattenburgh on the eighteenth (both died at Devils Harwar on 25 August). At this point with only
four common marines left, the *Cerberus* is retired. Stedman writes to the
commander, Colonel Fourgeoud, requesting relief but receives the response
that "we were Still to Continue on the cursed Station by his order who like a
true General was Relentless of our Misery and Complaints" (139). Increasingly, over the course of the narrative, Fourgeoud is seen as the ultimate cause
of Stedman's distresses, a focus for his frustration and fear in dealing with the
tropical environment. When on 22 August Stedman himself becomes sick, he
despairs of surviving. "I . . . was now truly in a Pitiful condition," he writes,
"deprived of both my Officers and my Serjeant, my Men upon the three Stations viz. the 2 barges, and Devils Harwar together melted down to only 15
from the 42 without a Surgeon or Refreshment surrounded with a black for-
rest, and exposed to the Mercy of a relentless Enemy should he be Inform'd of
our defenceless Situation" (140). Three days later, faced with a likely rebellion
among the remaining marines under his command (three more had by this
time fallen sick), Stedman concludes that "nothing else was now expected
more for me who was at this moment in a burning fever, forsaken by all my
Officers and Men, without a friend, or assistance of any kind" (145).

At this point Stedman finally receives an order from Fourgeoud to relieve
the station at Devils Harwar. Although his spirits initially recover, he soon
learns his optimism is premature: the place got its name from its "very great
unhealthiness" (124), proving to be a "Pest house of the human species"
(125). Fourgeoud provides Stedman with twenty more troops, but these are
"the refuge [refuse] of the whole Party, with agues, wounds, ruptures, and
rotten limbs most of whom next day were obliged to enter the Hospital"
(152). On 29 August two more of Stedman's men die, just as he learns that the
rebels are nearby and have burned three plantations. On hearing this news,
not only "the few that were well" but the sick also could be seen "crawling on
hands and feet to their Arms." Seeking to find a comparison for "such a Scene
of Misery and distress here lame, blind, Seek, and wounded, in the hopes of
preserving a wretched existance rushed upon certain Death," Stedman quotes
Thomson's description, in "Summer," of Admiral Vernon at Cartagena:

> You Gallant Vernon Saw
> The miserable Scene; you Pitying Saw.
> To infant weakness sunk the Warriors Arm,
> Saw the deep racking pang; the ghastly form,
> The lip pale quivering, and the beamless Eye,
> No more with ardour bright.   (152–53)

What might seem a sentimental identification with Vernon, however, is shortly thereafter undercut when Stedman speaks of the soldiers' persecutor, "the Gallant Fourgeoud," the allusion suggesting that there is no major difference between the two. Stedman describes how the troops spent the night expecting imminent attack: "No Enemy appearing in the morning we buried the dead in theyr hammocks, not a board to make a Coffin to be met with on the whole post." On 30 August he is left with twelve able-bodied men under his command. The next day he writes: "In the Morning found dead 2 more of my poor Soldiers on the Ground" (153). A day later another man is buried, and Stedman can hardly conceive how the remaining soldiers can even survive the toil of burying their dead. On 2 September "another man died" leaving him with "7 Marines" (154); the next day, "I buryed another of my Marines" (154). On 4 September "one died again," and none of his marines is well. "I began now to be reconsiled to putting my last Man under Ground, and to leap into the Grave after him myself—when finally arrived from Paramaribo a barge with the proper reinforcement, Ammunition, Provisions, Medicines—a Surgeon &c &c" (154–55). A week later, on 12 September, Stedman is finally given sick leave. "Stepping in the boat, I left this human butchery & where I had burried so many brave fellows, & row'd with 6 Negroes and my black boy to the Town of Paramaribo" (161).

Stedman's account of his ten weeks on the Cottica River establishes a pattern that would be repeated throughout the narrative as Fourgeoud, over the next three years, expanded the range of the expeditions into the wilderness without showing any greater success against the rebels. By 18 November, with Major Rughcopf "dead at last" (203), Stedman was now responsible for four hundred men (two hundred of them sick), so his understanding of the scope of military action and its epidemiological cost is much greater. With the same desire for scientific accuracy that characterizes his extensive descriptions of the flora and fauna of the region, he details the awful diseases that have affected his men, notably the prickly heat (which settlers believed was part of the "seasoning" to a new climate), ringworm, chigoes (a sand flea that burrows into the feet), belly-hatty or drygripes (probably caused by lead poisoning), putrid fever (malaria or yellow fever), agues, boils, consaca (a mycosa like athlete's foot, which Stedman avoided by not wearing shoes), and bloody flux (dysentery). Throughout, Fourgeoud is implacable in his desire to locate the rebel settlements. "March thro' a Swamp or Marsh in Terra Firma," a plate that was probably engraved by William Blake, captures the horror of these marches, as the men are shown wading up to their waists in the marshes, while the Urizenic Fourgeoud, through sheer will, points their direction (fig. 4). During this period Fourgeoud received reinforcements from Holland, bringing their overall numbers to somewhere between 1,200 and 1,650 men. Of these, fewer than one hundred returned. Writes Stedman: "Others were Ruin'd both in the frame of theyr *Body & mind* past all Recovery; . . . in Short out of a number of near twelve hundred Able bodied men, now not one hundred did return to theyr Friends at home Amongst whom Perhaps not 20 were to be found in perfect health, all the others a verry few of the Remaining Relief Excepted, being Repatriated, sick; discharged, past all Remedy; Lost; kill'd; & murdered by the Climate. . . . Amongst the dead were including the Surgeons betwixt 20 & 30 Officers, three of which number were Colonels, & one a Major, which were the Fruits of this Long & Disagreeable expedition in the marshes and woods of Surinam" (607). The frontispiece of Stedman's *Narrative* (fig. 5), which displays the white European standing over the body of a slain rebel, is a powerful indictment of colonial military victories, even though Stedman's guilt is registered sentimentally: " 'Twas *Yours* to fall—but *Mine* to feel the wound." One of the great ironies of this portrait of colonial military heroism is that by far the majority of deaths in this narrative are of Europeans—not by wounds, but by disease.

Stedman's *Narrative* has long been recognized for its importance in the antislavery debates of the 1790s, and most notably in the work of Blake.[16] What has not been recognized is its contribution to growing public concern, during the 1790s, about the epidemiological cost of colonialism. Stedman provides countless examples of the extreme violence of slaveowning societies and of the lack of any form of social justice for blacks. Yet it is equally obvious that European soldiers are hardly better off. In fact Stedman demonstrates that "to[o] often at least with some nations the Sailor the Soldier and the Slave but differ in the name" (78). He even suggests that common soldiers and sailors are "actually being used worse than the negroes in this Scorching Climate. . . . I have heard a poor Sailor wish to God he had been born a Negroe and beg to be imploy'd amongst them in Cultivating a Sugar or Coffee Plantation—all this is truly Shamefull and Calls loudly for imediate redress" (97). Modern criticism, interpreting such comments solely in terms of an apologetics for slavery, has also contributed to the silence that envelops European colonial disease.

Stedman's *Narrative* is a complex social document because it repeatedly suggests that "slavery" and "military service" are almost identical—both being structured by an enormous loss of life, by loss of liberty, and by lack of social justice—even as it continues to see "war" as fundamental to human life. Despite what he went through, Stedman continued to support both institu-

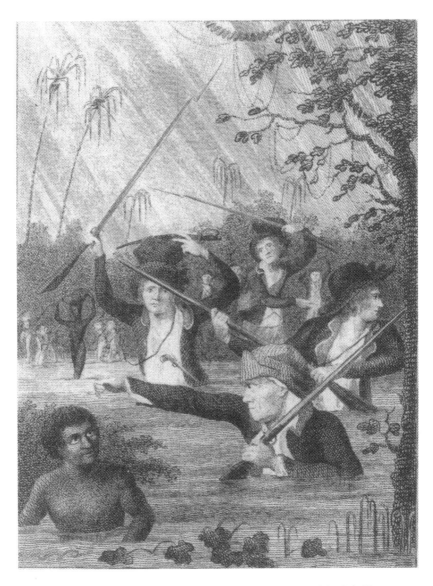

FIG. 4. William Blake (?), engraver. "March thro' a Swamp or Marsh in Terra Firma," in John Gabriel Stedman's *Narrative of a Five Year's Expedition against the Revolted Negroes of Surinam,* ed. Richard and Sally Price (Baltimore: Johns Hopkins UP, 1988).

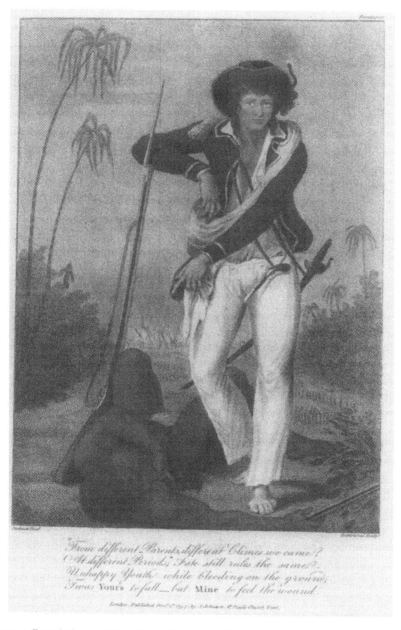

FIG. 5. Frontispiece to John Gabriel Stedman, *Narrative of a Five Years' Expedition against the Revolted Negroes of Surinam,* ed. Richard and Sally Price (Baltimore: Johns Hopkins UP, 1988).

tions. Thus he can be critical of Thomas Clarkson's abolitionist arguments not because his estimate of the number of blacks lost annually through slavery is incorrect, but because it pales beside the annual losses suffered by European servicemen. "These 100000 Spoke of to be transported yearly, are shurely but a very small proportion, to the Millions, that in all Europe annually expire under the name of Liberty, loaded with the pangs of want & disease, and crushed under the galling chains of oppression" (170). Nor are urban prostitutes much better off: "Above 50,000 helpless young Women, who independent of their genius, and beauty, must for the Sake of a loathsome temporary Subsistance, parade the Streets of our Metropolis in all Weathers, exposed to all thats Horrid, till they die unpitied upon a dunghill, in the middle of their own Countrymen, Starved, destested, kik'd, and wallowing in Corruption." Yet Stedman still maintains that "what happens in Africa, the same as what happens in Europe seems so perfectly necessary to me" (171). He consequently supports not only slavery, but also the high death rate of sailors.

As for the *Sailors* imployed in it [the slave trade] great numbers of them perish I acknowledge, but who if not died in this Way, would possibly have been obliged, to pick your Pockets for a Subsistance, and in Company with too many of theyr unfortunate Ship Mates, have been hang'd to keep them from Starving—it being very well known that these poor Men who are the props, and bulwarks of every Mercantile-Nation have no Provisions made for them in times of Peace, and that the brave Tar, who has escaped a watery Grave during the War to protect your Life and Property is often only saved to exchange it for an Airy one when it is over—thus better go to the Coast of Guinea to buy Negroes. (171)

Here the conservatism of Townsend and the cynicism of Stedman meet: the sailor must choose between war, the hanging tree, and the Guinea slave trade.

Even though many of Stedman's contemporaries would have been critical of his acceptance of the "state of war," they nevertheless would have recognized the close similarities between slaves and soldiers. Both, as Blake suggests in *Visions of the Daughters of Albion,* are "bound back to back" (pl. 2, line 5) by Theotormon. Elizabeth Bohls suggests that this close identity between slave and soldier produces in the *Narrative* a complex mimetic structure, as Stedman continually sees himself in the rebelling slaves that he is fighting; at one point he is even mistaken for Bony, the leader of the rebelling blacks ("Mimicry"). Similarly, the accounts of slaveowners' cruelty that are interspersed throughout the narrative are balanced by those decrying the cruelty of the commander Fourgeoud. Nevertheless, common soldiers remain anonymous in this text: it is the deaths of the officers that receive individual mention, especially the "Gentlemen Officers," who are specially listed.

The Ancient Mariner's "Ghastly Tale": Tropical Disease as Punishment

At the end of a century largely silent about the enormous number of servicemen being lost in military and colonial ventures, the 1790s saw the emergence of debate, especially with the greater public role being played by military physicians and the reports of the casualties in the British attempt to occupy St. Domingue. It should now be clear that the appearance of a literature focused on dead and dying soldiers and their abandoned wives may have less to do with literary fashion than with a growing need to understand and speak about the epidemiological cost of colonialism, especially when we realize that throughout most of the eighteenth century about one-quarter of British battalions were in or bound for the West Indies.[17] The ongoing warfare on the Continent was causing equally disastrous losses by disease, though public concern did not develop substantial momentum until the scandalous losses at Walcheren, where in six months, out of an original force of 39,000 men, almost 4,000 died of malaria and over 11,000 returned sick.

One gauge of the depth of this concern is that even the more conservative voices in the British Parliament were beginning to question the cost of colonial policy in the West Indies. Edmund Burke, for instance, was arguing that it was not military might but a combination of race and climate that was the true enemy of the British:

In carrying on the war in the West Indies, the hostile sword is merciful; the country in which we engage is the dreadful enemy. There the European conqueror finds a cruel defeat in the very fruits of his success. Every advantage is but a new demand on England for recruits to the West Indian grave. In a West India war, the Regicides have for their troops, a race of fierce barbarians, to whom the poisoned air, in which our youth inhale certain death, is salubrity and life. To them the climate is the surest and most faithful of allies. (9: 273)

Burke powerfully captures the growing public perception of the Sugar Islands as a deadly pathogenic space. It is not the people but the environment that the English are fighting, a gigantic graveyard or miasmatic space of death incessantly swallowing up new recruits. "It was not an enemy we had to vanquish, but a cemetery to conquer," he declares. Whereas throughout the eighteenth century the high mortality of Europeans in tropical regions was a justification for slavery in the New World, over the nineteenth century it raised more and more questions about the feasibility of empire.

Romantic poets, writing in the midst of this public debate, lacked neither knowledge nor examples of the terrible impact of war and colonial expansion on the lives of both indigenous peoples and the European "casualties" who served in the military.[18] On 5 May 1796, for instance, in a passage that anticipates the "Rime," Coleridge writes: "About 70 men of the 20th regiment landed at Plymouth on Tuesday last from on board a transport lately arrived from the West-Indies. Many of them are in an unhealthy state. They are the remains of 700 fine fellows, who have been thus reduced by the ravages of the yellow fever" (*Watchman* 332). As poets sought to respond to the staggering epidemiological cost of empire, however, they simultaneously faced the problem that by 1795 the discourse of protest was itself becoming commonplace. Sentimentalism's appeal to the generalized sympathy of an educated audience had lost its power. In the midst of suffering on an unprecedented scale, the rhetoric of the philanthropic observer seemed just that—rhetoric. Take, for example, the following passage from Coleridge's 1795 lecture "On the Present War":

We will now take a rapid survey of the consequences of this unjust because unnecessary War. I mean not to describe the distressful stagnation of Trade and Commerce: I direct not your attention to the wretches that sadden every street in this City, the pale and meagre Troop, who in the bitterness of reluctant Pride, are forced to beg the Morsel. . . . I will not frighten you by relating the distresses of that brave Army, which has been melted away on the Continent, nor picture to your imaginations the loathsome pestilence that has mocked our Victories in the West-Indies: I bid you not hear the screams of the deluded Citizens of Toulon—I will not press on your recollection the awful Truth, that in the course of this calamitous Contest more than a Million of men have perished—a MILLION of men, of each one of whom the mangled corse terrifies the dreams of her that loved him, and makes some mother, some sister, some widow start from slumber with a shriek! These arguments have been urged even to satiety—a British Senator has sneeringly styled them mere *common-place* against wars. I could weep for the criminal Patience of Humanity! These arguments are *hacknied;* yet *Wars* continue! (*Lectures* 59–60)

Employing a rhetoric that he disowns ("I mean not to describe," "I direct not your attention," "I will not frighten you by relating," "nor picture to your imaginations," "I bid you not hear," "I will not press on your recollection"), Coleridge stages an emotional fall into the "hacknied" language he has ostensibly rejected as he evokes the nightmare vision of a million dead men visiting the dreams of "some mother, some sister, some widow." He draws attention to the consequences of English colonialism; servicemen reduced to vagrancy on "every street," an army "melted away on the Continent," epidemic disease in the West Indies. A paragraph earlier, he notes the global nature of this destruction; after citing the "putrified fields of La Vendee," the "unnumbered Victims of a detestable Slave-trade," the starvation of people in Hindustan, and "scalping" in America, he declares that "the four Quarters of the Globe groan beneath the intolerable iniquity of this nation" (58). Yet he is also quite aware that his audience is no longer listening, that this style of rhetoric, even as he struggles to make it serviceable, has become "common-place" and that the scope of global crisis cannot be adequately conveyed by a sentimentalist vocabulary.

In this context Coleridge wrote the "Rime" not as a displacement of "history" but to express the enormous suffering produced by colonialism in a more imaginative and emotionally engaging language.[19] Like the sentimental magazine poetry of the day, the poem is structured as an encounter between a vagrant (one of those "wretches that sadden every street in this City") and an English gentleman. Coleridge, however, overturns the sentimentalist paradigm by giving us a Wedding Guest who feels he has better things to do than listen to a wandering, perhaps mad, vagrant. Nor are we asked to adopt the Mariner's point of view, even though his account dominates the poem. Their meeting is staged as a forced encounter: the Mariner cannot refuse to speak, nor can the Wedding Guest refuse to hear. The story must be told.

Jerome J. McGann has made a strong case for reading the "Rime" as an "imitation of a culturally redacted literary work" ("Meaning of *The Ancient Mariner*" 51). He argues that it is about the historical reception of salvific narratives, as the original story told by the Mariner in the early 1500s is made into a ballad by an Elizabethan minstrel and then published during the late seventeenth century as an edited text complete with a Neoplatonic prose gloss. According to McGann, the poem is an imitation of higher criticism's concept of Scripture; it "is, as it were, an English national Scripture; that is to say, the poem imitates a redacted literary text which comprises various material extending from early pre-Christian periods through a succession of later epochs of Christian culture, and the ultimate locus of these transmissions is England" (57).[20] It should be stressed, however, that the time frame of the narrative and its successive retellings, from the early sixteenth century to its publication as a literary imitation in 1798 (or to its revised form in 1817), is also that of the colonial period. The poem is very much a colonial narrative, "a supreme crystallization of the spirit of maritime expansion" (Ebbatson

175). Yet as an interpolated narrative, a story that has undergone interpretive transformations over three hundred years, it is more than simply an account of colonial experience—*it also enacts the historical reception of colonial narratives*. In the "Rime," Coleridge made his own frustration at representing colonial suffering—obvious in the lecture "On the Present War"—itself the subject of the narrative. For the Wedding Guest, who is but one of a long line of people who hear, sing, or read this tale, the events narrated are fantastic and frightening. They document an experience that is almost totally beyond comprehension, yet "he cannot choose but hear" (*Complete Poems* 38). As the final stanza of the poem suggests, the narrative has transformed him:

> He went like one that hath been stunned,
> And is of sense forlorn:
> A sadder and a wiser man,
> He rose the morrow morn.   (622–25)

The Ancient Mariner has been more than "stunned" by colonial experience; he has been traumatized. Recourse to the supernatural seems the only way to explain it. As Charles Lamb suggested, he has undergone "such trials as overwhelm and bury all individuality or memory of what he was—like the state of a man in a bad dream" (1: 266). Telling the tale thus becomes a partial means of expiating his own guilt:

> Since then, at an uncertain hour,
> That agony returns:
> And till my ghastly tale is told,
> This heart within me burns.
>   (582–85)

Even though the tale is told in Britain, the radical differences between the experience of the Mariner and that of the Wedding Guest seriously undermine the claim that the poem takes on the status of a "national Scripture" because a coherent interpretive community is lacking. Coleridge may have been attempting to write a Christian "saving history," one that would make sense of an otherwise pointless nightmare of suffering. Yet within the framework of the poem, the "salvific narrative" is itself another redaction, which does not fully displace the world and experience of the Ancient Mariner, whose conversion has been largely based on his sense of being in a world where "God himself / Scarce seemèd there to be" (599–600). What remains a priority throughout the poem is the necessity to tell the tale and to force someone to listen. Although in literal terms the "silent sea" (106) of the poem refers to the Pacific, it also evokes the silent world of death that the tropics had become by the end of the eighteenth century.

The "Rime" is typical of the kind of colonial narrative that Coleridge and Wordsworth were writing at this time because it is less about "colonial encounter" than about "colonial return." The epidemiological cost of colonialism returns in the form of "tropical invalids" who wander through the landscape as vagrants or frightening pariahs. Through his encounter with the Ancient Mariner, the Wedding Guest confronts colonialism registered not in the experience of indigenous populations, but in that of those Europeans who played a key role in the expansion of empire. He fears what he sees, and rightly so, because the Mariner embodies sickness and death. As in Glover's "Admiral Hosier's Ghost" the disease experience of the common sailor is anonymous and spectral, voiced by the background appearance of silent ghosts—"these mournful spectres sweeping / Ghastly o'er this hated wave" (Masefield 131). The Ancient Mariner's voice draws its being from this spectral world; it taps into the dark cultural unconscious of an England that recognized its fundamental link to these pariahs even as it disowned them. To the Wedding Guest he is almost a figure of the colonial landscape itself, the beaches of the New World—"thou art long, and lank, and brown, / As is the ribbed sea-sand" (226–27). "I pass, like night, from land to land" (586), the Ancient Mariner declares, as if he were death itself and a force that moves across the globe, recognizing no geographical boundaries. Sara Suleri suggests that "colonial facts are vertiginous," that "they move with a ghostly mobility to suggest how highly unsettling an economy of complicity and guilt is in operation between each actor on the colonial stage" (3–4). Coleridge's narrative of the encounter between the Wedding Guest and Britain's disowned son, the Mariner, profoundly enacts this economy of "complicity and guilt."

Like Smallpox in the legend of the Kiowas, the Ancient Mariner is mythologized. Nevertheless one should not ignore the social and historical reality he embodies. James C. McKusick has suggested that his "ominous, shadowy presence" (106) can already be seen in the 1795 "Lecture on the Slave-Trade," where Coleridge claims that the West Indian slave trade has been an epidemiological catastrophe not only for blacks, but also for the sailors engaged in it:

From the brutality of their Captain and the unwholesomeness of the Climate through which they pass, it has been calculated that every Slave Vessel from the Port of Bristol loses on an average almost a fourth of the whole Crew—and so far is this Trade from being a nursery for Seamen, that the Survivors are rather shadows in their appearance than men and frequently perish in Hospitals after the completion of the Voyage. . . . In Jamaica many rather than re-embark for their native Country beg from door to door, and many are seen in the streets dying daily in an ulcerated state—and they who return home, are generally incapacitated for future service by a complication of Disorder[s] contracted from the very nature of the Voyage. (*Lectures* 238–39)

In drawing attention to the many sailors invalided or reduced to beggary or "shadows" by the slave trade, Coleridge was greatly indebted to the work of Thomas Clarkson, who made the high mortality rate of sailors a key justification for abolishing it. Although the British had long recognized the high mortality suffered by blacks—in Africa, during the "middle passage," and after their arrival in the West Indies—it was not until the late 1780s that attention was drawn to slavery's cost in sailors' lives. Not surprisingly, sailors had a good idea of the dangers, for despite the offer of higher wages, merchants had difficulty filling their ship complements and frequently resorted to subterfuge. It was a common saying among sailors:

> Beware and take care
> Of the Bight of Benin
> For one that comes out,
> There are forty go in.
> (qtd. in Rawley 286)

Clarkson, working for the Society for the Abolition of the Slave Trade, made the health of sailors working in the trade a public issue. To support his arguments, he did something extraordinary for the time: by personally interviewing sailors in the major slaving ports of London, Bristol, and Liverpool and examining ship muster lists, he attempted to compile a detailed record of what happened to *every* sailor employed in the trade. He notes that by 1788 "I had already obtained the names of more than 20,000 seamen, in different voyages, knowing what had become of each" (*History* 1: 412).[21] Clarkson was thus able to demonstrate, for instance, that "of 5000 sailors on the triangular route in 1786, 2320 came home, 1130 died, 80 were discharged in Africa and unaccounted for and 1470 were discharged or deserted in the West Indies" (Wilson 40). In the *Essay on the Impolicy of the African Slave Trade* (1788), in a passage cited by Coleridge, Clarkson asserted that contrary to prevailing opinion the slave trade was not "a nursery for [British] seamen" but "a Grave" that destroyed "more in one year, than all the other trades of Great Britain when put together destroy in two" (53–54). "If we refer it to the number of seamen employed" in each slave-trading voyage, Clarkson concluded, "more than a fifth perish" (the rates for Bristol, Coleridge notes, were higher) (57). Clarkson also pointed out another surprising fact: mortality rates for seamen on the middle passage were higher than those of slaves! As the

French trader P. Labarthe remarked in 1805, with some exaggeration, some "parts of the Guinea Coast were so unhealthy that the slave trade there was 'an exchange of whites for blacks'" (qtd. in Hartwig and Patterson "Disease Factor" 7).

Although Clarkson's disease statistics may appear extreme, they have been confirmed by recent historians. Curtin observes that "the death rate per voyage among the crew was uniformly higher than the death rate among the slaves in transit at the same period" (*Atlantic Slave Trade* 282–83).[22] He adds another surprising statistic, that even as the death rates for slaves fell throughout the eighteenth century, those "of the crew remained fairly at the same level" (284). Marcus Rediker explains this difference by pointing out that "the merchant who gave the captain a bounty for every slave delivered alive in the New World offered no such reward for a sailor still living at voyage's end" (43). Merchants had less investment in sailors than in slaves.

This historical context informs the Mariner's story as it explores how the racial violence directed toward blacks recoils on the enslavers. In Shelvocke's *Voyage* (1726), from which the central event in the poem was taken, it is the color of the albatross that disturbs Hatley, the second captain and justifies his destruction of it: "a disconsolate black *Albitross* . . . accompanied us for several days . . . till *Hatley* . . . imagined from his colour, that it might be some ill omen. . . . [He] at length, shot the *Albitross*, not doubting (perhaps) that we should have a fair wind after it" (73–74). Agreeing with Clarkson, Coleridge recognizes that although sailors seem to have greater control over their destinies, they are treated no better than those they victimize.[23] The "Rime" produces a similar symbolic conflation of these two groups, as many images used to describe the Ancient Mariner's disease experience could just as easily have been drawn from descriptions of slaves during the middle passage. The Mariner undergoes a symbolic "blackening" throughout the poem. There is a striking emphasis on his brown skin: "I fear thee, ancient Mariner . . . thou art long, and lank, and brown . . . I fear . . . thy skinny hand so brown" (224–29).[24] In describing the Ancient Mariner's entrance into the "tropical Latitude of the Great Pacific Ocean" (Argument), Coleridge reinforces the contemporary expectation that such spaces are pathogenic, for it is a depopulated world of corruption, disease, and death. Yet he also asserts that the institution of slavery has made this space what it is. The old sailor does not come upon an "other" but instead, as William Empson has observed, meets the "naked hulk" (195) and "rotting planks" of a European slaver ("Introduction" 28–32).[25] What the Mariner sees, he sees through the eyes of the slaves of the middle passage:

> With throats unslaked, with *black lips* baked,
> We could nor laugh nor wail;
> . . . .
> I bit my arm, I sucked the blood
> And cried, A sail! a sail!
>
> (157–61, emphasis added)

Thus the Mariner's experience extends across the determinacies of race, as it draws parallels between the maritime experience of sailors and slaves; through his own violence he has been given the ability to see the world differently.[26] Where the Kiowas personified disease in the figure of Smallpox, Coleridge locates it in a slave ship, whose reach now extends to the limits of the known world. "There was a ship" (line 10) are the Mariner's first words.

As the hulk approaches, it is portrayed as a force that imprisons, its naked ribs appearing like a "dungeon-grate" (179) standing "Betwixt us and the Sun" (176). On board are two allegorical figures, who represent the two primary aspects of colonialism—"Death" and "Life-in-Death." The latter is described as a prostitute:

> Her lips were red, her looks were free,
> Her locks were yellow as gold:
> Her skin was as white as leprosy,
> The Night-mare Life-in-Death was she,
> Who thicks man's blood with cold.
>
> (190–94)

Although prostitution, in a colonial context, has a massive range of meanings, Coleridge is here drawing extensively on the discourse on luxury, which plays such a key role in his understanding of colonial slavery. "The pestilent inventions of Luxury," he argues, are the fundamental basis of the West Indian slave economy (*Lectures* 236):

Perhaps from the beginning of the world the evils arising from the formation of imaginary wants have been in no instance so dreadfully exemplified as in the Slave Trade & the West India Commerce! We receive from the West Indias Sugars, Rum, Cotton, log-wood, cocoa, coffee, pimento, ginger, indigo, mahogany, and conserves—not one of these are necessary—indeed with the exception of cotton and mahogany we cannot with truth call them even useful, and not one is at present attainable by the poor and labouring part of Society. (236–37)

Coleridge consistently employs the metaphors of disease and contagion to describe the slave trade, whose source is to be found in the European "imaginary." He speaks of "the contagion of European vice" and of the West Indies as "the hot-bed of their [the Europeans'] pestilent luxuries" (240).

Coleridge portrays Life-in-Death as having "leprosy," a disease that was associated not only with the Middle East and Africa but also with the impact of European colonialism on the people of the Pacific.[27] Writing less than a decade after Captain James Cook's Hawaiian voyage, a surgeon describes their deplorable condition:

The beauty of the climate, and fertility of the soil, might render the inhabitants extremely happy, if the leprosy and venereal disease prevailed among them less generally, and with less virulence. These scourges, the most humiliating and most destructive with which the human race are afflicted, display themselves among these islanders by the following symptoms: buboes, and scars which result from their suppurating, warts, spreading ulcers with caries of the bones, nodes, exostoses, fistula, tumors of the lachrymal and salival ducts, scrofulous swelling, inveterate ophthalmiae, ichorous ulcerations of the tunica conjunctiva, atrophy of the eyes, blindness, inflamed prurient herpetic eruptions, indolent swellings of the extremities, and among children, scald head, or a malignant tinea, from which exudes a fetid and acrid matter." (Pérouse 2: 337)

Since the sailors themselves were also afflicted by many of the same diseases, Life-in-Death is the allegorical embodiment of colonial epidemiology.[28] Leprosy also brings into focus the importance of race and skin color within the economics of colonialism. "Her skin was as white as leprosy" suggests both an artificial whitening of the skin and a disease of "white" society.[29] In the *Watchman* essay "On the Slave Trade," Coleridge emphasizes the link between luxury, cosmetics, and leprosy when he writes that the various reasons that have been brought forward to justify the slave trade "have been the cosmetics with which our parliamentary orators have endeavored to conceal the deformities of a commerce, which is blotched all over with one leprosy of evil" (136). Coleridge's Life-in-Death represents this "leprosy of evil." Like the "painted ship" and the "painted ocean" (*Complete Poems* 117–18), she personifies what the world the Mariner moves in has become.

This encounter produces one of the most vivid representations of tropical death in British literature. In "On the Slave Trade," Coleridge speaks of the West Indian trade as "more often a losing than a winning trade—a Lottery with more blanks than prizes in it" (*Watchman* 135). In the poem this gamble is literalized, as the mariners watch Death and Life-in-Death rolling dice to decide their fate. Although Life-in-Death wins the Mariner, the other two hundred sailors will die with the rapidity frequently ascribed to epidemic fevers:

> Four times fifty living men,
> (And I heard nor sigh nor groan)
> With heavy thump, a lifeless lump
> They dropped down one by one.
>
> (216–19)

They die silently, cursing the Ancient Mariner with their eyes, their only sound the "heavy thump" of their bodies falling to the deck, which is made even more gruesome by the "homely" diction in which it is purveyed (J. Jackson 75). Conditions on the ship evoke the worst in contemporary descriptions of slave ships:

> I looked upon the rotting sea,
> And drew my eyes away;
> I looked upon the rotting deck,
> And there the dead men lay.
>
> (240–43)

A passage like this one, for instance, might be compared to Olaudah Equiano's description of the "stench" in the hold of the slave vessel: "Now that the whole ship's cargo were confined together, it became absolutely pestilential. The closeness of the place, and the heat of the climate, added to the number in the ship . . . almost suffocated us. This produced copious perspirations, so that the air soon became unfit for respiration, from a variety of loathsome smells, and brought on a sickness among the slaves, of which many died" (78–79).

Coleridge hoped the imagination would cure itself, that the faculty that creates the desire for West Indian luxuries would also lead human beings beyond them, as "sensual wants / Unsensualize the mind" ("On the Slave Trade," *Watchman* 131). Telling the tale serves a similar purpose in the "Rime," as the vagrant sailor's account of the horror and the guilt connected with the death of the albatross makes the Wedding Guest (and through him, contemporary readers) realize the cost of colonial commerce. It demonstrates that living in harmony with nature is inseparable from living in harmony with each other. In one of the more extraordinary episodes of the poem, which might be said to enact "the psychopathology of empire,"[30] the dead mariners are brought to life, as if, indeed, they have been redeemed:

> The mariners all 'gan work the ropes,
> Where they were wont to do;
> They raised their limbs like lifeless tools—
> We were a ghastly crew.

> The body of my brother's son
> Stood by me, knee to knee:
> The body and I pulled at one rope,
> But he said nought to me.   (337–44)

In this image of the mariner working alongside the dead, "knee to knee," we are once more in the haunted world of "Admiral Hosier's Ghost." The viewpoint, however, is no longer that of the Admiral, appealing for patriotic retribution, but instead is that of the spectral Mariner. The episode might seem to recover the voices of the forgotten, yet they remain silent throughout: these corpses are no longer inhabited by the guilty spirits of the mariners but are occupied by a new "troop of spirits blest" (349) who produce "sweet sounds . . . slowly through their mouths" (352). Eventually their voices will be symbolically dissolved into the "sweet jargoning" (362) of nature. The horrors of the slave trade, the deaths of innumerable sailors and slaves, are thus poetically transformed into a utopian image of nature under divine protection, though even here the gruesomeness of these spectral warblers powerfully emphasizes the tensions within this poetic recovery. When the Mariner returns to his native home the dichotomy between the abjected corpses of the sailors and the drive for a salvific conclusion is once more apparent. "Each corse" continues to "lay flat, lifeless and flat" (488), yet on each stands "A man all light, a seraph-man" (490), and the light from this angelic crew guides the ship into the harbour:

> This seraph-band, each waved his hand,
> No voice did they impart—
> No voice; but oh! the silence sank
> Like music on my heart.   (496–99)

Now, not only the voices of the anonymous crew but also the angels that have displaced them are silent, yet Coleridge hopes this silence will speak as music to the heart of a transformed Mariner and reader.

Throughout history, disease has frequently been understood as a *punishment* for sin, from biblical explanations of the link between leprosy and lust, through Renaissance explanations of syphilis as a divine retribution for sexual promiscuity, to contemporary accounts of AIDS as a punishment for homosexuality. The "Rime" powerfully suggests how far colonial disease and death were understood as fitting retribution for the crime against nature (both human and natural) implicit in colonialism. The experience of the sailors remains unredeemed, for they can speak only once their bodies have been taken over by new recruits, the "troop" of angelic spirits. Nevertheless, their experience continues to be articulated as narrative, through the pariah Mariner whose frightening tale continues to exert its power over listeners long after the voices of his fellow crew members have become silent. Indeed, Coleridge seems to be suggesting that if there is any redemption at all, it lies in telling the tale. Our relation to the "Rime," as modern readers, is not significantly different from that of Coleridge's audience. Through retelling the tale, these events are repeated over and over, the "silent sea" is "burst" into again, thus demanding that readers take a stance in regard to the actions recounted. The poem narrativizes the meeting of worlds, as we are asked to confront the colonial world and to understand the trauma that continues to lie within its silence. The "Rime" is among the first great Romantic narratives to question colonialism by interrogating not a colonized other but the "otherness" that colonialism produced within Britain itself. The Mariner is a hybrid double, at once a phantasmic other who voices colonial experience as in a glass darkly and also the most common of colonial others, the vagrant and displaced sailor. Homi Bhabha describes how colonial authority is structured and subverted in the scene of the "discovery [and reading] of the English Book" (102). The "Rime" presents a similar yet opposite scene, as those at "home" are taught the text of colonialism, in a reading in which identities are riven by difference and anxiety.

The Salisbury Plain *Poems and* "The Discharged Soldier"

In seeking to understand colonialism in terms of the disease experience of a group of people who had been largely ignored, Coleridge was responding not only to historical events but also to the poetry of Wordsworth, who, as an original collaborator on the "Rime," first suggested the killing of the albatross and the reanimation of the sailors. The writings of the two poets during this period are very much a "lyrical dialogue," as each found his voice in relation to the other's work (Magnuson 16–32).[31] How to represent colonial disease was also a central concern of Wordsworth's, giving rise to a series of experimental narratives, each based on the same story yet all strikingly different in their approach to the problem.

Salisbury Plain, composed in 1793–94, arose from a walk Wordsworth took across this dreary plain shortly after seeing the British fleet preparing for war off the Isle of Wight. The poem tells of the encounter between an anonymous, homeless male traveler and a Female Vagrant, whose tale was later included in *Lyrical Ballads.* An extraordinary aspect of the poem is the alien landscape of Salisbury Plain, which is portrayed as a huge burial ground, a haunted wasteland where "warrior spectres of gigantic bones, / Forth-issuing from a thousand rifted tombs / Wheel on their fiery steeds amid the infernal glooms" (*Salisbury Plain Poems* 97–99). It is also a space of human sacrifice where " 'Mid priests and spectres grim and idols dire, / Far heard the great flame utters human moans" (93–94). As a field of death and violence, Salisbury Plain mirrors revolutionary France (Liu 193–97). Stonehenge, a "sacrificial altar fed / With living men" (184–85), speaks of the continuance of England's barbaric, primitive past in modern warfare. Yet the violence Wordsworth is describing is not localized in France but instead is global, and thus inflected across a colonial register. The plain is both a desert and a sea, " 'Twas dark and waste as ocean's shipless flood / Roaring with storms beneath night's starless gloom" (109–10), and it is portrayed as a socially constructed space:

> When men in various vessels roam the deep
> Of social life, and turns of chance prevail
> Various and sad, how many thousands weep
> Beset with foes more fierce than e'er assail
> The savage without home in winter's keenest gale.
>
> (32–36)

As a primitive burial ground for unnumbered dead warriors, Salisbury Plain mirrors the watery wastes that Britain has created, "more fierce than e'er assail / The savage," in its struggle for empire; indeed the Female Vagrant, instead of finding her "ready tomb" in the "ocean-flood," is all but buried on this plain (*Salisbury Plain Poems,* "Adventures" 465). Early Wordsworth employs gothic elements to portray the haunted world of colonialism. In the midst of this terrible environment, struggling against the "watery storm" (102) and seeking shelter, the solitary traveler comes upon Stonehenge but is warned by a supernatural voice to avoid it. Instead he seeks refuge in a "lonely Spital" (hospital) (123), which evokes times past when the "lazarettos" or "plague houses" were built to house people suffering from contagious diseases, especially leprosy. Lepers, the most feared of social outcasts during the Middle Ages, could not inherit property and passed through a church ritual that formally pronounced them dead. The traveler is thus linked directly to disease and to those cut off from society by it. In this less generous age, the hospital has become a ruin. Yet even so it remains "the dead house of the plain" (126), reserved for a new kind of social pariah, those marked by colonial violence.

The watery landscape of Salisbury Plain is a "spatial corollary" of the colonial world, yet rather than using this parallel to represent colonial space, Wordsworth uses colonial geography to understand English rural society and the impact British expansionary policies were having on it. He reads colonialism into the English landscape, and this strategy gives these landscapes their uncanny alien quality. Throughout the 1790s, Wordsworth questioned the assumption that English rural society was somehow removed from the changes that were transforming other regions of the globe. In *Salisbury Plain*, he even doubts whether there is any substantial difference for the poor between living on the ocean and living on the plain, between an external and an internal colonialism.

Salisbury Plain is an ironic reworking of the "serviceman's return," poems that dealt with the problems discharged soldiers and sailors faced as they sought to recover the life disrupted by war. Most focus on the encounter in the cottage between a soldier and his former lover. In the anonymous "The Soldier's Return," published in the *Scots Magazine* (1804), Harry nears his family's cottage yet fears the effect his sudden appearance might have on those who have long considered him dead. He disguises himself, like Odysseus, to soften the emotional blow of his return. In a complex theatrical doubling, which combines the negative and positive images of the homecoming serviceman, he appears as a crippled soldier:

> What could I do?—If in I went,
> Surprize might chill each tender heart;
> Some story, then, I must invent,
> And act the poor maim'd soldier's part.

> I drew a bandage o'er my face,
> And crooked up a lying knee,
> And found that e'en in that blest place
> Not one dear friend knew ought of me.
> (B. Bennett 322–24)

Given the finest food the cottagers can offer—"best hung meat," "curds and cheese"—the soldier informs his family that their son, Harry Goodman, is still alive. After an appropriate delay to allow his family to adjust to this news, Harry takes off his eye patch and adopts his normal voice. A celebration of the recovery of the rural cottage ideal ensues:

> "My Jessy, dear!" I softly said:
> She gaz'd, and answer'd with a sigh:
> My sisters look'd as half-afraid;
> My mother fainted quite for joy.

> My father danced round his son;
>> My brothers shook my hand away;
> My mother said, Her glass might run,
>> She car'd not now how soon that day.

> "Hout, woman!" cry'd my father dear.
>> "A wedding first I'm sure we'll have;
> I warrant we'll live this hundred year—
>> Nay, may be, lass, escape the grave."

In the "Effects of War," which appeared in the *Cambridge Intelligencer* (16 November 1793), the emphasis is placed on recovery:

> Not e'en the sickly face and mangled limb,
> Checks the pure joy that glows at his return.
> Terror had long suggested he was lost:
> He is once more at home, and all seems well.
>> (B. Bennett 96)

Both poems suggest the darker side of such homecomings, for they portray, if only to deny, the vagrancy, sickness, broken bodies, and alienation that frequently accompanied such returns.

Although this literature offers numerous examples of patriotic defenses of war and of the maintenance of domestic happiness, most recount failed homecomings. In Robert Merry's "The Wounded Soldier," a discharged soldier, his strength gone, fears that his lover, Lucy, will shun him and that his parents will "curse the hour that gave me birth" that "I should gloom for e'er your homely mirth, / Exist upon the pittance ye procure" (B. Bennett 242–45). For a moment readers are allowed to believe that his fears are unfounded, for when he calls to them from the doorway of the cottage:

> A ray of rapture chas'd habitual care:
> "Our HENRY lives—we may again rejoice!"
> And LUCY sweetly blush'd, for she was there.

Such happiness, however, is only temporary:

> But when he enter'd in such horrid guise,
>> His mother shriek'd, and dropp'd upon the floor:
> His father look'd to heav'n with streaming eyes,
>> And Lucy sunk, alas! to rise no more.

Here the soldier's return destroys the rural cottage life that he sought to recover. In R. T.'s "The Worn Soldier," published in the *Scots Magazine*

(1808), a veteran returns to find "the dear cottage a tenantless waste, / And his kindred all sunk to the grave." His "visions of bliss" shattered, he is reduced to the status of a beggar: "helpless and poor, / And, forc'd to solicit a slender relief, / He wanders from door to door" (B. Bennett 382).

Wordsworth's most extensive reworking of the genre of the serviceman's return is to be found in "The Brothers," where he questions the possibility of any homecoming. (Ironically, when John Wordsworth arrived in Grasmere, he too was afraid to knock on his brother's door, so he returned to his hotel and announced his arrival from there.) In *Salisbury Plain* the vision of a return is structurally less sophisticated, but it may even be darker: Wordsworth's traveler, who is identified in the later *Adventures on Salisbury Plain* as a sailor, returns to a cottage that has now become the "dead house of the plain" and to a lover, or at least a potential one, who has been reduced to vagrancy. In a perceptive discussion of the poem, Paul Sheats suggests that a characteristic feature of Wordsworth's poetry at this time is that he uses narrative as "a means of suppressing subjectivity and of dramatizing and objectifying feelings that are implicitly contradictory and probably in large part unconscious. Each of the three characters in the poem—the narrator, the vagrant, and the traveler—exemplifies a different aspect of Wordsworth's recent experience and a different response to it" (85). Such a view of the poem is valuable, because it suggests that his poetry responds to colonial death and disease not by attempting to establish a univocal position or a consensus, but by dramatizing different positions in regard to it and setting them in often contradictory relation to each other. In *Salisbury Plain* the narrative focus is on the Female Vagrant's story, based on an actual case, Wordsworth claimed, of dispossession, sickness, death, and alienation.[32] She recounts how, after losing her childhood home through oppression, she married a weaver and had three children. With the American War of Independence, her husband lost his employment. Now a "casualty," yet unwilling to beg or starve, he joined the army. Wordsworth was well aware of the tacit administrative policy of using the army to rid English society of the poor and unemployed, for the Female Vagrant tells us that "the noisy drum / Beat round, *to sweep the streets of want and pain*" ("Adventures" 300–301, emphasis added).[33] Having arrived with many others on the seacoast and embarked on the ships, the family suffered as the "crowded fleet" lay anchored for "months and months" in sight of the "green fields" of their "native shore." This delay invites an epidemic: through "foul neglect" and "By fever, from polluted air incurred, / Ravage was made" (361–65). The dead, one learns, were buried without any ceremony—"no knell was heard" (365)—and still the fleet lay at anchor. Eventually it departs for the West Indies, where Spain, France, and England in the early 1780s were all seeking to expand their empires.[34] Typical of the Admiralty, delay causes the fleet to arrive in the West Indies, the "equinoctial deep" (371), at the wrong time of year, during the height of the hurricane season and just before the wet season, when yellow fever is at its height. Since the following passage is not included in the original 1793–94 version of the poem, it is likely that Wordsworth had a very specific event in mind when the woman describes those drowned in the storm: "We gazed with terror on the gloomy sleep / Of them that perished in the whirlwind's sweep" (373–74). In a letter written in late November 1795, Dorothy mentions that "my brother saw the West India fleet sailing in all its glory before the storm had made such dreadful ravages" (*Letters* 1: 162).[35] The editor notes that "a fleet commanded by Rear-Admiral Sir Hugh Christian (1747–1798) sailed from Spithead for the West Indies. It consisted of eight naval vessels and some 200 transports and merchantmen. During the night of 17 Nov. it was struck by a hurricane. . . . By 26 Nov. the shore between Abbotsbury and Bridport, a dozen miles east of Racedown, had been strewn with hundreds of corpses" (*Letters* 1: 162n). Worse, however, awaits the Female Vagrant. In a short year she loses her entire family, "one by one, by sword / And ravenous plague, all perished" (393–94). Madness ensues, and she awakens, like the Ancient Mariner, on "a British ship . . . as from a trance restored" (396). Better by far, she says, to have starved "unseen, unheard, unwatched," or to have "obtrude[d]" her family's "dying bodies" on the notice of "proud men," than "dog-like," to wade "at the heels of war, / Protract a curst existence, with the brood / That lap (their very nourishment!) their brother's blood" (382–87). Whatever sympathy the reader might feel for her, she feels that she has committed a crime against herself and others. "Oh! dreadful price of being," she says, "to resign / All that is dear *in* being!" (379–80).

Wordsworth here articulates a central feature of the culture of colonialism, already noted in the "Rime": those who played the most important role in the military expansion of British society were themselves viewed as less than human. Their deaths, whether from disease or war, were seen as an appropriate punishment for their actions. "The man that is merely a soldier," Godwin writes, "must always be uncommonly depraved" (*Enquiry* 523). Paralleling the experience of a returning soldier, the woman discovers on reaching England that she has nowhere to go: "Homeless near a thousand homes I stood, / And near a thousand tables pined, and wanted food" (467–68). Without government support, she has been reduced to vagrancy. Throughout his writings Wordsworth explores, in often contradictory ways, the intimate social and economic relation between colonialism, disease, and vagrancy.[36] Here he is responsive to his times. As A. L. Beier has noted, one of the principal problems with conscription was that it "uprooted the young and unpropertied, who then had nothing to which to return" (94). If they survived military duty, soldiers and sailors would frequently come back to England as invalids or vagrants, a continuing source of anxiety for property owners. Afraid that these men were likely to be violent, governments often allowed them to beg their way home, if there still was a "home." Many, especially those who had been disabled, headed for cities, where they could beg, like the London sailor whom Wordsworth describes as lying "at length beside a range / Of written characters, with chalk inscribed / Upon the smooth flat stones" (1805 *Prelude* 7.221–23).[37] The Female Vagrant follows a similar course. "Helpless as sailor cast on desart rock" (470), she says, yet unwilling to become a beggar, she passes four days without food, only to find herself again in a hospital. Once released, she briefly lives with a band of Gypsies, who show her the only kindness she has known in England. Since then, because she is unwilling to engage in petty thievery, she has been a wanderer cut off from human society. When the traveler meets her, she is living in both a hospital and a death house: in social terms, she is at once a pariah, a leper, and one of the walking dead. Her tale comes to an end when she literally runs out of words to describe the horror of her life: "she had no more to say / Of that perpetual weight which on her spirit lay" (557–58). Words remain insufficient to her experience.

Whereas the Female Vagrant's history ends in a silence that speaks of self-destroying trauma, we know almost nothing about her auditor. Except for the information that sometime in the past "he too had withered young in sorrow's deadly blight" ("Salisbury Plain" 405), we learn little about him. Only once do we hear him speak directly (334–35), though he is portrayed, through "third person" narration, as being both horrified by his surroundings and eager to console the woman. In striking contrast to these two is the relatively well-developed figure of the narrator of the poem, whose satisfaction with an overtly ideological rhetoric is very much out of place, given the world inhabited by the two wanderers. His rhetoric, as Sheats has observed, "measures his psychological distance from them. He is a poised and controlled spectator; they are his *exemplum*" (86). He turns the experience of these two outcasts into a celebratory "return" poem. Their journey toward "a lonely cot" (349), for instance, occasions the following celebration of English cottage life:

Adieu ye friendless hope-forsaken pair!
Yet friendless ere ye take your several road,
Enter that lowly cot and ye shall share
Comforts by prouder mansions unbestowed.
For you yon milkmaid bears her brimming load,
For you the board is piled with homely bread,
And think that life is like this desart broad,
Where all the happiest find is but a shed
And a green spot 'mid wastes interminably spread.
(415–23)

Wordsworth's revisions to the poem indicate that he was unsatisfied with this kind of rhetoric, which had very little to do with the reality of rural labor in the 1790s.

Sheats's argument that Wordsworth's contradictory attitudes toward his subject matter are dramatized across his characters can be extended to include the composition history of the *Salisbury Plain* poems, suggesting that these attitudes were unstable and shifted with each new revision over the course of the decade. In the 1797–98 revision of the poem, *Adventures on Salisbury Plain,* the language of the distanced and moralizing narrator disappears. Just as significantly, Wordsworth shifted the focus from the Female Vagrant (whose story—about to be published separately in *Lyrical Ballads*—was to have been replaced with another) to the male traveler, who now appears as a discharged sailor. The poem now begins with an act of charity, as the sailor assists an old and sick soldier ("his ragged coat scarce showed the Soldier's faded red" [9]) across the plain. We learn that after serving two years as a sailor, he was on his way home when he was seized by a press-gang. Forced to serve in the navy for many years, he was finally released, yet denied payment for his service. Returning home in rage, the sailor killed a traveler and "fled, a vagrant since, the murderer's fate to shun" (99). His has also been a failed return. Wordsworth's revision thus expands the range and complexity of his representation of colonial servicemen and vagrancy to include not only the "soldier's widow" (629) but an invalided soldier (whose name, "Robert Walford," recalls a man who murdered his wife in Dodington Common, Somersetshire) and a criminal sailor.[38] Where the threatening aspects of discharged servicemen were displaced in the earlier version by employing the perspective of a female vagrant who fears that it is she who is about to be murdered when the traveler enters her ruined shelter, *Adventures* brings to the fore the dangers of dehumanization and the guilt produced by war. Also, more powerfully than the first version, it examines the psychology of the sailor. At its conclusion he confesses his guilt, not because he has come to accept the English legal system, which he continues to recognize as oppressive, but because he has adopted a higher moral code; yet this conclusion shows none of the optimism that shaped the earlier narrative. The sailor, like many others before him, is hanged and gibbeted, but his sacrifice to a higher moral justice is perverted in that shopkeepers make money from his death, having opened up "their festive booths beneath his face" (822).[39] In his silence, whatever terror he produces is reserved for the next sailor who "upon his swinging corpse his eye may glance / And drop, as he once dropp'd, in miserable trance" (827–28). *Adventures* establishes a cycle of violence with no end. Whatever we make of the concept of moral justice that stands above the internal violence shaping English colonial activity, it is a justice that exists more at the level of gesture than of social reality; furthermore, it is a notion reserved for those Europeans most affected by colonialism and is ignored by the shopkeepers who benefit from it.

Even here Wordsworth appears not to have been satisfied with this attempt to represent "distress and misery beyond all possible calculation" (*Salisbury Plain Poems* 217), for the poem, after many significant revisions, was not published until 1842, and then it appeared under the title *Guilt and Sorrow*. The poet explained his reluctance, saying that "the mariner's fate appeared to me so tragical as to require a treatment more subdued and yet more strictly applicable in expression than I had at first given to it" (221). This struggle to find a satisfactory means of representing the larger tragedy represented by these individual histories continued to be a troubling source of narrative and poetic experiment. In late January or early February 1798, at the time Coleridge was completing the "Rime," Wordsworth composed the fragment titled "The Discharged Soldier," which he later incorporated into book 4 of *The Prelude*. The encounter is carefully staged:

> a sudden turning of the road
> Presented to my view an uncouth shape
> So near that, stepping back into the shade
> Of a thick hawthorn, I could mark him well,
> Myself unseen. He was in stature tall,
> A foot above man's common measure tall,
> And lank, and upright. There was in his form
> A meagre stiffness. You might almost think
> That his bones wounded him.
>
> . . . .
>
> His arms were long and lean; his hands were bare;

His visage, wasted though it seemed, was large
In feature; his cheeks sunken; and his mouth
Shewed ghastly in the moonlight.
(*William Wordsworth* 37–51)

Rewriting the encounter between the Wedding Guest and the Ancient Mariner, Wordsworth fuses gothicism with a kind of photographic realism that
radically revises how this "tropical invalid" is seen. It is not fear alone that
structures this encounter, however, but a complex "mingled sense / Of fear
and sorrow" (68–69). More than the Ancient Mariner, the soldier personifies
disease and death, as his body itself has become the site of wounding. And
even more strongly than in his earlier poems, Wordsworth reverses the pattern of colonial encounters. For rather than describing a Death that comes to
the New World from Europe, the poet—himself hiding behind a hawthorn—
describes the Death that has returned. What critics have taken to be the
soldier's "otherworldly" qualities, however, need not be understood in spiritual terms; even more powerfully, this emaciated soldier brings the hunger,
malnutrition, and disease of the colonial world home. He is truly an "uncanny" figure, in whom the *heimlich* reappears as a threatening *unheimlich*.
Hybridity is uncanny, as his presence in England questions the notion that
"tropical disease" is located somewhere else. Complex, contradictory feelings
of "fear and sorrow" are produced as Wordsworth looks on this individual
whose body is marked by violence and disease. The soldier is indeed an
allegory of Death, drawn from Milton, Dante, and Spenser, "clad in military
garb, / Though faded yet entire" (54–55). Yet this should not deflect one
from recognizing that allegory makes possible, in a way that the gothic psychological portraiture of the *Salisbury Plain* poems does not, the articulation
of the anonymous suffering of thousands of soldiers and sailors who did not
return to England. To the extent that the soldier is a specter, a ghost from the
past, he reevokes the colonial tropics as a haunted burial ground.

Wordsworth represents the soldier as suffering from alienation almost beyond imagining, as "a man cut off / From all his kind, and more than half
detached / From his own nature" (58–60). At first all that can be heard from
him are "murmuring sounds as if of pain / Or of uneasy thought" (70–71).
Later Wordsworth, still in hiding, describes these sounds as "a murmuring
voice of dead complaint, / A groan scarce audible" (79–80). As in the earlier
poems, the fundamental problem of the narrative is how to find words to
convey what the soldier has undergone. Finally the poet subdues his "heart's
specious cowardice" (85) and hails the soldier. Asked his history, he recounts

what we can now recognize as a common social narrative of the time, heightened by Wordsworth's recent reading of Bryan Edwards's account of recent military disasters in the West Indies:[40]

> he in reply
> Was neither slow nor eager, but unmoved,
> And with a quiet uncomplaining voice,
> A stately air of mild indifference,
> He told a simple fact: that he had been
> A Soldier, to the tropic isles had gone,
> Whence he had landed now some ten days past;
> That on his landing he had been dismissed,
> And with the little strength he yet had left
> Was travelling to regain his native home.
>
> (95–104).

Celeste Langan has claimed that the soldier is simply conforming to the requirements of the vagrancy statute by giving only the information required to avoid being prosecuted: "all further communication is superfluous" (206). The major problem with this strictly legalistic reading of this exchange is that the soldier, though reticent, *does* say more than is legally necessary. More important, I believe, is Wordsworth's own suggestion that some experiences are "so tragical as to require a treatment more subdued." The Discharged Soldier's history is reduced to the sparest details. It stands almost as an epitaph, yet as such it reaches beyond the individual to encompass the "simple fact[s]" of an entire population lost to history. Read in the context of the "indignant realism" of the earlier poems, Wordsworth's focus on the "quiet uncomplaining voice" and the "mild indifference" of the soldier may seem to be signs of a weakening political focus (Sheats 85). Yet to my mind the poem achieves more by adopting this language than did the overtly politicized rhetoric of the earlier poems. The soldier's silences and hollow words are more troubling than the confident rhetoric of the narrator of *Salisbury Plain*. The poem provides, indeed, a striking contrast to the "Rime," where the colonial experience has produced an obsessive need to tell the tale. At the same time, despite Wordsworth's emphasis on the soldier's dignity, we are just as conscious that the paucity of speech reflects a maimed and exhausted state, as if the colonial experience has affected not only his body, but his very being. The soldier's apparent inability to take any interest in his past suggests an alienation beyond narrative, as if the social world implied by telling tales, the interchange of sympathy and the sharing of worlds implied by the relationship of speaking and listening, is no longer even possible:

> in all he said
> There was a strange half-absence and a tone
> Of weakness and indifference, as of one
> Remembering the importance of his theme,
> But feeling it no longer.   (142–46)

The past has been so traumatic that he can no longer even respond to it. Thus the tale is spare because the experience itself is so deadly that it has killed the man who would speak it. There is no celebration of the glory of battle or the extension of empire. Like those soldiers "neglected and ungratefully thrown by / Even for the very service they had wrought" (1805 *Prelude* 1.544–45), the man tells a tale of "war and battle and the pestilence" (138) and of military authorities who "dismissed" him when his health was destroyed and he could no longer serve them. Instead of finding hospitable shores on his return to England, he encounters a world that sees him as a threatening outsider. Only "an arrow's flight" (76) from a village (in one of Wordsworth's allusions to the "Rime"), he tells of being unable to proceed in his journey because of the howling of a dog: "the village mastiff fretted me, / And every second moment rang a peal / Felt at my very heart" (131–33).

Wordsworth's "ill-suppressed astonishment" at walking alongside this "tall and ghostly figure" can serve as an image of contemporary criticism's relation to such characters. Like the mariner working "knee to knee" with the dead sailors, it captures powerfully the ambiguous way Wordsworth increasingly responded to these figures of colonial return. Instead of attempting to voice their experience, he explores their speaking silence. Where Goldsmith portrayed the private centinel ironically, as someone who, despite his victimizing, remains a card-carrying "Brit," Wordsworth allows the soldier's silence and his emphasis on maintaining social decorum in spite of his intense suffering to function as a form of resistance. At the same time, the discharged soldier's life has proved unsatisfactory both to himself and to those who encounter him. His concluding declaration, "My trust is in the God of heaven, / And in the eye of him that passes me" (164–65) may be read, Mary Jacobus argues, "as an instance of sublimely self-negligent faith in providence."[41] My view is that it encapsulates a social demand by someone who has not yet made it home and may never do so.

"The Ruined Cottage"

While composing "The Discharged Soldier" and revising *Adventures on Salisbury Plain,* Wordsworth was also writing "The Ruined Cottage." Having already discussed in chapter 1 how the pathogenic landscape of the poem reflects the framing practices of colonial medical geography, I want now to see it in terms of Wordsworth's ongoing reflection on how colonialism affected the rural poor of Britain. Once again Wordsworth articulates a range of contradictory attitudes toward his subject by employing differing viewpoints— those of the narrator, the Pedlar, and Margaret. As in the previous poems, the extensive revisions the poem underwent before finally being published as book 1 of *The Excursion* suggest a continuing struggle and dissatisfaction with how these events are to be understood.[42] Here Wordsworth shifts his view from the diseased bodies of English servicemen returning from the tropics to demonstrate that colonialism produces disease landscapes at home just as easily as elsewhere. For Wordsworth, colonialism was not restricted to "somewhere else" but was also actively reshaping British landscapes and dispossessing the English rural population.

Although the poem presents three biographies, only two usually receive attention. In its early stage, from 1797 to 1798, as "the story of Margaret,"[43] the poem was about the psychology of loss. Margaret's decline leads with tragic inevitability to a stark conclusion, as if there were nothing to say in the face of such suffering: "in sickness she remained, and here she died, / Last human tenant of these ruined walls" (*"Ruined Cottage"* 527–28). In 1798 the poem doubled in size as Wordsworth increased the role of the Pedlar, who now provides a philosophy of nature that makes healing sense of this tragedy. Dorothy Wordsworth writes, on 5 March 1798, "The Pedlar's character now makes a very, certainly the *most,* considerable part of the poem" (*Letters* 1: 199). In this version the emphasis has shifted to how to interpret these events. A third biography nevertheless resides at the heart of the poem—the story of Margaret's husband, Robert. This history remains a fragment, for we never learn what happened to him.

Robert's story follows a familiar pattern. A weaver, after a long illness he falls among the ranks of "casualties" in the 1780s, when war and drought combined to make employment scarce. He is forced to search for "any casual task" (219), "pointing lame buckle-tongues and rusty nails," "braiding cords or weaving bells and caps / Of rushes" (226–29). David Simpson remarks that Wordsworth shows "a complex awareness of the terrible effect of unemployment on the moral and domestic life" (192). Poverty leads to erratic behavior and aimlessness. Eventually Robert enlists with "a troop of soldiers going to a distant land" (327–28), leaving behind a "purse of gold" (323) to support his family. This is the last that is ever heard of him.

In the face of these events Margaret's grief is natural, but the intensity of her suffering and her inability to relinquish the need to know what happened to Robert constitute an enigma. In depicting Margaret's inability to forget Robert, Wordsworth drew on contemporary literary sources, such as the Crazy Kate episode in Cowper's *The Task,* which tells of a maid who fell in love

> With one who left her, went to sea and died.
> Her fancy followed him through foaming waves
> To distant shores, and she would sit and weep
> At what a sailor suffers . . .[44]   (1.538—41)

Through Margaret readers are forced—like Coleridge's Wedding Guest—to address what they might otherwise prefer to forget. From the Pedlar's first encounter with the abandoned Margaret, when "she inquired / If I had seen her husband" (315—16), to our final image of her, she is obsessed with learning what happened to Robert:

> Yet ever as there passed
> A man whose garments shewed the Soldier's red,
> Or crippled Mendicant in Sailor's garb,
>
> .   .   .   .
>
> she with faltering voice,
> Expecting still to learn her husband's fate,
> Made many a fond inquiry.   (498—504)

For the Pedlar, Margaret's questioning is a *psychological* enigma, a "fond" "sickness" (527) or madness. Its very persistence disturbs him: "any heart had ached to hear her [beg] / That wheresoe'er I went I still would ask / For him whom she had lost" (480—82). Unable to learn whether Robert is dead, Margaret lives in a state of permanent paralysis, in "unquiet widowhood, / A wife, and widow" (483—84) until she finally dies. Like the contemporaneous "Baker's Cart" passage, Margaret's is a case study in psychopathology, an example of "a mind / Which being long neglected and denied / The common food of hope was now become / Sick and extravagant" (*"Ruined Cottage"* 463, lines 18—21). Unable to bury the dead, she joins them.

De Quincey was indignant. For him Robert was not dead and could hardly be considered a victim. Not only was he a coward for deserting his family when life became difficult, De Quincey thought, he continued to shirk his responsibilities by denying them support, for which he "forfeits his last hold upon our lingering sympathy" (*De Quincey as Critic* 408). As for Margaret, she could have learned her husband's whereabouts by asking the War Office, which would have relieved her of the cause of her distress in "one fortnight" (409). As an alternative to De Quincey's own fictional account of what actually happened to Robert, one might place the naval physician Thomas Trotter's remarks on what frequently did happen to these men. For people employed in manufacturing, he remarks, "it is the first effect of a war to throw many of them out of employment. The only resource is the navy and army." They frequently are forced to abandon their families, and their situations do not require "the language of romance to find its way to feeling hearts; but must now and then be aggravated to the most poignant distress, by resigning wives and children to beggary and want, and a thousand ills of which I can form no idea." This "dejection of spirits" makes them the "first subjects for the scurvy, and the earliest victims to contagious diseases." Trotter concludes that "many a melancholy story is thus related to the medical attendant of a sailor or soldier, and it begets a sympathy that interests us the more in their recovery: under this species of mental affliction we know that numbers perish, without any apparent disorder" (1: 46). For Trotter as for Wordsworth, such individuals endure a context of suffering so great that he "can form no idea" of it.

Even without introducing Trotter's account of what typically happened to uprooted laborers, it is clear that Margaret, the Pedlar, and De Quincey give us contradictory views about Robert's life and character, as well as about how to respond to the silence that envelops them. For the Pedlar, the nagging questions raised by Robert's disappearance die with Margaret: "Be wise and chearful. . . . She sleeps in the calm earth, and peace is here" (MS D 510–12). De Quincey eliminates anxiety by reinforcing the stereotypical link between soldiers, immorality, and social irresponsibility, while affirming the wise guardianship of military authorities. Margaret's unwillingness to bury Robert suggests a problem within the narrative that remains unresolved. Its openness lies not only in the historical gap within which these characters move, but also in the ways we as readers are forced to respond to that silence. "The Ruined Cottage" is quite clearly "the story of Margaret," but even more, it worries about the history of an entire range of people whose lives and actions many readers would prefer to forget. Read from a social rather than a psychological perspective, Margaret's questions produce an unsettling *unease,* because we cannot but feel they do deserve an answer. "Forget Robert," the Pedlar seems to say, even as he recognizes his own impotence in the face of a narrative whose very openness suggests a final indignity directed toward Robert. One of the strengths of the poem, a strength that postcolonial criticism can learn from, is that it idealizes neither Margaret's resistance nor Robert's status as a subaltern, nor does it forget Robert because he supposedly *deserves* oblivion.

Margaret's answer to Robert's disappearance, her continuing state of critical grieving, is shown to be just as unsatisfactory. We are left, then, not with an answer to the problematic link between colonial disease and forgetting, but with a dramatic structuring of the problem. Wordsworth simultaneously asks readers to occupy a position between grief and its denial, between acceptance of the past and a continuing critique of it, between the absence of a recoverable history for a large number of colonial victims and our insistence on the need to know. Denied the "last rites" provided by burial and narratives, Robert haunts this text, and Margaret takes on his ghostly status. The Pedlar seeks to bury both these ghosts by burying one of them. One of the strengths of the narrative, however, is that it recognizes their continuing presence, the unwillingness of those who have suffered indignity during life to rest easy in death.

Like the *Salisbury Plain* poems, "The Ruined Cottage" examines the social production of English "casualties." Yet even more powerfully, it talks about colonialism and British social space, arguing that the separation between colonial and British life is both unstable and no longer valid. Even as it represents a specific "domestic tragedy" (p. 14), its link to other narratives about dead soldiers and abandoned women suggests that Wordsworth was seeking to depict more than an isolated tragedy. It should be read as a "depopulation narrative," in which the ruin of a single cottage is intended to stand for a general social situation. How many Roberts and Margarets were there? As I have suggested, there were many. In an article in the *Watchman* for 17 March 1796, Coleridge reached a similar conclusion. There he uses statistics drawn from the *Monthly Magazine* to argue that wars over the previous century have produced a major depopulation crisis:

> In 1690, the number of Houses in England and Wales was — 1, 319, 215
> In 1759, the number was reduced to — 986, 482
> In 1777, the number did not exceed — 952, 734
> And it is extremely probable that the American war and the present has still further reduced them. The above are the reports made by the Collectors of the House and Window Taxes; so that allowing five persons to each house, the number of inhabitants has decreased two millions, or almost one-third of what it was at the time of the Revolution. (*Watchman* 109)

For many recent demographers, eighteenth-century population debates are something of an enigma, for just at the very moment when England was undergoing a population boom, many contemporary writers—among them, Richard Price, Oliver Goldsmith, John Brown, Robert Wallace, and James

Steuart—believed it was undergoing a severe decline. These population pessi-mists, among whom we must include Coleridge and Wordsworth, have been proved wrong in their general assessment of the situation. Undoubtedly moral and political assumptions shaped their interpretation of relevant data, though the same can be said for the other side, which included Thomas Malthus. More significant for this discussion is that eighteenth-century de-population narratives reflect a perception of enormous change and crisis. Even if their demographic conclusions were incorrect, their demography itself articulates a perceived social reality. For instance, Goldsmith, in his dedication of "The Deserted Village" to Joshua Reynolds, admits that for many "the depopulation it deplores is no where to be seen, and the disorders it laments are only to be found in the poet's own imagination." Yet he answers: "I sincerely believe what I have written; that I have taken all possible pains, in my country excursions, for these four or five years past, to be certain of what I alledge, and that all my views and enquiries have led me to believe those miseries real, which I here attempt to display" (4: 285). Romantic poetry of the 1790s should be read in the same light, since the notion of depopulation is a powerful form of social criticism, giving a shape to "mis-eries real" understood on a profound scale.

Coleridge rightly recognized that population growth is not necessarily uniform across all classes of society. The general population can increase even as one group within it suffers a major decline. He notes the decrease in the number of "cottages" in England:

> In 1689, the number of Cottages was — 554, 631
> In 1777, the number was reduced to — 251, 261
> So that between these two periods the decrease was more than one half, that is above 300,000 Cottages, which, at five to a Cottage, make 1,500,000 labourers less than a century ago. What can this be ascribed to, but the difficulty of procuring subsistence by labour? (109)

There are many reasons for this decline, not all of them related to population decrease. Coleridge's comments, however, suggest that we need to go beyond simply seeing the "cottage" as a glorification of "old England." The "ruined cottage" is itself a figure of the tremendous changes that took place in English society, which were of major consequence to the British rural poor. As such, Wordsworth's "ruined cottage," with its "four clay walls / That stared upon each other" (30–31) should be seen not only in terms of the discourse of the picturesque, but also as part of that "alien" landscape of death that first emerged in his poetry with *Salisbury Plain*. Its symbolic links are much closer to the "dead house of the plain" and Coleridge's spectral ship than to the middle-class aesthetics of William Gilpin.

History is largely written by the healthy. The people who suffered most from the changes brought by colonial expansion were also those who left the fewest traces of their experience. Consequently "The Ruined Cottage" is valuable in allowing a modern reader to understand what colonialism meant to the British "casualties" of the imperial age, those who were displaced in this era of expansion and disease. Rather than reading Wordsworth's poetry as an affirmation of British cultural dominance, a position I believe is deeply mistaken if it is made without substantial qualification, it is more relevant to read poems such as "The Ruined Cottage" as documents of a nativist resistance to colonialism. Instead of looking to Gilpin, I would compare it with descriptions such as the following one of the desolation that met the eyes of travelers in western Canada in the nineteenth century:

In whatever direction you turn, nothing but sad wrecks of mortality meet the eye; lodges standing on every hill, but not a streak of smoke rising from them. Not a sound can be heard to break the awful stillness. . . . It seems as if the very genius of desolation had stalked through the prairies, and wreaked his vengeance on everything bearing the shape of humanity. (Qtd. in Stannard, *American Holocaust* 127–28)

The English rural poor may not have undergone anything approaching the kind of social collapse experienced by American indigenous populations. Nevertheless, famine, disease, social uprooting, and family dissolution were an ongoing part of their existence, and they were even more extreme in Irish and Scottish rural society.

In arguing that these poems constitute successive revisionary retellings of the same narrative, I have sought to demonstrate the instability within Wordsworth's struggle to understand the cost of colonialism to British society. This reflection is further complicated by "Ruth," which tells of the abondonment of a young English woman by a soldier from Georgia whose tribal dress and wild morality reflect both his life among the "Indians in the West" and "the tumult of a tropic sky" (*Lyrical Ballads* 114–16). The personal and private side of these revisions should not be ignored; for instance, Wordsworth's own ambivalence about the role of war in forcing him to abandon Annette Vallon and his child Caroline. In a rich analysis that cannot be summarized here, Peter Manning has suggested how far the various perspectives of "The Ruined Cottage" and their intensity express Wordsworth's private effort to grapple with the loss of his mother. (She and Margaret both appear to have died of pneumonia.) Manning traces one set of the poem's images back to a passage in *An Evening Walk,* in which Wordsworth juxtaposes European and colonial space as he describes a dying woman's struggle:

> [She] bids her soldier come her woes to share,
> Asleep on Bunker's charnel hill afar;
> For hope's deserted well why wistful look?
> Choked is the pathway, and the pitcher broke.
> (*William Wordsworth* 253–56)

Conclusion

To read colonialism through European servicemen is to recognize that colonial disease experience was not homogeneous but was structured in multiple ways along class and national lines. This large subaltern population was present everywhere in England during the colonial period, because its members played such a key role in the expansion and commerce of empire, yet their story has largely been forgotten, even though it was largely catastrophic. Romanticism emerged when attention was finally being given to their difficult lives. Thus the following comment in 1791 by Charles Fletcher is typical of a changing public perception: "That we have so few writers upon a subject so important as the health of seamen, is to me truly amazing" (xvii). He notes the irony that though John Howard had significantly improved the health conditions of prisoners, sailors (many of them drawn from jails) had been ignored. By the 1790s, in the antiwar and antislavery debates, an increasing number of military physicians began to point out the economic cost attached to these deaths. A different system of accounting emerged as the commercial interests of a new form of imperialism replaced the earlier strategies of the landed gentry. The naval surgeon Frederick Thomson argues, for instance, that the health of seamen should be preserved even if they are considered "merely as a commodity" (xiii). As military officers accepted the notion that it was their duty to maintain their subordinates' health, the mortality rates of sailors declined, especially after 1796, when the Admiralty finally introduced lemons into their diets to prevent scurvy. Changes had not come too soon. In comparing the mortality and morbidity rates of sailors during the Napoleonic Wars with those during the American War, Blane concluded in 1822 that if these rates had continued "the whole stock of seamen would have been exhausted" ("Comparative Health" 188). By 1811 naval commanders were finally ordered to provide an annual account of all deaths on their ships.

The health conditions of soldiers improved more slowly. It was not until the 1820s and 1830s that the British Parliament began to inquire into the health and well-being of soldiers in colonial service, and it was not until the late 1830s and early 1840s that detailed studies were done of the mortality and morbidity of soldiers in colonial service. As late as the 1850s James Martin could still speak of the deplorable condition of soldiers in camps. Indignant that so little had been done to improve their lives, Martin notes that it is "but another instance out of many of the utter disregard of the subject by the authorities of the state, both civil and military, who for ages regarded the soldier as but a red-coated pariah" (405). Martin nevertheless felt that the life of servicemen was about to improve: "We are said to have acted hitherto as if armies had been made for generals, and not generals for armies; but let us hope that the time is not distant when soldiers and seamen shall cease to perish without necessity, and without results" (415). In the wake of the controversy caused by the public recognition of the deplorable waste of lives caused by administrative negligence during the Crimean War, a Royal Commission on the Sanitary State of the Army in India was established. The report, published in 1863, is an extraordinary medical study, which contributed substantially to a significant decline in the deaths of soldiers through disease in the remaining decades of the nineteenth century. By the time the Cantonments Manual was published in 1909, the shift in perspective is clear: "It should be carefully borne in mind that the cardinal principle underlying the administration of cantonments in India is that the cantonments exist primarily for the health of British troops and to considerations affecting the well-being and efficiency of the garrison, all other matters must give place" (qtd. in A. King 118).

Between 1821 and 1870, the hulks of three ships—first the 48-gun HMS *Grampus,* then the 104-gun *Dreadnought,* and finally the 120-gun *Caledonia* (renamed *Dreadnought*)—lay moored in the Thames at Greenwich. Coleridge would have appreciated the significance of these ships, especially the words painted on the side of the first *Dreadnought:* "Seamen's Hospital, Supported by Voluntary Contributions, for Seamen of All Nations."[45] As the fruits of a voluntary subscription raised by a group of philanthropists, among them William Wilberforce and Zachary Macaulay, who formed the Seamen's Hospital Society, these ships represent the first hospital exclusively devoted to the care of all seamen, regardless of their country of origin.[46] Significantly, the medicine practiced on board was not typical of other British hospitals, for these sailors frequently suffered from diseases that would over the course of the century be classified as "tropical"—malaria, beriberi, liver abscess, dysentery, guinea worm, filariasis, and plague. The London School of Tropical Medicine would not be established until 1899, but its origins can be traced back to the Seamen's Hospital Society, which has been called "the Foster Mother of Tropical Medicine in London" (Manson-Bahr 15).

These hospital ships and the population they sought to care for constitute a fitting emblem of one aspect of British colonial experience in that they suggest how often the diseases thought to exist elsewhere returned to England through its commercial navy and in people invalided by service abroad. Colonialism produced a global disease pool, and though many writers continued to believe that tropical diseases were largely restricted to specific geographical regions, most also feared that perhaps it was not physical geography but other factors—moral, hygienic, economic—that defined the world's disease geographies. Within the context of the expansive exchange of pathogens opened up by colonial expansion and travel, the English were no longer so secure. Tropical medicine not only aimed to preserve British colonial administrators and military personnel in other parts of the globe, it also sought to deal with an increasing number of people who suffered from tropical diseases in England itself. In his study of hybridity within English culture, Robert C. Young uses the brass strip that marks the prime meridian at Greenwich as an emblem that "the sameness of the West will always be riven by difference" (1). For me the *Dreadnought* serves as a more powerful emblem of the inability of England to remain immune to the new epidemiological world opened up by its marine commerce and military power. The colonial world was always moored in the very heart of the metropolis or figured in its depopulated countryside.

Colonialism has frequently been read as a discourse of the "other," resting on the cultural and biomedical construction of "other" races and peoples. The history of colonial servicemen demonstrates that those who colonized were not immune to such othering. The pathologies associated with tropical regions were transmitted to them too, not only in biological, but in symbolic terms. Our own relation to this history, even in its polemical and apologetic modes, has much in common with past attitudes. Postcolonial criticism, despite its claim to provide a critical understanding of subaltern populations, continues to see European colonial servicemen through colonial eyes.

Epilogue: Missolonghi

I have been primarily examining the disease experience of a large, anonymous, and mostly forgotten social group for whom colonial expansion generally proved a disaster rather than an opportunity. Servicemen were not, of course, the only military personnel who encountered sickness. The higher ranks also suffered, though to a lesser degree because their world was different from that of common servicemen. In closing a chapter devoted to the link between disease and military activity during the Romantic period, I would be remiss, therefore, not to mention one of the most famous of Romantic deaths. On 5 January 1824 Lord Byron arrived at Missolonghi with a view to commanding six hundred Suliotes in the Greek War of Independence. Eileen Bigland, in her biography of the poet, powerfully captures the pathogenic topography of the place:

The little town rises crazily, on rotten piles and mud-banks, above a three-mile-wide lagoon of filthy, scum-covered water; and is protected most effectively from the clear and lovely Gulf of Patras by a sandy bar. The houses are dilapidated affairs of stone and plaster. . . . All around the town stretch stagnant, colourless marshes. . . . A sort of miasma broods over Missolonghi. A week—even a day—in the place induces an apathy hard to describe. The very air is thick and sluggish; the mists rise from the marshes till the sun shows only as a distant lemon-coloured ball; the ground is so dank that even in summer the muddy open spaces never quite dry up. (247)

A place less suitable for a military camp can hardly be imagined, and Byron, despite the recent catastrophe at Walcheren, displayed the typical attitude of an early nineteenth-century commander in being largely unconcerned about the dangers of such an environment. He was quartered in a large house at the edge of the lagoon. "At high water or on rain-soaked days the ground about the house was a morass," Leslie Marchand notes, "and it was approachable only by water" (3: 1155). By 26 January Byron was already showing signs of malaria, for James Forrester, surgeon of the *Alacrity,* remarks that his "hand shook as if under the influence of an ague fit" (3: 1168). On 15 February Byron suffered a violent convulsion similar to an epileptic fit. By the end of February, anxious about his health, impatient in the face of constant wet weather, and frustrated by his failure to achieve any military success, Byron sought to regain his health by leading his men on daily marches across the marshy plains behind Missolonghi and by continuing a regimen of riding and exercise. As noted by Colonel Lester Stanhope, who seemed more cognizant of the dangers of the place than the poet, it would have required "some great impetus to move Lord Byron from that unhealthy swamp" (qtd. in Marchand, 3: 1189). On 9 April the poet came down with a severe fever. He did not have much faith in doctors, and the history of criticism, following Leslie Marchand's lead, has been severe in accusing those who attended him. Following the accepted practices of the day, they tried pills, cathartics, quinine, and extensive bleeding. On 19 April, however, a little over three months after arriving at Missolonghi, Byron was dead—one more name added to an already frightening list of sick and dead soldiers, which over the first half of the nineteenth century showed little signs of ending.

THREE

Colonial Dietary Anxieties

In a 1709 issue of the *Tatler,* Joseph Addison describes a dinner party he attended at the house of a friend who was "a great admirer of the French cookery, and (as the Phrase is) 'eats well'" (2: 108–9). Two principles appear to govern French cookery, says Addison: no food can ever appear in "its natural form, or without some disguise," and nothing must be eaten that would be "agreeable to ordinary palates; . . . nothing is to gratify their senses, but what would offend those of their inferiors." Caught in a dietary space where food no longer shows any link to nature and where eating is primarily an affirmation of class identity, Addison portrays himself as a modern-day Tantalus: food is everywhere, but he cannot find anything to eat. Looking at the various dishes, he remarks, "I was mightily at a loss to learn what they were, and therefore did not know where to help myself. That which stood before me I took to be a roasted porcupine; however, did not care for asking questions; and have since been informed, that it was only a larded turkey. I afterwards passed my eye over several hashes, which I do not know the names of to this day; and hearing that they were delicacies, did not think fit to meddle with them." At this point, having reached a nadir of "hunger and confusion," Addison "smelled the agreeable savour of roast-beef, but could not tell from which dish it arose, though I did not but question that it lay disguised in one of them. Upon turning my head, I saw a noble sirloin on the side-table, smoking in the most delicious manner. I had recourse to it more than once, and could not see, without some indignation, that substantial English dish banished in so ignominious a manner, to make way for French kickshaws." Addison's anecdote usefully illustrates how profoundly notions of cultural identity are linked to diet. You become what you eat in more than a biological sense, for foods are ingestible signs: through eating, people assimilate culture into themselves and in turn become part of a culture. Addison's story conveys the deep discomfort caused on both a physical and a cultural level when one cannot find the right kind of food: what prolongs one's *cultural* as much as *biological* being. If for some eighteenth- and nineteenth-century writers the contact of cultures was the source of new dietary opportunities, for many it produced anxiety—cultural and national dislocation felt at the very primary level of the body. Addison's patriotic defense of "roast-beef," his indignation over its being sidelined in favor of "French kickshaws," that is, "French somethings" (*quelque choses*), points up that food—what we eat or how we cook what we eat—plays a powerful role both in the affirmation of national identities and in the perception of cultural differences. As Ross Leckie observes, "The stomach is an instrument of culture as important as the brain" (7).

There are many ways of approaching the cultural politics of food and diet during the colonial period. As Addison's anecdote shows, they were instrumental in defining class identities. Haute cuisine is exactly that—the cookery of the French upper class. Class affiliations are established not only by what one eats but by how it is cooked. In the numerous satiric portrayals of the fat, gluttonous, and gouty English gentry of the period, epicures with gigantic bellies and expansive butts sitting at tables amid an oversupply of food, the portrayal of aristocratic diet was a powerful medium of social criticism. James Gillray's *Temperance Enjoying a Frugal Meal* (28 July 1792) (fig. 6), for instance, satirizes the miserliness underlying the domestic simplicity of the reigning king: as George III eats a soft-boiled egg while Queen Charlotte chews on salad. (The bilious Mr. Woodhouse in Austen's *Emma* would later declare, perhaps in emulation of the king, "An egg boiled very soft is not unwholesome" [55]). Against this extreme parsimony in the midst of great wealth, Gillray paired the equally damning portrait of the Prince of Wales. In a *Voluptuary under the Horrors of Digestion* (2 July 1792) (fig. 7), the excesses of the prince are portrayed in dietary terms—his huge stomach occupies the center of the engraving. In contrast to these might be set the representations, sometimes idealized, often satiric, of poor people at dinner, as in Burns's "A Cotter's Saturday Night": "now the Supper crowns their simple board, / The healsome *Porritch*, chief of SCOTIA's food" (1: 148). Contemporary anthropological theories also influenced colonial ideas about diet: savages, it was believed, were prone to eating meat raw, and they also had a nasty fondness for human flesh. Yet these two areas of dietary writing should not be read in isolation from the even more extensive role that the contemporary medical literature on diet played in establishing cultural identities and differences during this period. Environmental medicine made diet a primary factor in main-

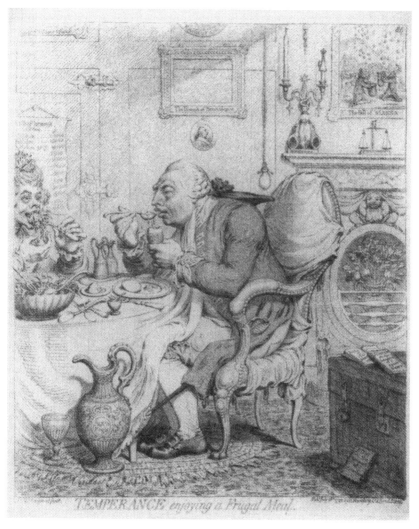

F I G . 6. James Gillray, *Temperance Enjoying a Frugal Meal* (28 July 1792).

taining health. By the end of the eighteenth century it had became a central
term in an emerging biopolitics of health, which focused on colonial diet.

Addison's anecdote also demonstrates that eating cannot be separated from
geographical considerations, since disorientation and anxiety ensue when the
dietary space one occupies makes one conscious of cultural or political differ-

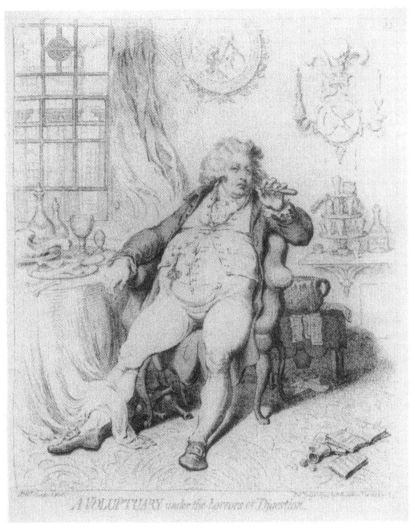

FIG. 7. James Gillray, *Voluptuary under the Horrors of Digestion* (2 July 1792).

ences. Colonial discourse developed a powerful "geography of diet," largely inflected across the three discourses mentioned above: the political, the anthropological, and the medical. Eating was intrinsically understood as a geographical event, as ideas about who one is and what one eats were linked to concerns about where one does the eating. An affirmation of biological and cultural identity, diet in a colonial context was a complex business, not easily separable from larger imaginative and sociopolitical debates concerning territorial expansion and the anxiety that attended it.

Consuming a Local and National Identity

Before discussing colonial dietary anxieties, I must give some attention to local (or nativist) and nationalistic conceptions of diet. Local diets usually produce local identities. One of the most powerful expressions of this idea, one that also served as the standard for an English national ideal, is given by Matt Bramble in Smollett's *Humphry Clinker* as he extols the benefits of country life over city living. "At Brambleton-hall," he declares,

I have elbow-room within doors, and breathe a clear, elastic, salutary air. . . . I drink the virgin lymph, pure and crystalline as it gushes from the rock, or the sparkling beveridge, home-brewed from malt of my own making . . . my bread is sweet and nourishing, made from my own wheat, ground in my own mill, and baked in my own oven; my table is, in a great measure, furnished from my own ground; my five-year old mutton, fed on the fragrant herbage of the mountains, that might vie with venison in juice and flavour; my delicious veal, fattened with nothing but the mother's milk, that fills the dish with gravy; my poultry from the barn-door, that never knew confinement, but when they were at roost; my rabbits panting from the warren . . . my sallads, roots, and pot-herbs, my own garden yields in plenty and perfection; the produce of the natural soil, prepared by moderate cultivation. The same soil affords all the different fruits which England may call her own, so that my desert is every day fresh-gathered from the tree. (117–18)

Bramble is describing what I would call an "eating spot," a space where cultural identities are affirmed or called into question by the very act of eating. As his repeated emphasis on "my" and "own" indicates, he celebrates not only the self-sufficiency of English rural society but also his possession of it as a member of the landed gentry. Brambleness as an identity is, quite literally, inseparable from the social and dietary space denominated by Brambleton. The landed gentry become the places they consume.

From the health benefits of a rural estate, Bramble turns to the unhealthy environment of London, where one is forced to "breathe the steams of endless putrefaction" and drink water that comes from "an open aqueduct, exposed to all manner of defilement." Even worse is the water from the Thames: "Human excrement" is the least of one's worries, since it is infused with "all the drugs, minerals, and poisons, used in mechanics and manufacture, enriched with the putrefying carcases of beasts and men; and mixed with the scourings of all the wash-tubs, kennels, and common sewers, within the bills of mortality" (118–19). The food is no better. Wine has been adulterated, as has the bread, which has been whitened through the addition of "chalk, alum, and bone-ashes." (In the polemical literature of 1756–58, it was also feared that the bones of the London poor were being added to the mixture, recalling the famous phrase in "Jack and the Beanstalk," "I'll grind his bones to make my bread.") Bramble goes on to describe the contaminated meat and vegetables of London, concluding with a description of "that table-beer, guiltless of hops and malt, vapid and nauseous; much fitter to facilitate the operation of a vomit, than to quench thirst and promote digestion; the tallowy rancid mass, called butter, manufactured with candle-grease and kitchen-stuff; and their fresh eggs, imported from France and Scotland" (121). Bramble celebrates the health merits of the *local* "eating spot" over the much more complex dietary economy of London. His is an affirmation of the positive relation between a local diet and a local identity, a self composed of what can be grown or raised close by: homemade, homegrown, homebody. These ideas shaped contemporary debates over the merits of rural and commercial environments.

William Hogarth's two prints titled *Beer Street* and *Gin Lane* (1 February 1751) (figs. 8 and 9) demonstrate the increasing importance of diet in articulating a national ideal. The first anticipates modern beer commercials in its celebration of the benefits of drinking beer. As its caption suggests:

> Beer, happy Produce of our Isle
> Can sinewy Strength impart,
> And wearied with Fatigue and Toil
> Can chear each manly Heart.

> Labour and Art upheld by Thee
> Successfully advance,
> We quaff Thy balmy Juice with Glee
> And Water leave to France.

> Genius of Health, thy grateful Taste
> Rivals the Cup of Jove,
> And warms each English generous Breast
> With Liberty and Love.
> (Paulson, *Hogarth's Graphic Works* 2: 197)

All the elements that compose the picture reinforce the notion that English national prosperity—"strength," "manl[iness]," "health," "liberty," and "love"—ultimately flow from beer. In the foreground a fat and happy butcher (a crucial figure in the land of "John Bull") looks on as two fishwives (one with her hand on a flagon of beer) read "A New Ballad on the Herring Fishery by M^r

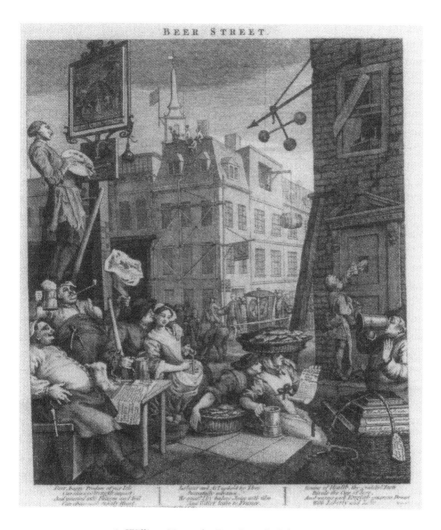

FIG. 8. William Hogarth, *Beer Street* (1 February 1751).

Lockman." Beside him stands a blacksmith holding a mug of beer in his right hand, while in his left he hoists a shoulder of mutton, an image that echoes Hogarth's earlier painting *The Roast Beefe of Old England,* where we see a man carrying a beef quarter on his shoulder. Significantly, in an earlier version of the plate, rather than the piece of mutton, the portly blacksmith lifts a French-man by the belt, a sign not only of "sinewy strength" but also of how little the man weighs compared with a flagon of beer. This dark, cadaverous, threatening figure was removed in the later print, to be replaced by a street pavior, with one hand on his mug and the other on a young servant girl's breast. To reinforce the link between sexual reproduction and diet, she is shown beside a basket of fresh vegetables. This is more than simply a place where people consume beer: the space itself and the people within it derive their very life and character from this pastime. Inasmuch as food makes labor possible, it also produces the spaces within which it is consumed. In the many images of construction, notably the paving of roads and the erecting of buildings, Hogarth is claiming that the culture of beer drinking makes this space what it is, in the same way as the culture of stock trading makes a "Wall Street." Even the fat woman in the sedan chair, representing the gentry, depends for her transport on the flow of beer that her chairmen are drinking.[1] Meanwhile the flag above St. Martin-in-the-Fields shows that this scene takes place on George II's birthday.

I will not dwell on Hogarth's companion print titled *Gin Lane* (fig. 9), apart from pointing out that the consumption of gin produces a radically different "eating spot." The "street," symbolically associated with public space and progressive commerce, is replaced by the "lane," with its pathogenic associations. Here we see the decay of society, registered not only in the numerous images of diseased, dying, or dead people, but also in buildings that have fallen into disrepair. On the left side a carpenter sells his coat and saw to S. Gripe, the Pawnbroker, while a housewife with her cooking utensils waits her turn. Everywhere one sees the effects of an entire culture reduced to drinking gin. Only in one instance, on the left side of the print, is something other than gin being consumed: there a man and a dog fight over a bone.

In his 1751 advertisement, Hogarth indicated that the subject matter of the two prints was "calculated to reform some reigning Vices peculiar to the lower Class of People." The engravings are thus explicitly aimed at reforming the dietary behavior of the lower classes, at making them understand their "true" dietary identity. Hogarth popularized the idea that Englishness is fundamentally linked to beef and beer. Gin, a relatively inexpensive intoxicant, was a foreign import, so the representation of Gin Lane is as much about the economic impact of this foreign trade as about its effect on the health, productivity, and reproduction of the English working class. Foreignness, like the Frenchman originally portrayed in *Beer Street,* is a disease invading England through lower-class diets. Hogarth is worried that the English are drinking themselves out of existence. The contrast between these two "eating spots" points up Hogarth's view that food is basic to defining social spaces and the people who inhabit them. The plates represent two different "geographies of diet." People do not simply occupy "abstract spaces" in his work: they eat

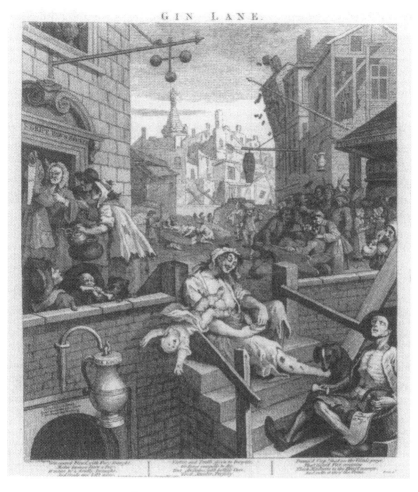

FIG. 9. William Hogarth, *Gin Lane* (1 February 1751).

there, deriving their character from them in the same manner as plants express the soils in which they are cultivated.

Hogarth's prints are just one indication of the way diet during the eighteenth century was radically politicized, as differences between nations and peoples were articulated through ideas about differences in diet and its impact on culture. The geography of diet was easily marshaled for nationalistic propaganda. In the magazine poems of the period, for instance, David Garrick's "France," dietary disparities are exaggerated as a rallying point for such propaganda:

> With lanthern jaws and croaking gut
> See how the half-starv'd Frenchmen strut,
>   And call us English dogs;
> But soon we'll teach these bragging foes,
> That beef and beer give heavier blows,
>   Than soup and roasted frogs.
>
>   (B. Bennett 97)

Once again the French are portrayed as a "half-starv'd" people reduced to eating "soup" and "frogs." You are what you eat, so not surprisingly, the French, called "frogs," have "croaking gut[s]." In Garrick's companion "England," even though English servicemen at this time could hardly claim to be better fed than the French, in this conflict of dietary identities "beef and beer give heavier blows."

> See John, the soldier, Jack, the tar,
> With sword and pistol arm'd for war,
>   Should Mounseer dare come here!
> The hungry slaves have smelt our food,
> They long to taste our flesh and blood,
>   Old England's beef and beer!
>
>   (B. Bennett 98)

Note that French imperialist expansion is encoded in terms of physical hunger. Territorial struggles are rewritten in dietary terms, as a form of eating—as consuming somebody else's place. In its most excessive rhetorical form, French imperialism is cannibalism: "They long to taste our flesh and blood, / Old England's beef and beer!"

In James Gillray's work, the nationalistic politics of eating are taken to even greater extremes. In *French Liberty, British Slavery* (21 December 1792) (fig. 10), Gillray contributes to the political geography of diet. On the left side a starving Frenchman, in the midst of a meal of leeks and snails, reflects on a "Map of French Conquests" and a future Utopia: "Vat blessing be de Liberté vive le Assemblé Nationale!—no more Tax! no more Slavery!—all free Citizen! ha hah! By Gar how ve live!—ve swim in de Milk and Honey!" On the other side, a corpulent Englishman, his face inflamed by a diet rich in fat, makes a meal of a huge roast while complaining that the British government is "Starving us to Death!"

A sign of Gillray's ambivalence is that both spaces produce sickness, though of different kinds: one feeds on a diet of ideas while the other is the heavy embodiment of stupidity. As Ronald Paulson notes, Gillray typically "will

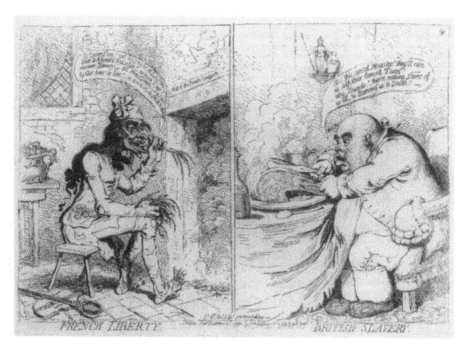

FIG. 10. James Gillray, *French Liberty, British Slavery* (21 December 1792).

attack more than one side at once," so that even as this plate draws on nationalistic conceptions of the link between diet and identity, it does not idealize them (*Representations of Revolution* 185). In *Dumourier Dining in State at St. James's* (30 March 1793) (fig. 11), a satire that encapsulates fears of a French invasion, Gillray returns to the idea that French imperialism is driven by a hunger that is ultimately cannibalistic. Here the tall, skeletal French general (he was actually short and stocky) is served the head of Pitt on a dish heavily ornamented with frogs. A year earlier Gillray engraved the even more extreme *Un Petit Souper à la Parisienne* (20 September 1792) (fig. 12), in which he drew on popular images of native cannibalistic feasts in order to portray the French *sans culottes* ravenously eating human body parts—eyes, hearts, kidneys, arms, and intestines. As the caption suggests, "Here as you see, and as 'tis known / Frenchmen mere Cannibals are grown; / On *Maigre Days* each *had* his Dish / Of Soup, or Sallad, Eggs, or Fish; / But *now* 'tis human Flesh they gnaw, / And ev'ry Day is *Mardi Gras*." French imperialism has made possible a regressive change of French dietary identity for the carnivorous French are finally able to quit their vegetables in favor of meat, even if it is human.

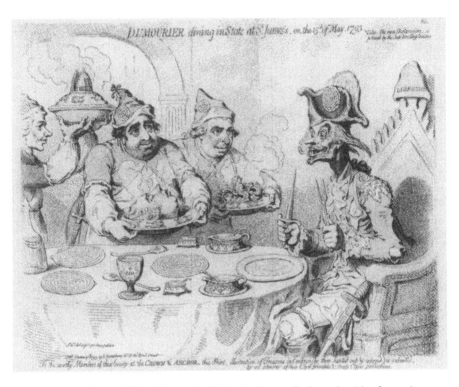

FIG. 11. James Gillray, *Dumourier Dining in State at St. James* (30 March 1793).

By the 1790s the geography of diet had become a powerful term in nationalistic rhetoric and in the articulation of ideas (both celebratory and critical) of imperial conflict and territorial expansion. At its most extreme this fear is expressed in images of cannibalism. Losing one's identity, understood in either local or national terms, is represented as being eaten up. An interesting aspect of Gillray's work is his demonstrating that the construction of a "cannibalistic other" is to a great extent a self-projection. In *John Bull Taking a Luncheon, or British Cooks, Cramming Old Grumble-Gizzard with Bonne-Chére* (24 October 1798) (fig. 13), he is shown gorging on "frigasees." The appetizer is a plate of "Soup and Bouilli" (or boiled beef), while beside John Bull is a huge jug of "True British Stout." John Bull's appetite, his capacity to consume a huge number of ships at a single sitting, is viewed as a sign of strength. By shifting attention from eating bodies to eating ships, Gillray moderates the cannibalistic shock of this print, yet the point is nevertheless made by Sheridan, Fox, and Priestley, who had served Dumourier dining in state, as

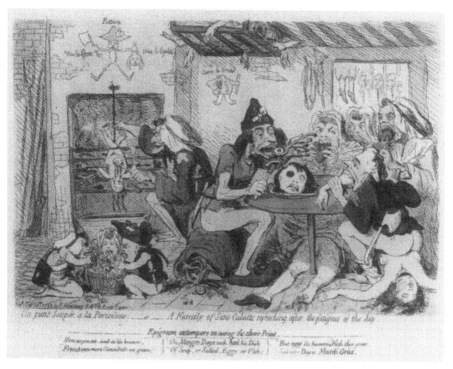

FIG. 12. James Gillray, *Un Petit Souper à la Parisienne* (20 September 1792).

they curse Bull's "gut," which is about to turn them into "chops": "Oh, Curse his Guts, he'll take a chop at Us, next." Isaac Cruikshank's *General Swallow Shown Destroying the French Army* (1 June 1799) (fig. 14) provides another example of the celebration of English cannibalism. The point is made quite clearly by one of the fleeing officers when he says, "O Begar if he once get to Paris the Directory will scarce serve him for a Breakfast."

In Gillray's *The Plumb-Pudding in Danger; or State Epicures Taking un Petit Souper* (26 February 1805) (fig. 15), there seems little difference between the two rival nations in their dietary ambitions. Here Pitt and Napoleon are shown carving up the world for lunch. Local and national dietary differences—"plumb-pudding" versus "petit souper"—matter little within the context of imperial *geophagy:* in both the capacity to rule the world is signified by one's ability to consume it.

Although simplified by the requirements of satire, Gillray's subject—the "imperial banquet"—has a long history. From the classical period onward, the

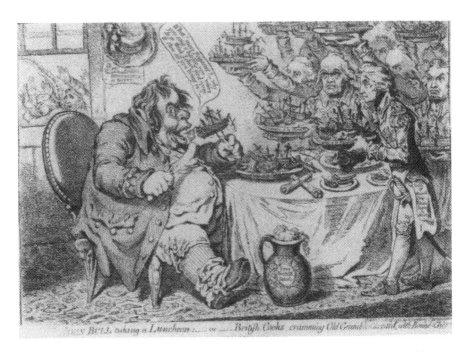

FIG. 13. James Gillray, *John Bull Taking a Luncheon, or British Cooks, Cramming Old Grumble-Gizzard with Bonne-Chére* (24 October 1798).

power of an empire has been symbolically conveyed in its rulers' ability to go beyond a local diet by eating, at a single sitting, foods from all the regions that lie within their control. There is not, therefore, that great a difference between the overt gestures of Pitt and Napoleon and the assumptions that govern the drinking of coffee in Pope's *The Rape of the Lock:*

> For lo! the Board with Cups and Spoons is crown'd,
> The Berries crackle, and the Mill turns round.
> On shining Altars of *Japan* they raise
> The silver Lamp; the fiery Spirits blaze.
> From silver Spouts the grateful Liquors glide,
> While *China's* Earth receives the smoking Tyde.
> At once they gratify their Scent and Taste,
> And frequent Cups prolong the rich Repast.
>   (3.105–12)

If one cannot afford to consume the entire world at a sitting, one can at least eat a selection of foods whose origins suggest the global reach of empire:

thus coffee, cocoa, chocolate, sugar, and tea came to be staple foods on eighteenth-century imperial tables. In this regard the critique of empire often was articulated as a critique of its foods. The use of sugar—the mainstay of the slavery economies of the West Indies—provided a rallying point for the abolition movement during the 1790s. As Samuel Taylor Coleridge thundered in his 1795 "Lecture on the Slave-Trade," genteel ladies who drink tea with sugar while tearfully reading sentimental novels were drinking the blood of black slaves. "At your meals you rise up and pressing your hands to your bosom ye lift up your eyes to God and say O Lord bless the Food which thou hast given us!" he writes. "A part of that Food among most of you is sweetened with the Blood of the Murdered. Bless the Food which thou hast given us! O Blasphemy! Did God give Food mingled with Brothers [*sic*] blood! Will the Father of all men bless the Food of Cannibals—the food which is polluted with the blood of his own innocent Children?" (*Lectures* 248). In 1792 Gillray addressed this issue in *Barbarities in the West Indias* (23 April 1791) (fig. 16), which shows an overseer, looking very much like contemporary illustrations

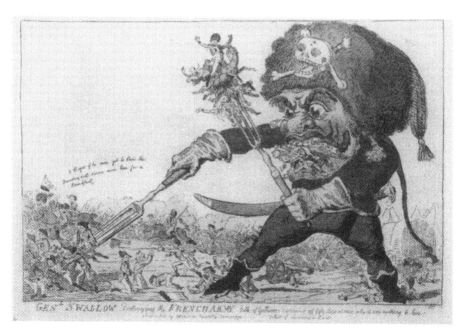

FIG. 14. Isaac Cruikshank, *General Swallow Shown Destroying the French Army* (1 June 1799).

of a "savage," simian Irishman, stirring a pot in which a slave is being boiled. "Blast your black eyes!" he says. "I'll give you a warm bath to cure your Ague, & a Curry-combing afterwards to put Spunk into you." Here Gillray inverts the popular stereotypes of black cannibalism, in the setting of Montaigne's "cannibals." That the slave is being cooked in "sugar juice" rather than soup further supports the idea that the print portrays British cannibalism in its most abject form—as an Irish plantation manager who has replaced the absentee British owner. Yet even here Gillray's position is not fully clear, since the caption suggests he may be portraying West Indian slavery less as it *is* than as it is *represented* in the discourse of abolitionists.

In a collection of *Riddles,* Jonathan Swift presented the following:

> Ever eating, never cloying,
> All devouring, all destroying,
> Never finding full Repast,
> Till I eat the World at last.
> (*Poetical Works* 630)

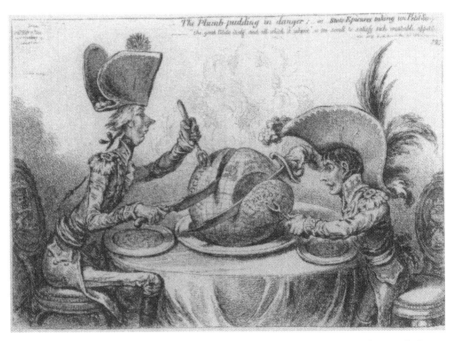

FIG. 15. James Gillray, *The Plumb-Pudding in Danger, or State Epicures Taking un Petit Souper* (26 February 1805).

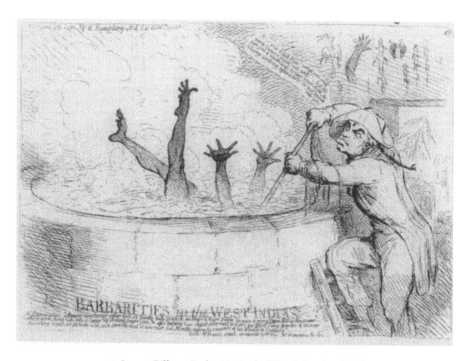

FIG. 16. James Gillray, *Barbarities in the West Indias* (23 April 1791).

Swift's answer was "Time": in the 1790s the response "Colonialism" would have been just as appropriate.

Colonial Dietary Anxieties

In the literature I have discussed so far, diet affirms local, class, or national identities. In the "local" diet the relation between place and identity is not problematic because each is seen as an expression of the other: local diets produce local people. Similarly, imperial diets express an imperial confidence in a nation's capacity to consume the "space" of others without being determined by it. Transcending local dietary regimes suggests a transcendence of geographical constraints. Read in terms of a center-periphery model, the imperial center defines itself by its ability to draw on and consume at will the local or national diets that define people on the periphery. Colonial expansion, however, produced another dietary situation. For eighteenth- and nineteenth-century colonists, those who left Europe to live for long periods in colonial regions as settlers, colonial administrators, or servicemen, the pos-

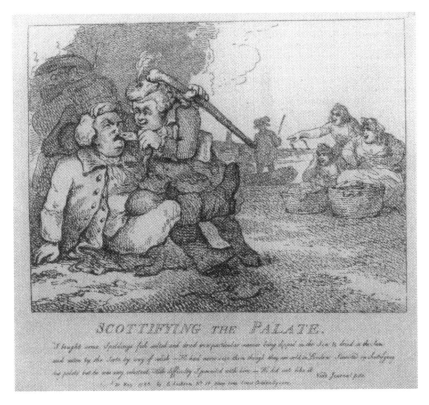

FIG. 17. Thomas Rowlandson, *Scottifying the Palate at Leith* (30 May 1786).

sible long-term effect of a change of diet and a change of place on physical and cultural identity was more frequently a source of anxiety than of confidence.

Dietary predicaments, springing from the conflict of cultures implicit in the ingestion of foods, are easily found in the literature of travel. Thomas Rowlandson's engraving *Scottifying the Palate at Leith* (30 May 1786) (fig. 17) offers a good example, as it shows Boswell force-feeding Johnson with a "spelding," a salted and dried fish that, he says in his *Life of Johnson,* is "eaten by the Scots by way of a relish. He had never seen them, though they are sold in London. I insisted on *scottifying* his palate; but he was very reluctant. With difficulty I prevailed with him to let a bit of one of them lie in his mouth. He did not like it" (5: 55). In the illustration one sees more than dislike. Johnson contorts his body and face as he struggles to resist ingesting the material signs of Scottish culture. Rowlandson infantilizes the great hero of eighteenth-century culture, representing him as a child refusing to take his medicine. In this struggle for power the force-feeding of the fish suggests rape. The promulgator of English taste is being give a taste of what it means to be a Scot, as three fishwives look on, enjoying the spectacle of an outsider's being forced to deal with their culture on far more intimate terms than he had bargained for. Perhaps some cultural revenge is also taking place, for what Scot could forget Johnson's definition of "oats" in his *Dictionary:* "A grain, which in England is generally given to horses, but in Scotland supports the people."

Eating at once affirms and threatens cultural and biological boundaries. It takes place at the boundary between the self and the exterior world. Mary Douglas notes that "we cannot possibly interpret rituals concerning excreta, breast milk, saliva and the rest unless we are prepared to see in the body a symbol of society" (115). In Johnson's struggle to maintain his own "proper self" in the face of exterior circumstances, one can recognize that eating in a colonial context threatened cultural identities. Refusing to eat expresses the desire to maintain boundaries by refusing to become "scottified." Travel and eating thus articulate cultural ambivalence perceived at a fundamental level of existence. Such ambivalence, however, was far more profoundly raised within the context of colonial settlement, where this conflict went well beyond taste to touch on primary fears about whether the physiology and health of the European body itself might be changed through diet. One might mistakenly continue to eat what one normally did in a new geographical situation (the right food in the wrong place), or one might change the food one ate and thereby risk becoming what one eats. The enormous quantity of literature arguing for the need to adopt highly regulated colonial dietary regimens, some of it reflecting the important place that diet, as a nonnatural, occupies in the Hippocratic tradition, reveals the anxiety the topic produced among colonists. In the tropics, the optimism raised by success in colonizing temperate regions of the globe was substantially modified as the British struggled with doubt about the biological or medical capacity of human beings to travel anywhere and eat anything. The powerful metaphoric understanding of the politics and anthropology of diet is very much a part of the medical discourse on colonial diets and drew much of its sustenance from it. Colonialism raised new questions about the impact of diet on the body's constitution. Dietary differences between people were expressive of underlying constitutional differences, themselves reflective of the changing impact of geography on human bodies. A change of place would seem to require a change in diet, yet it was not at all clear what the consequences of this change might be.

One of the most important reasons diet was so closely bound up with colonial anxiety was that it appeared to explain the extraordinary mortality and morbidity rates of Europeans in tropical climates. As early as the seventeenth century physicians had recognized that scurvy was connected with dietary change. "This change of character in the European who quits his country," writes the abbé Raynal, is "a phenomenon of so extraordinary a nature, the imagination is so deeply affected with it, that while it attends to it with astonishment, reflection tortures itself in endeavouring to find out the principle of it, whether it exist in human nature in general, or in the peculiar character of the navigators, or in the circumstances preceding or posterior to the event" (5: 2). The horrific example of scorbutic sailors inhabiting bodies that seemed to be literally rotting away provided ample illustration of the dangers of dietary change long before physicians knew which foods might forestall the malady. Physicians also believed that a European's constitution had to undergo a significant change to adapt to a new climate. They spoke of "seasoning," as sickness helped the body to become accommodated to a new environment. If one did not die from the change, then one's chances for a relatively long life were much better. James Lind, for instance, writes,

Men who thus exchange their native for a distant Climate, may be considered as affected in a manner somewhat analogous to plants removed into a foreign soil; where the utmost care and attention are required, to keep them in health, and to inure them to their new situation; since, thus transplanted, some change must happen in the constitutions of both.

Some Climates are healthy and favourable to European constitutions, as some Soils are favourable to the production of European plants. But most of the Countries beyond the limits of Europe, which are frequented by Europeans, unfortunately prove very unhealthy to them. (*Essay on Diseases* 2)

Just as plants frequently suffer from being transplanted to new environments, so too "European constitutions" are susceptible to the dangerous effects of geographical change. Special precautions are required if health is to be preserved. Lind follows Hippocratic tradition in arguing that a change of climate requires a change of diet. "In an intended voyage to the coast of Guinea, the East or West Indies," he observes, "the first point of consequence to the future health of the men seems to be to make such a change in the diet or ship's provisions, as may prepare the body for the alteration it must necessarily undergo, by passing from a cold to a warm climate." The geography of diet is largely a reflection of climatic differences. Whereas "the natives between the tropics . . . live chiefly on a vegetable diet, on grains, roots, and fruits; with plenty of thin diluting liquors," a "full animal diet, and malt liquors" are "better adapted to the constitution in our own, and other northern countries." The enormous loss of life associated with colonialism, Lind suggests, occurs primarily because newcomers fail to accommodate their diets to new geographical environments. Although a full diet "of hard salted meats, and the coarsest food" suits the sailors of Greenland, it is "pernicious to health" in the West Indies. Thus, he remarks, "it is, indeed, a truth evinced by most fatal experience, that their devouring of large quantities of flesh meats, and using the same heavy food in the West Indies, or upon the Coast of Guinea, and in other warm countries, as they were accustomed to at home, have proved the destruction of many thousand English in those climates" (*Essay on the Most Effectual Means* 39). In his study of an outbreak of yellow fever in the West Indies, Leonard Gillespie draws a similar conclusion: "The abuse of spirituous liquors, and the too plentiful use of animal foods, are amongst the first causes of creating dangerous fevers among strangers on their arrival in the West Indies. During the passage from Europe, it would be highly adviseable to retrench the usual quantity of animal food made use of, and to drink little or no spirits" (3). To retain normal habits in a colonial environment was foolhardy. Eating the right European food in the wrong place could be fatal. In tropical regions, where meat decays rapidly, the tendency of the body to keep animal foods inside too long produced bodily "plethoras," one of the most common causes of putrid diseases.

To a great extent, colonial medical practice affirmed the relation between local diets and local peoples. Colin Chisholm's *Essay on the Malignant Pestilential Fever Introduced in the West Indian Islands from Boullam* (1795) draws a correlation between a region's climate and the properties of the plants found there. His representation of Grenada as an earthly paradise is little different from Matt Bramble's.

Every human want, except those introduced by European luxury, is here amply provided for, almost without exertion. The most wholesome food is the spontaneous production of the country. The various species of the banana, of the potatoe, of the pea, of the bean, of the cassada [i.e., cassava], stand unrivalled in salubrity and native elegance of taste. To these may be added a variety of pot-herbs and greens, unknown in Europe; and at least sixty kinds of fruit, chiefly natives of the country, of the most delicious flavour and taste. To strengthen and give tone to the stomach, diminished by debilitating causes continually present, various peppers and grateful stimulating plants spontaneously present themselves. Is the traveller in the woods parched with heat, and languishing for diluting drink, the kindly water-withe and wild pine, are on every tree ready to assuage his thirst. Do the chilling northerly winds of winter check the perspiration and excite catarrhal complaints, many hundred plants well suited to

remove them, are everywhere furnished by Nature. Do fevers prevail, the same kind
Provider has amply bestowed on us the means of relief. (23–24)

Given such a complimentary view of the merits of the island, Chisholm had
some difficulty explaining why so many Europeans were dying there. He
admits that in those areas where marshes are abundant, the annual death rate is
an extraordinary 180 per thousand; however, in other regions, in common
years, he claims it is only about 20 per thousand, comparable to Europe's. The
main cause of disease is foreign luxuries. In Grenada, he argues, nature goes to
great lengths to assimilate "the European constitution to the tropic climate"
so that "diseases, mild among the indigenæ, or the assimilated of the country,
become fatal to the imprudent stranger." Consequently Chisholm will claim
that people who confine themselves "to the wholesome indigenous aliment
of the country, with occasionally the addition of the least injurious of the
European delicacies, live to an age uncommon even in the temperate regions
of the old continent" (28–29). Trotter, remarking on the increase in epidemic
fevers in colonial America, similarly warns Americans to "forego the luxury
of European banquets, and return to your primitive simplicity of living" (2:
69). In India, Charles Curtis concluded it was essential that Europeans "ac-
custom themselves to what are called the native dishes, which consist for the
most part of boiled rice, and fruits, highly seasoned with hot aromatics, along
with meat items and sauces, but with a small proportion of animal matter."
Unfortunately, most colonists fell prey to "a kind of false bravado and the
exhibition of a generous contempt for what they reckon the luxurious and
effeminate practices of the country" (280–81).

The dangers of a luxurious or "imperial" diet are a constant theme in these
texts. Just as colonists were encouraged to keep the tropics at a distance by
emphasizing a moral regimen, so too dietary advice was largely spartan in
character. For instance Edward Long, in his *History of Jamaica* (1774), argues
that Europeans are especially prone to ill health because they "unthinkingly"
persist "in those habits of life to which they were long used in Europe, and
chuse not to leave off, although by no means proper in the West-Indies. . . .
[T]he European keeps late hours at night; lounges a-bed in the morning;
gormandizes at dinner and supper on loads of flesh, fish, and fruits; loves
poignant sauces; dilutes with ale, porter, punch, claret, and madeira, frequently jumbling all together; and continues this mode of living till, by
constantly manuring his stomach with such an heterogeneous compost, he
has laid the foundation for a plentiful crop of ailments. . . . They who have
attained to the greatest age here were always early risers, temperate livers in

general, inured to moderate exercise and avoiders of excess in eating" (1: 375). Colonial dietary literature thus constituted a powerful discourse warning that eating local foods and avoiding excess were crucial to maintain one's health in such regions. Bodies from "temperate" climates, it seems, faced with the extremes of a tropical environment, needed to reassert that identity through diet. In a temperate environment intemperance was intrinsically held in check; in the tropics it was fatal. As Anna Maria Falconbridge remarks, dietary restraint was a matter of prudence: "Our dinner was very good, and I had prudence enough to be temperate, having often heard of fatal consequences from indulgencies in similar cases" (99). Do not depend on tonics and stimulants to resist disease, Edward Laing remarks, "depend upon evacuations and temperance" (qtd. in Trotter 2: 83).

So far I have focused on dietary anxiety relating to new colonists. An even deeper level of anxiety emerged in regard to the long-term impact of diet on physiology and identity, fear about whether a European constitution could be maintained in the new tropical environments where settlers found themselves. Rousseau, in *Emile,* was doubtful:

Our own body is constantly being used up and needs constantly to be renewed. Although we have the faculty of changing other bodies into our own substance, the choice among them is not a matter of indifference. Everything is not food for man; and, of the substances which can be, there are ones more or less suitable for him according to the constitution of his species, according to the climate he inhabits, according to his individual temperament, and according to the way of life prescribed to him by his station. . . . The man who is not yet of any country will adapt himself without difficulty to the [dietary] practices of any country whatsoever, but the man of one country can no longer become the man of another. (150–51)

Even if in the short term one could maintain one's health and "Englishness" through a strict dietary regimen, the long-term impact of colonial environments on human physiology and reproduction remained unclear, since European plants and animals usually were seen to "degenerate" in nontemperate climates. Most colonial physicians would have agreed with the Calcutta surgeon Adam Burt that human beings, "no less than vegetables," are "materially changed by transition from their native to a different soil" (9–10). Benjamin Moseley notes in his *Treatise on Tropical Diseases:* "European animals in general degenerate in the West-Indies; and, as they descend in a few generations, retain but little resemblance of their original stock. How far this extends to the human race, as relative to natural endowments, is a subject of nice inquiry, and foreign to my present pursuit." Nevertheless, he goes on to declare that

"European dogs lose their scent, horses their speed, and human beings, of delicate structure and fine feelings, sink into a wearisome existence, deprived of power and inclination to move" (102–3). To consume a colonial environment, in other words, is ultimately to risk being consumed by it.

The "English Opium Eater"

Colonists were, by and large, engaged in a form of dietary hybridity, not simply because they felt they had to accommodate their dietary habits to a new situation, but because they believed their cultural identities as well as their bodily constitutions were being changed. Yet the cultural anxiety raised by diet was not restricted to colonial regions. Boswell, when he introduced Johnson to speldings, knew something Johnson did not: that this Scottish delicacy was now available in London shops. Colonial diets were not restricted to the colonies. They were available in the heart of the British Empire, and for hybrid Scots like Boswell, whose presence in London was a sign of empire's reach, these new London diets were a sign of a change within the imperial center. The colonial expansion of England's commercial borders raised the prospect that it could no longer isolate itself from the larger dietary identities its expansion had made possible.

John Barrell, Nigel Leask, and Barry Milligan have recently shown how much Thomas De Quincey, during the high phase of English imperial expansion, feared that England was becoming another Orient. In *Confessions of an English Opium Eater* these fears are articulated in dietary terms, in De Quincey's anxious account of the pleasures and pains of opium eating. Admittedly opium is a drug rather than a food, yet in talking about the dangers of making opium eating a habit, De Quincey employs the language of colonial medical dietetics, especially on its impact on one's health and cultural identity. Empire has made it possible for the English to consume the East: De Quincey fears that in so doing the English are being consumed by it.

The "English opium eater" is, of course, a dietary hybrid, an orientalized Englishman. The *Confessions* are thus both the delineation of the etiology of a disease and the autobiographical account of the sequence of events that have conspired to produce this new kind of person. The addiction had its origins, De Quincey tells us, in the recurrence of a childhood stomach ailment. "In the twenty-eighth year of my age," he declares, "a most painful affection of the stomach, which I had first experienced about ten years before, attacked me in great strength. This affection had originally been caused by extremities of hunger, suffered in my boyish days" (*Confessions* 35). Interestingly, his diseased stomach can be traced back to his childhood wanderings in Wales. One sign of the cultural ambiguities of the narrative is that De Quincey blames his disease on the combined effects of a healthy climate and regular exercise on a hungry stomach. "From the keen appetite produced by constant exercise, and mountain air, acting on a youthful stomach," he writes, "I soon began to suffer greatly on this slender regiment. . . . I subsisted either on blackberries, hips, haws, &c., or on the casual hospitalities which I now and then received, in return for such little services as I had an opportunity of rendering" (43). In an irony that pervades De Quincey's text, a healthful British regimen—of good air and frequent exercise—combines with poverty and perhaps a "Hindoo" vegetarian diet to produce his illness. Even here, however, he adds layer on layer of dietary ironies, for the reason he ran away from the Manchester Grammar School in the first place was that he had developed a chronic liver complaint because he was *not* allowed enough exercise. He writes that "far better, as acting always upon me with a magical celerity and a magical certainty, would have been the authoritative prescription . . . of seventy miles' walking in each week" (166). It appears that De Quincey's quest for health and the very means by which it would normally be preserved have instead made him susceptible to the lifelong perils of opium. Exercise combined with a healthful quantity of British country air have led, through a perverse system of ironies and the lack of money, to the emergence of an Oriental Englishman.

De Quincey's is a hybrid style. The stabilities of European disease geographies, in which the East is equated with contagion, sickness, and death and the West with health, continually merge into each other, producing a deeper sense of their fundamental identity and interaction. He states the obvious: "There are, as perhaps the reader knows by experience, no jaguars in Wales—nor pumas—nor anacondas—nor (generally speaking) any Thugs." This differentiation of space, however, is only momentary, for the narrative immediately populates the Welsh countryside with "Brahminical-looking cows" that threaten to destroy him because he has an "English" face (187). This hybridity is also clear in the passages describing the origins of his stomach complaint. De Quincey begins by presenting the journey to rural Wales in the conventional language of a health retreat, yet Wales is contrasted not only with the urban confinement of a Manchester, Liverpool, or London, but also with the disease-ridden populations of the East. "No huge Babylonian centres of commerce towered into the clouds on these sweet sylvan routes: no hurricanes of haste, or fever-stricken armies of horses and flying chariots, tormented the echoes in these mountain recesses," he writes. Wales is separated from the contagion of urban populations, either those of the East or their contemporary British urban equivalents. Vagrancy is celebrated, yet it is not without its risks, as De Quincey contrasts this "most delightful of lives" with the punishment imposed on the Wandering Jew: "Here was the eternal motion of winds and rivers, or of the Wandering Jew liberated from the persecution which compelled him to move, and turned his breezy freedom into a killing captivity" (186). The language of the pariah is not far distant from this apparently stable system of geographic dichotomies. How a "breezy freedom" can be turned into a "killing captivity" is not yet clear, but one senses that the difference between a healthful West and a disease-ridden East cannot be easily maintained.

De Quincey's employment of the conventions of English medical dietetics reaches its apex with his assertion that he is "never thoroughly in health unless when having pedestrian exercise to the extent of fifteen miles at the most, and eight to ten miles at the least" (187). He thus seems to be another Wordsworth, and the journey to Wales seems to reenact the opening of *The Prelude,* with its evocation of the health-giving and inspirational powers, the "blessing in this gentle breeze" (1.1), "the mild creative breeze / A vital breeze" felt by the poet who has long been pent in the city (1.43–44). Yet one learns that De Quincey differs from Wordsworth because he literally *cannot afford* this health regimen: "The flagrant health, health boiling over in fiery rapture, which ran along, side by side, with exercise on this scale, whilst all the while from morning to night I was inhaling mountain air, soon passed into a hateful scourge" (*Confessions* 187). The speed with which De Quincey moves from the world of Wordsworth to the fevered world of the East is extraordinary, as he speaks of "flagrant health" that becomes fevered ("boiling over in fiery rapture") and of mountain air as a "hateful scourge." With remarkable rapidity the healthful landscape of temperate England becomes its pathogenic double, as if the East were always already there in England, needing only the proper conditions to become a virulent reality. Whereas most "colonial invalids" recount how they lost their youthful health, often through a liver complaint, by going to the tropics, De Quincey loses his in Wales. The narrative is the same, but the geographies, differentially distinguished, have collapsed into each other.

De Quincey's analysis of the "science of happiness" in the introduction to "The Pains of Opium" even more powerfully destabilizes conventional disease geographies. He begins with a parody of God's creation of the world, "Let there be a cottage," suggesting ironically that what follows is the recovery of Eden. Since he describes not just any cottage, but Dove Cottage,

Wordsworth's previous home, what follows is in many ways a deconstruction of the cultural heart of England. Happiness has its own season, De Quincey declares: it must be neither spring, summer, nor autumn, but "winter, in his sternest shape," at least a Canadian winter, if not a Russian one. In the climatological ideologies governing the description of the virtues of an English climate, cold weather plays a key role in distinguishing the northern character from its more tropical alternatives, so it is in keeping with conventional expectations that the ideal of English domestic happiness will be achieved by balancing the warmth of the cottage with the coldness outside. Into this setting, happiness arrives with the entrance of the tea tray. Parody is hard to separate from wish fulfillment as De Quincey has recourse to what by this time was a sacred English ritual: "Near the fire, paint me a tea-table; and (as it is clear that no creature can come to see one such a stormy night,) place only two cups and saucers on the tea-tray: and, if you know how to paint such a thing symbolically, or otherwise, paint me an eternal teapot." Even if one overlooks the fact that this most English of drinks is a product of the Orient and thus itself part of the hybrid dietary culture of imperial England—a "spelding" so successful in infiltrating English culture that it ultimately was thought the epitome of Englishness—De Quincey does not allow one to rest long with this comfortable image of English rural domestic happiness, removed from the dangers of metropolitan commerce. In the midst of this cultural ideal, probably at the very table where Wordsworth produced his own celebration of native English culture, De Quincey introduces himself, the "picture of the Opium-eater" (*Confessions* 93–95). For him Englishness seems to produce its opposite; the hybridity implicit in the very idea of an "English opium eater" is not eccentric to the culture but seems to be born from it. As if to emphasize this point, it was "in that very northern region," De Quincey says, "even in that very valley, nay, in that very house to which my erroneous wishes pointed, that this second birth of my sufferings began" (68). De Quincey's addiction to opium, his hybrid dietary self, was born in the very heart of an English national ideal. Just as the very healthfulness of the British environment produces fever, so too Dove Cottage summons up its foreign hybridized other, through its very insistence on its isolation from the world of colonial commerce. De Quincey is indeed Wordsworth's abjected other.

Through opium eating De Quincey articulates the threat that the East poses to English culture. In the *Confessions* this struggle is internalized; it is presented as a psychomachia of identity, as a struggle within the hybrid body of the English opium eater, a body whose very constitution is threatened by a steady diet of opium. Insofar as De Quincey claims he eventually learned how to untwist "the accursed chain which fettered me" (30), the narrative seems to provide readers, at least superficially, with a positive account of the ultimate victory of the Western mind and body over the East. Yet such a reading overlooks how De Quincey's identity as an author and the fantastic imaginary resources that he draws upon are inseparable from his addiction. Indeed, it is his Eastern imagination that has been unlocked by opium, and it is this imagination, so unusual in a disciple of the English Lake poets, that he believes distinguishes him from Wordsworth. Even his struggle with opium gains much of its expansive power from Eastern imagery and Oriental landscapes, as if the opium eater's nightmares were somehow equivalent to the dreams Fuseli claimed he had from eating raw meat. De Quincey thus struggles with the medical geography that his imagination has drawn on and augmented. Even as he assures readers that the disease of the imagination produced by opium addiction has been cured, and that the physiology and mind of the opium eater can be returned to their original English character, the text provides far fewer assurances. As De Quincey notes in his introduction: "those eat now, who never ate before; / And those who always ate, now eat the more" (32).

De Quincey was not simply describing a unique dietary and cultural problem but was also suggesting—as did Hogarth in his attack on importing gin—that opium is a disease that is transforming English society. De Quincey's "East" is a figural displacement of the populous facelessness of the urban working class. That he believed parts of London were becoming a hybrid Orient is clear in the *Confessions*. Note, for instance, the way he describes his navigation of London's streets:

And sometimes in my attempts to steer homewards, upon nautical principles, by fixing my eye on the pole-star, and seeking ambitiously for a north-west passage, instead of circumnavigating all the capes and headlands I had doubled in my outward voyage, I came suddenly upon such knotty problems of alleys, such enigmatical entries, and such sphinx's riddles of streets without thoroughfares, as must, I conceive baffle the audacity of porters, and confound the intellects of hackney-coachmen. I could almost have believed, at times, that I must be the first discoverer of some of these *terræ incognitæ*, and doubted, whether they had yet been laid down in the modern charts of London. (81)

Working-class London is here portrayed as a foreign space, an alien world that has emerged in the very heart of the imperial center. Poverty and Eastern geographies are fused in De Quincey's mind, and the *Confessions* presents the possibility that the English class system is producing a dangerous foreign population within itself. The greatest fear is that England is becoming "Oriental"; opium might be "more in request with us than the Turks themselves" (32).

These anxieties are given their most powerful figurative expression in De Quincey's encounter with the Malay, whose "disturbing figure" is introduced, Charles Rzepka asserts, "in order to 'exorcise' it" (8). What adds to its uncanny disruptiveness is that it takes place in Dove Cottage. The viewpoint of the narrative is also unstable, since the encounter is described through the eyes of the "opium eater," whose imagination has already been contaminated by the East. De Quincey tells us that "one day a Malay knocked at my door" (90). Since a Malay would seem to have no "business" (De Quincey also uses the word "transact") "amongst English mountains," De Quincey concludes that he is a sailor "on his road to a sea-port" forty miles distant. Initially the encounter is between the Malay and a young girl, "born and bred amongst the mountains," who had never before seen anything Asian. Not only is she the emblem of a noncolonial England, supposed to be uncontaminated by global commerce, but she is also Barbara Lewthwaite, the speaker in Wordsworth's "The Pet-Lamb." Critics have already noted that much of the tension in the episode derives from racial anxieties and from the overt sexual threat the Malay embodies: "He had placed himself nearer to the girl than she seemed to relish; though her native spirit of mountain intrepidity contended with the feeling of simple awe which her countenance expressed as she gazed upon the tiger-cat before her." Yet one should not miss the further suggestion of epidemiological threat implicit in the comparison of the two figures: "The beautiful English face of the girl, and its exquisite fairness . . . contrasted with the sallow and bilious skin of the Malay" (90–91).[2] For De Quincey, the Malay is a figure of the disease of the East, of tropical fever and its threat to a domestic England. Sex, disease, and cultural otherness are superimposed as De Quincey describes the embodiment of a nightmare encounter made possible by colonialism.

Whereas the meeting of Barbara Lewthwaite and the Malay is shaped by naïveté, that between the opium eater and the Malay is even more complicated because they seem to have a secret understanding of each other, partly because the Malay parodies the wanderings and sicknesses of the young De Quincey, but also because they share the same disease of diet—the love of opium. They know each other because they eat the same food. John Barrell suggests that De Quincey sought to protect himself from the infection embodied by the East through the metaphor of inoculation, of "taking something of the East into himself, and projecting whatever he could not acknowledge as his out into a further East, an East *beyond* the East" (16). De Quincey uses the fluidity of a margin that links him to the Malay to assert the bound-aries. In an extraordinary scene, he reverses the dynamics of opium eating by giving the Malay enough opium "to kill three dragoons and their horses," only to see him bolt it down in one gulp. We never learn what happened to the Malay. De Quincey tells us that for many days he felt anxious, but since he "never heard of any Malay being found dead," he concluded that he had done him a good service (91–92). With De Quincey's characteristic ambivalence, the same act that possibly benefits the Malay also possibly has killed him. By forcing the Malay to eat the food that he himself eats yet also denies as being part of himself, De Quincey is able to abject the otherness within himself. It is as if Johnson were to force-feed Boswell with his own "speldings" in order to assert his Englishness—to give Boswell some of his own medicine. In a final irony, the anxiety about how to preserve the self that is consumed by eating finds and affirms itself in watching an abject colonial other eat the food reserved for oneself.

FOUR

Keats and the
Geography of Consumption

On 5 September 1819, two weeks before composing "To Autumn," Keats wrote to his publisher, John Taylor, about the respective healthiness of different kinds of air. "You should no[t] have delay'd so long in fleet Street; leading an inactive life as you did was breathing poison," he writes. "You will find Country air [can] do more for you than you expect. But it must be proper country air; you must choose a spot" (*Letters* 2: 155–56). The right kind of air is crucial to good health, but finding it is not so easy. Keats draws on medical topography. "You should live in a dry, gravelly, barren elevated country open to the currents of air, and such a place is generally furnnish'd with the finest springs." The air of urban environments, not surprisingly, is especially poisonous, as William Farr notes when he claims that the air produced by "the foul untrapped sewers and the ground areas of the best streets" is "as fatal as arsenic to a certain number of persons" (*Ninth Annual Report* [1847–48], xxi). Yet Keats stresses that rural spaces can be just as bad: at Shanklin on the Isle of Wight, the air was "almost as bad as the smoke of fleetstreet," because it was in "the neighbourhood of a rich inclosed fulsome manured arrable Land." Closed off except to the southeast, Shanklin's damp air had "an unhealthy idiosyncrasy altogether enervating and weakening as a city Smoke," Keats writes. "I felt it much." At Winchester, on the other hand, he has been steadily "improving in health—it is not so confined—and there is on one side of the city a dry chalky down where the air is worth six pence a pint." Since health has less to do with *who* than *where* you are, Keats advises Taylor that if his constitution does not improve "impute it [not] to your own weakness before you have well considered the nature of the air and soil—especially as Autumn is encroaching: for the autum fogs over a rich land is like the steam from cabbage water."

Medical topography provides Keats with the conceptual vocabulary for establishing both a sociology and a geography of human temperaments. "What makes the great difference between valemen flatland men, and Mountaineers?" he asks. "Our hea[l]th temperament and dispositions are taken more . . . from the air we breathe than is generally imagined. See the difference between a Peasant and a Butcher. I am convinced a great cause of it is the difference of the air they breathe—The one takes his mingled with the fume of slaughter the other with the damp exhalement from the glebe." Breathing is ingestion: the butcher who inhales the minuscule particles that rise with the fume of slaughter develops the same aggressive, hot temperament associated with eating flesh. "All savages are cruel," writes Rousseau, "and it is not their morals which cause them to be so. This cruelty comes from their food. . . . Even in England butchers are not accepted as witnesses, and neither are surgeons" (153). The rural laborer is no less affected by the environment, yet in this case the air he breathes is like "mother's milk." "The teeming damp that comes from the plough furrow," writes Keats, "is of great effect in taming the fierceness of a strong Man more than his labour—let him be mowing furze upon a Mountain and at the days end his thoughts will run upon a withe axe if he ever had handled one, let him leave the Plough and he will think qu[i]etly of his supper—Agriculture is the tamer of men; the steam from the earth is like drinking their mother's milk—It enervates their natures." Whether in the sedentary confined spaces of a London publisher, the hot, bloody world of the butcher, or the soporific damps of a field, air is an occupational hazard. From sociology Keats shifts to a global perspective, speculating that the air rising from agricultural fields might be "a great cause of the imbecillity of the Chinese."

That Keats was accustomed to using a sophisticated and comprehensive discourse on air, climate, and regimen not only to address questions of health but also to explain differences in the character and behavior of social classes and peoples is hardly unexpected, given his extensive medical training.[1] "The connection between poetry and medicine," Hermione de Almeida argues, "was thoroughgoing, obvious, traditional, and ever present in his consciousness" (18). To understand his writing one needs to be similarly sophisticated in diagnosing air—seeing a pathogenic link between the "steams" that derive from cabbage water and autumnal fogs; recognizing the lactic qualities of the air rising from newly plowed fields; discriminating the different airs that rise from limestone gravels, manured fields, and urban streets; differentiating between breezes and the "unhealthy idiosyncrasy" that can develop when air stays put too long. Keats's letter belongs to a burgeoning literature that sought to provide medical advice to a growing number of invalids who were seeking to recover their health through a "change" of climate or air. In his frequently reprinted work *The Sanative Influence of Climate,* Sir James Clark, later the physician to Queen Victoria, remarks that "for the prevention and cure of a numerous class of chronic diseases, we possess in change of climate, and even in the more limited measure of change of air in the same climate, one of our most efficient remedial agents; and one, too, for which, in many cases, we have no adequate substitute" (3).[2] One reason Clark's book was so popular was that he was an authority on the treatment and prevention of consumption (or tuberculosis, as it is now called), a disease that was epidemic in England during the early nineteenth century. It was also to a younger Clark that Taylor eventually turned for medical assistance, not for himself but for Keats, who lay dying in Rome.

Taylor's decision to take a holiday in the country was probably motivated by fear that his physical constitution, combined with his bookish occupation, heightened his risk of developing consumption. Compare, for instance, Keats's remarks with those of George Barrell to his brother-in-law Nathaniel Cheever, a publisher and bookseller living in Hallowell, Maine, who came down with a chronic cough at age thirty-nine. "Let me advise you my dear friend and don't slight my advice," Barrell writes. "The climate is the most wretched in creation where you now are, and altogether unfit for human beings much less for invalids. . . . Leave it for a season, take your passage at once for a warmer and better air—take a trip to sea—go to Madeira, to Bermuda, Savannah. . . . Take passage for it will add thirty years to your life and give happiness to your wife and children. . . . A change of air is necessary for you and you must not neglect this imperious duty" (qtd. in Rothman 59). For those labeled invalids, improving one's health was not simply a value in itself, it was a social and familial duty. Sheila Rothman notes that "the term was as much a social as a medical category, defining the responsibilities of the sick even as it freed them from fault. Invalids were obliged to seek cures . . . In the language of the day, they had a lifelong obligation to improve—with all the nuances of the phrase intended" (4).

Keats's medical advice to his publisher might be taken as disinterested but for the fact, rarely adequately recognized, that throughout most of his writing career he himself was in dangerously poor health. The confirmation of consumption came on the night of 3 February 1820, with the first pulmonary hemorrhage, yet even as early as March 1817 Keats writes that his brothers were "anxious that I sho^d go myself into the country . . . that I sho^d be alone to improve myself. . . . Jack Health—honest Jack Health, true Jack Health, banish health and banish all the world" (*Letters* 1: 125). A month later he was on the Isle of Wight, one of the many "health spots" and "seaside resorts" he would visit during the next thirty months. That year Keats also moved his lodgings from Cheapside to Hampstead, which was then gaining a reputation for the quality of its air.[3] In 1818 he went on a walking tour of northern England, Scotland, and Ireland. Carol Kyros Walker voices the common mistaken view that "the price of this lively journey was Keats's health and span of life" (1). Although Keats was forced to halt his travels when he developed a sore throat, a sign of the onset of consumption, one reason for taking the walking tour in the first place must have been to stave off the disease by improving his health through exercise. By 1819 Keats was clearly in poor health. The reference to Shanklin, a popular health retreat of the time, and his assertion of the benefits of his stay in Winchester ("Since I have been at Winchester I have been improving in health") reveal that he is giving medical advice less in the capacity of a doctor than as an invalid, providing whatever medical advice he can, and recommending places based on personal experience. The idea that certain kinds of air might be "worth six pence a pint" aptly captures the mythology that underlay an entire commerce in salubrious airs. Keats's ideas about the relation between geographical land-scapes and disease are culturally determined abstractions, but they also helped him make sense of his own experience of illness. Rather than reading Keats's poems under the banner of a healthy life unexpectedly cut short by dis-ease, therefore, one should recognize that they represent an anxious struggle against an illness he had already been exposed to. They are dominated by the quest for health. Writing to Fanny Keats, one week before the letter to Taylor, Keats declares that "the delightful Weather we have had for two Months is the highest gratification I could receive . . . no need of much exercise—a Mile a day being quite sufficient—My greatest regret is that I have not been well enough to bathe though I have been two Months by the sea side. . . . Still I enjoy the Weather I adore fine Weather as the greatest blessing I can have" (2: 148–49).[4]

Poetry, Power, and Disease

Climates and landscapes in Keats's poetry are thoroughly medicalized, read within the context of an emerging biogeographical and medical discourse that divided the world into regions of health and sickness. Take, for instance, his description of the dismal climate of America in "What can I do to drive away remembrance," verse that is contemporary with "To Autumn." "Where shall I learn to get my peace again?" writes the poet:

> To banish thoughts of that most hateful land,
> Dungeoner of my friends, that wicked strand
> Where they were wreck'd and live a wretched life;
> That monstrous region, whose dull rivers pour
> Ever from their sordid urns unto the shore,
> Unown'd of any weedy-haired gods;
> Whose winds, all zephyrless, hold scourging rods,
> Iced in the great lakes, to afflict mankind;
> Whose rank-grown forests, frosted, black, and blind,
> Would fright a Dryad.   (*Complete Poems* 30–40)

Keats describes America as a "monstrous region," whose icy winds and "rank-grown forests" "afflict mankind." Here his indebtedness to the Comte de Buffon's and William Robertson's descriptions of America as an inferior habitat are clear. For Buffon, America's cold and damp climate had had a profound impact on its flora and fauna by significantly reducing their overall reproductive capacity. All species, he claimed, including humankind, suffered degeneration in America. As Keats describes it, America's

> harsh herbaged meads
> Make lean and lank the starv'd ox while he feeds;
> There flowers have no scent, birds no sweet song,
> And great unerring Nature once seems wrong.
>
> (40–43)

Here diet functions within the context of colonial biogeography. Since eating recycles the vital germs that compose life, the problem is not that there is nothing to eat in America, but that the ox is "starv'd" "*while he feeds*" because the food itself is degenerate.[5] Keats recalls Goldsmith's claim, in "The Deserted Village," that in the "matted woods" of America "birds forget to sing," as he adds his own characteristic voice to the catalog of complaints against the American environment: "there flowers have no scent."

Although Keats often equates sickness with regions of extreme cold, he more commonly focuses on tropical environments. The Titans of *Hyperion*, patterned on a fusion of the ancient druids and the gigantic Eastern sculptures that Keats saw at the British Museum, inhabit a disease landscape of monumental proportions. These superannuated beings, born "when sages look'd to Egypt for their lore" (1.33), inhabit a world "far sunken from the healthy breath of morn" (1.2). They seem to be caught in a space of death that reflects not only their mortality—even gods must die—but also their inability to understand their new being. We hear of "regions of laborious breath" (2.22);

of monstrous spaces where agony and sorrow are "portion'd to a giant nerve" (1.175); of "big hearts / Heaving in pain" (2.26–27), of "palsied tongue[s]" (1.93), "aspen-malady" (1.94), and "hectic lips" (2.250). The "nerveless, list-less, dead, / Unsceptred" (1.18–19) Saturn struggles to understand his loss of both physical and political power, a struggle represented by fever:

> This passion lifted him upon his feet,
> And made his hands to struggle in the air,
> His Druid locks to shake and ooze with sweat,
> His eyes to fever out, his voice to cease.
> . . . .
>   "But cannot I create?
> Cannot I form? Cannot I fashion forth
> Another world, another universe,
> To overbear and crumble this to nought?"
>   (1.135–44)

Saturn's struggle to recover his past being is structured as that of an invalid seeking his previous healthy identity: "I have left / My strong identity, my real self. . . . Thea! Thea! Thea! where is Saturn?" (1.113–34). At the same time, Keats makes health inseparable from creativity, suggesting that questions of identity, power, and disease cannot be divorced from artistic creation: "cannot I create? / Cannot I form?" Suffering suffers more when it lacks a voice.[6]

Whereas Saturn is already a fallen god at the beginning of the poem, Hyperion sees a god-sickening epidemic around him and knows that he too is becoming ill. Anger and fear color in feverish flushes the court of this Oriental god:

>   His palace bright,
> Bastion'd with pyramids of glowing gold,
> And touch'd with shade of bronzed obelisks,
> Glar'd a blood-red through all its thousand courts,
> Arches, and domes, and fiery galleries;
> And all its curtains of Aurorian clouds
> Flush'd angerly.   (1.176–82)

As with Saturn, disease is manifested as a loss of linguistic power. Words leap out of Hyperion's mouth "despite of godlike curb" (1.226), while others lie struggling in "his throat but came not forth" (1.252). Anticipating Shelley's later posthumous account of his being killed by a review, Keats portrays the epidemic as being invoked and symptomized by words:

> So at Hyperion's words the Phantoms pale
> Bestirr'd themselves, thrice horrible and cold;
> And from the mirror'd level where he stood
> A mist arose, as from a scummy marsh.
> At this, through all his bulk an agony
> Crept gradual, from the feet unto the crown.
>
> (1.255–60)

Here sick words rise like a miasmatic mist from a "scummy marsh." In representing the space of the fallen Titans, these "effigies of pain" (1.228), the poet drew extensively on the geography of *Paradise Lost,* yet Keats's hell is primarily an epidemiological state, patterned on the "disease landscapes" he learned to diagnose through his medical training:

> many more, the brawniest in assault,
> Were pent in regions of laborious breath;
> Dungeon'd in opaque element, to keep
> Their clenched teeth still clench'd, and all their limbs
> Lock'd up like veins of metal, crampt and screw'd;
> Without a motion, save of their big hearts
> Heaving in pain, and horribly convuls'd
> With sanguine feverous boiling gurge of pulse.
>
> (2.21–28)

The silence of these gods, dungeoned in worlds of "laborious breath," their bodies fevered and contorted, is a reminder that history is mostly written by the healthy.

Critics have long linked the presence of disease metaphors in *Hyperion* to its immediate biographical context: Keats nursing his brother Tom, who was dying of tuberculosis. In a letter to Charles Dilke, Keats indicates that the poem represents a struggle to create a symbolic alternative to living in the same space as his dying brother. "I wish I could say Tom was any better," he writes. "His identity presses upon me so all day that I am . . . obliged to write, and plunge into abstract images to ease myself of his countenance his voice and feebleness" (*Letters* 1: 369). Poetry is here understood as an escape from diseased space, akin to the speaker's attempt, in the "Ode to a Nightingale," to fade into the "forest dim" and "quite forget . . . The weariness, the fever, and the fret . . . Where youth grows pale, and spectre-thin, and dies" (20–26). Such a view, however, is a good reading neither of the "Ode," whose forest is a direct translation of Dante's *selva oscura,* nor of *Hyperion.* It is more useful to see it as a symbolic attempt to cure such spaces by creating a habitable literary space, a cultural alternative to real space. Yet Keats also sought to understand and gain some control over the diseased space within which he lived by projecting it into the monumental pathogenic spaces of the East. The East thus provided him with a geography for representing and dealing with the feverish space around him. This is why the hell of the fallen Titans frequently looks more like England than the Middle East or North Africa. In describing this "nest of woe" (2.14) where no light "glimmer[s] on their tears" and "their own groans / They felt, but heard not" (2.6–7), Keats draws on the idea of the "fever-nest," those impoverished, overcrowded places that were believed to be the breeding grounds of fever, especially typhus.[7] The world of the fallen Titans is actually Cheapside in the tropics, a fever-nest of an expansive order of magnitude. Mythological syncretism—with its fusion of the classical, Eastern, and druidic gods—finds its counterpart in a form of *epidemiological syncretism,* as the Titans frequently become the sick spaces they inhabit. At one point these Oriental gods clearly manifest their hybridity when they appear as a set of druid stones marking out a space of fever:

> Scarce images of life, one here, one there,
> Lay vast and edgeways; like a dismal cirque
> Of Druid stones, upon a forlorn moor,
> When the chill rain begins at shut of eve,
> In dull November.   (2.33–37)

Here the only difference between England and the East is in the magnitude of the disease formations. The fallen Titans' suffering is more terrible in that it takes place among those whom history ignores, those who are powerless to speak. Tom's "voice and feebleness" pressed on Keats even as he sought to find an alternative to the diseased space in which he found himself. Tom, of course, was dying not from fever, but from tuberculosis, but within the unstable hybrid disease geography of the poem East and West are mutually inflected.

Elsewhere I have argued that the "war in heaven" serves as an allegory of a larger historical conflict between East and West articulated politically and aesthetically in what was to have been a narrative about the displacement of the rude sublimity of Egyptian sculpture by the art of Greece ("Political Implications"). *Hyperion* was to have celebrated Western progress, a history in which medicine would have played an important role. "Receive the truth and let it be your balm" (2.243), declares Oceanus, as he asserts that "first in beauty should be first in might" (2.229). The advent in book 3 of Apollo, "the

Father of all verse" (3.13), of medicine, and ironically, of disease, is first registered by the appearance of a new environment:[8]

> Rejoice, O Delos, with thine olives green,
> And poplars, and lawn-shading palms, and beech,
> In which the Zephyr breathes the loudest song,
> And hazels thick, dark-stemm'd beneath the shade:
> Apollo is once more the golden theme!
>
> (3.24–28)

Hyperion was intended to celebrate the Apollonian cure of the East, as the pathogenic world of the Titans, linked to Egypt and its monuments, was replaced by the Apollonian ideal—a landscape identified as European by its lawns, poplars, beeches, and hazels. What about the sick Titans? Keats writes, "Leave them, O Muse! for thou anon wilt find / Many a fallen old Divinity / Wandering in vain about bewildered shores" (3.7–9).

That the East needed curing by Western medicine is, as I have proposed, one of the grand narratives of nineteenth-century imperialism. *Hyperion* was originally planned to be a paean to such a liberal expansionary ideal. In a letter to Benjamin Haydon, Keats even suggests that his Apollo is a new and improved Napoleon: "The nature of *Hyperion* will lead me to treat it in a more naked and grecian Manner—and the march of passion and endeavour will be undeviating—and one great contrast between them will be—that the Hero of the written tale [Endymion] being mortal is led on, like Buonaparte, by circumstance; whereas the Apollo in Hyperion being a fore-seeing God will shape his actions like one" (*Letters* 1: 207). The displacement of the disease environment of the Titans with the healthy space of Greek poetry and medicine embodied in Apollo can be seen, then, as a symbolic acting out of what the poem itself was supposed to do for the young, aspiring Keats by ushering in a new healthy poet, replacing the sickness of soul exhibited by the poet of *Endymion*. The advent of Apollo was to have enacted the coming into being of a healthy authorial voice through the cure of the poet as much as of the physical and symbolic spaces he inhabits. What is nevertheless arresting about the poetic fragment is that its imaginative center is not Apollo, but the sick Titans. Keats may well have wanted to cure himself by curing the East, he may have wished to become a poetic Apollo, but instead he identified imaginatively with the world of the Titans.

Keats's letters suggest that this concern about disease and creation responded imaginatively not only to Tom's illness, but also to his own recurring low fever. In the letter I quoted from earlier, the poet provides a more complex perspective on his difficulty in displacing the Titans in favor of a healthy Apollo: Tom's "identity presses upon me so all day that I am . . . obliged to write, and plunge into abstract images to ease myself of his countenance his voice and feebleness—so that I live now in a continual fever—it must be poisonous to life although I feel well. Imagine 'the hateful siege of contraries'—if I think of fame of poetry it seems a crime to me, and yet I must do so or suffer" (1: 369). Underlined by the allusion to Milton's Satan, the hell endured by the Titans is within Keats himself, as he concludes that the contradiction between poetry and life itself produces disease, a "poison" that causes a "continual fever." That Keats is not speaking metaphorically is clear, because he also thinks this fever might derive from "a nervousness proceeding from" a mercury medication. Interestingly, he fears that writing itself might be unhealthy. Next day he seems to have recovered slightly, for he declares that "the feverous relief of Poetry seems a much less crime—This morning poetry has conquered—I have relapsed into those abstractions which are my only life—I feel escaped from a new strange and threatening sorrow—And I am thankful for it—There is an awful warmth about my heart like a load of Immortality" (1: 369). Yet even if poetry offers relief, it is nevertheless "feverous," and there is still something anxious in Keats's mention of the "awful warmth about my heart."

In a period that saw a close link between illness and the nervous strain caused by passion and imagination, writing poetry could be a dangerous occupation, especially for those predisposed to consumption. Before Robert Koch's discovery of the tubercle bacillus in 1882, consumption was not believed to be contagious. The predisposition toward it, the "consumptive diathesis," as it was called, was thought to be inherited, so the thrust of medical prevention and treatment was toward minimizing the "irritants" that were believed to play a role in the onset of the disease.[9] Some had to do with individual behavior; others were environmental, such as poverty, overcrowding, poor diet, and impure air. As Rothman notes in regard to the middle class, "Among the most 'irritating' occupations were such sedentary and bookish ones as law, ministry, and teaching" (4) (writing was, of course, just as dangerous), while for the lower classes, those who worked in the vitiated air of cramped workplaces, especially shoemakers and seamstresses, were most prone to the disease.[10] In 1817, having taken some mercury to improve his health, Keats declares, "I feel from my employment that I shall never be again secure in Robustness" (*Letters* 1: 171). A great poet, he claims, must have "a free and healthy and lasting organization of heart and Lungs—as strong as an ox's—so as to be able [to bear] unhurt the shock of extreme thought and sensation without weariness." Keats's constitution, on the other hand, was "too weak to support [him] to the height," forcing him continually to check himself "and strive to be nothing" (*Letters* 2: 146–47). Even after suffering the first hemorrhage, he still believed that poetry contributed to his ill health: "The Doctor [Clark] assures me that there is nothing the matter with me except nervous irritability and a general weakness of the whole system which has proceeded from my anxiety of mind of late years and the too great excitement of poetry" (*Letters* 2: 287).[11] In his last letter, written when the disease had spread to his stomach, Keats still speaks of poetry as dangerous: "The knowledge of contrast, feeling for light and shade, all that information (primitive sense) necessary for a poem are great enemies to the recovery of the stomach" (2: 360). The struggle between language, creation, and disease thematized in *Hyperion,* in the sick words and bodies of Saturn and Hyperion and the would-be healthy authority of Apollo, was thus a problem closely linked to Keats's anxiety about his own health, as he sought to deal with the prospect that words, working on a weak physical constitution, might kill him. Keats looked to the East to understand his own disease experience. Most poignant is the possibility, integral to the suffering articulated in *The Fall of Hyperion,* that the poet, rather than being a balm to the world, might be no more than "a dreaming thing; / A fever of thyself" (1.168–69).

Another reason disease and poetry are inflected across geographical and colonial lines in Keats's poetry is that he did not simply write poems but sought to live in them. But since he increasingly portrays the alternative environment of a poem as a pathogenic space, the attempt to live in poems seems to produce fevers analogous to those faced by tropical settlers. "I have the choice as it were of two Poisons (yet I ought not to call this a Poison)," Keats writes in May 1819; "the one is voyaging to and from India for a few years; the other is leading a fevrous life alone with Poetry—This latter will suit me best—for I cannot resolve to give up my Studies" (*Letters* 2: 112–13). Even as he notes how odd it is to speak of poetry as a poison, Keats compares it to the dangers of the maritime trade with India.[12] Both produce fevers. He adds: "Yes I would rather conquer my indolence and strain my ne[r]ves at some grand Poem—than be a dunderheaded indiaman." Shortly thereafter he seems, at least briefly, to have opted for the latter alternative. "I have my choice of three things—or at least two—South America [to write a poem on liberty] or Surgeon to an I[n]diaman—which last I think will be my fate" (2: 114).

Tropical Verse

Although Keats's health anxieties reflect the Romantic association of poetic genius with disease, itself a growing part of the discourse on consumption,[13] they are also not unrelated to the kind of poetic spaces he was creating—the tropical qualities of his verse. Contemporary responses to his poetry
reflect how medical ideas about the dangers of inhabiting tropical regions
were transposed into debates about literary style. For many readers Keats's
poetry was too hot, too exotic. The reviewer for the *North British Review,* for
instance, argues that "as all must feel, there is an excess of greenth and vegetable imagery; in reading his description, we seem either to breath the air of a
hothouse, heavy with the moist odours of great-leaved exotics, or to live full-
stretched out at noon in some shady nook in a wood, rank underneath with
the pipey hemlock, and kindred plants of strange overgrowth. In Wordsworth . . . there is no such *unhealthy lusciousness*" (494–95, emphasis added).
The idea that Wordsworth's is a healthier poetic environment than Keats's
world of "green-leaved exotics" and "plants of strange overgrowth" shows
that geographical ideas about the relative merits of the different regions of the
world shaped attitudes toward literary style: literary spaces were seen as akin
to physical spaces, through the same biomedical grid that was dividing the
world into healthy and unhealthy regions.

In his strident criticism of the *Poems* of 1817, George Felton Mathew
identifies Keats directly with an "oriental" poetic (435), as he warns readers
not to "roll the name of Byron, Moore, Campbell and Rogers, into the milky
way of literature, [just] because Keats is pouring forth his splendors in the
Orient" (436). Associating Asia with luxury, disease, and ruin, Mathew warns
that "the mere luxuries of imagination, more especially in the possession of
the proud egotist of diseased feelings and perverted principles, may become
the ruin of a people—inculcate the falsest and most dangerous ideas of the
condition of humanity—and refine us into the degeneracy of butterflies that
perish in the deceitful glories of a destructive taper" (437). Reading Keats is a
dangerous form of fiery immolation. Although sympathetic to *Endymion,*
Leigh Hunt also sees it as suffering from "unpruned luxuriance" (*Lord Byron*
1: 418). Coventry Patmore evokes contemporary estimations of the East as he
argues that Keats's "verses constitute a region of eye-wearying splendour,
from which all who can duly appreciate them, must feel glad to escape, after
the astonishment and rapture caused by a short sojourn among them" (72).
Visit the poetry, he seems to say, but don't plan to stay long. For the reviewer

of *Baldwin's London Magazine, Endymion* "is not a *poem,* at all. It is an ecstatic dream of poetry—a flush—a fever" (381).

In drawing out the analogies between Keats's poetic spaces and tropical environments, Romantic and Victorian reviewers were primarily concerned with moral, rather than physical, health. Thus Josiah Conder complains that "there is a sickliness about his productions, which shews there is a mischief at the core" (171). William Hazlitt also drew this connection, suggesting that Keats's poetry combined "an effeminacy of style, in some degree corresponding to effeminacy of character" (254). Since recent criticism has noted that colonial regions were frequently gendered as female, the geographical valances of "effeminate style" do not require argument.[14] As an attribution applied to males, however, effeminacy has an even more specific geographical connotation, for it was strongly associated with Asian men. In the *Enquiry concerning Political Justice,* for instance, William Godwin notes the commonplace that where luxury combines with "certain warm and effeminate climates" it is "impossible to establish a system of political liberty" (147). Thomas Salmon's popular *New Geographical and Historical Grammar* argues that "the warmth of these Eastern climates has doubtless ever contributed to the indolence and effeminacy of its inhabitants" (430). James Rennell agrees: the people of Hindustan suffer from the "softness and effeminacy induced by the climate, and the yielding nature of the soil, which produces almost spontaneously" (xxi). Indolence reigns in such places. Worst of all, at least for Robert Orme, is India, where the debilitation produced by the climate has weakened its people to an "effeminacy and resignation of spirit, not to be paralleled in the world. . . . Breathing in the softest of climates; having so few wants; and receiving even the luxuries of other nations with little labour, from their own soil; the Indian must become the most effeminate inhabitant of the globe; and this is the very point at which we now see him" (471–72). Asia is lazy, effeminate, and sensual, enslaved by pleasure. As Hazlitt wrote of Keats, "All is soft and fleshy, without bone or muscle" (255).

For a society that insisted on the value of labor and moral temperance, there was a threat in a poet who could write in "Ode on Indolence" about being unable to "raise / My head cool-bedded in the flowery grass" (*Complete Poems* 51–52). These concerns, powerfully articulated in the controversy that emerged with the criticism of Keats's first two volumes of poetry in the *Quarterly* and *Blackwood's,* have received extensive attention already, so here I will concentrate on the ways John Gibson Lockhart's construction of the "cockney school of poetry" derives much of its metaphoric power from its pervasive employment of a colonial geography of disease. Drawing on the anxiety that English poetry was being invaded by poetic foreigners, writers of low birth, sensuality, and urban depravity, Lockhart portrays them as the followers of Leigh Hunt, the "potent and august King of the Cockneys." The urban geography shaping this critique is clear, for *cockney* refers both to effeminate urbanites and to lower-class Londoners, but one should not miss the suggestion of Gypsy culture through the echo of the "King of the Gypsies." Lockhart portrays Hunt's writings as a contagious poison that will be counteracted by the reviewer's medicine. Metaphors of dirt, sex, impurity, immorality, and disease proliferate. Hunt is described as "the filthiest, and the most vulgar of Cockney poetasters" ("Cockney No. 4" 520), an infected poet whose filthy language breeds disease in his readers. His is a "prostituted" muse: "with her, indecency seems a disease, she appears to speak unclean things from perfect inanition" ("Cockney No. 1" 40).[15] As in *Hyperion*, sick language is both a symptom and a medium of disease. Elizabeth Jones has suggested that Lockhart's criticism draws on an earlier literature that portrayed the suburban regions of London as sites of pestilence and promiscuity ("Suburb Sinners").[16] Lockhart also questions the Englishness of Hunt and his followers. He finds it as inconceivable that the author of *Rimini* could ever admire Wordsworth as "for a Chinese polisher of cherry-stones, or gilder of tea-cups, to burst into tears at the sight of the Theseus or the Torso" ("Cockney No. 1" 40). Hunt's poetry is tropicalized, filled with a luxurious vegetation that has no counterpart in the English countryside. "A tree in the hands of Leigh Hunt," Lockhart claims, "is a very odd affair. No such tree as he is in the habit of describing grows in the British isles; nor is any description of it to be found in Evelyn's Silva" ("Letter" 198). The reason such plants would be absent from John Evelyn's great compendium of British arboriculture is that Hunt's nature is almost completely artificial, a social construction. Such plants, Lockhart argues, really belong in a Turkish bath or brothel. The temple in which Paolo and Francesca meet in *Rimini* ("Never, be sure, before or since was seen / A summer-house so fine in such a nest of green") is no more than a "bagnio," "its furniture conceived in the very spirit of the place" ("Cockney No. 2" 199).

Lockhart's criticism of "cockney poetry" can be seen, then, as having a very specific colonial inflection, since it portrays it as being not so much a representation of tropical nature as the expression of a new mode of British urban vulgarity, a tawdry tropicalized urbanism, the product of an effeminizing commerce with the East. To the Tory establishment, Keats and Hunt represented the worst consequences of imperial contact. They were dangerous because they produced an artificial East suited to "cockney" tastes—a foreignness within English literature and society. Even after his death, *Blackwood's* continued its attack on the "cockneys" as a "pestilent sect," the vectors of plague, "vermin to be crushed." Keats remains a poet who "outhunted Hunt in a species of emasculated pruriency, that, although invented in Little Britain, looks as if it were the product of some imaginative Eunoch's muse within the melancholy inspiration of the Haram" (Preface xv, xvi, xxvi). His poetry is seen as orientalist pornography, a combination of sensual excess and commercialized exoticism, analogous to the culture that Malek Alloula has analyzed in his study of French colonial postcards of Algerian women.

The Quest for Autumn

In 1832, in the preface to his *Poetical Works,* Leigh Hunt argued that one reason recent criticism had been so critical of his writing was that it had understood its "tropicalisms" as a personal *affectation* rather than an expression of his cultural background, his father having been born in Barbados. "It was the mistake of the criticism of a northern climate," he writes, "to think that the occasional quaintnesses and neologisms, which formerly disfigured the *Story of Rimini,* arose out of affectation. . . . While I was writing them, I never imagined that they were not proper to be indulged in. I have tropical blood in my veins, inherited through many generations, and was too full of impulse and sincerity to pretend to anything I did not feel" (xv–xvi).[17] The production of the "cockney school of poetry," it seems, arose from a criticism that mistook authentic tropical excess for social mannerism. In distancing himself from this colonial style, suggesting that the "formerly disfiguring" aspects of his verse derived from cultural differences and from inexperience with the demands of a literature of a "northern climate," Hunt was following the lead of his previous protégé, for in "To Autumn" Keats also sought to write against the dangerous tropicalism of his earlier verse. The subject of the poem is deceptively simple. What could be more natural, one might think, than for an English poet walking through the Winchester countryside in September 1819 to write a poem on autumn? Only a month later, Shelley did the same thing in "Ode to the West Wind."

Yet at a time when colonialism had made apparent the connection between health and climate, the seasonal cycle of spring, summer, fall, and winter was not taken for granted. As James Thomson well knew when he wrote *The Seasons,* this cycle was what tropical regions lacked, and over the course of the eighteenth century it had become a basis for claims about the epidemiological superiority of England over other regions of the globe. "To Autumn" is a veritable catalog of national imagery—the vines, apples, gourds, and hazelnuts, and the "thatch-eves," "moss'd cottage-trees," "cyder press[es]," "stubble-plains," and "garden-croft[s]" of English landscape painting. In what remains a classic analysis, Geoffrey Hartman suggests that "To Autumn" is "an ideological poem whose very form expresses a national idea." Delineating a geography of literary form, he points out that its ideological commitments are registered not in thematic, but in formal terms, as the "English or Hesperian" lyric, the product of a westering consciousness, "overcomes not only the traditional type of sublime poem but the 'Eastern' or epiphanic consciousness essential to it." He notes its unfevered quality: " 'To Autumn' seems to absorb rather than extrovert that questing imagination whose breeding fancies, feverish overidentifications, and ambitious projects motivate the other odes" (126). It is indeed a poem in which Keats sought to create a poetic space that would no longer bring on fever. Geography, medicine, and aesthetics are thus profoundly allied. Most treatments of the impersonality of the poem, which speak of its "transhistorical" subject and the complete absence of the poet from the poem, emphasize the universality of its climate and its landscape, thus ignoring its embodiment of the national ideal of "temperate space."[18] Climate and landscape thus are not a repression of the political but are instrumental in articulating this ideal, for a primary assertion of the poem is that the best environments exhibit a balance of extremes. As the season between summer and winter, moderating both the cold "mists" of America and the hot "fruitfulness" of the tropics, autumn in England is portrayed as a space of "mellow" fruition, for both places and poets.

More successfully than *Hyperion*, "To Autumn" enacts a curing of space by tempering pathogenic extremes. These extreme geographical environments, linked imaginatively to colonial spaces, are not removed from the poem, however, but instead enter its almost classical balance as elements to be moderated. The poem does not simply represent and celebrate a detropicalized England; it enacts its coming into being as the clearing of the landscape in the harvest combines with the cooling weather to temper a space that would otherwise risk overabundance, disease, and decay. To understand the construction of this healthy landscape, therefore, one must also register the pathogenic geographies that not only inhabit the borders of the poem but enter into and are transformed within it, as the "cold" and the "hot" are remade as the "warm."[19] By examining Keats's references to tropical environments, which constitute one pole of a geography of pathogenic extremes, I hope to show how the idea of a healthy, unfevered English environment during this period was always constructed in relational terms, as a hybrid tempering of the dangers of colonial environments. The landscape of "To Autumn" constitutes a kind of biomedical allegory of the coming into being of English climatic space out of its dangerous geographical alternatives.

The opening lines epitomize the differential patterning shaping the entire poem:

> Season of mists and mellow fruitfulness,
>   Close bosom-friend of the maturing sun;
> Conspiring with him how to load and bless
>   With fruit the vines that round the thatch-eves run . . .
>
>   (1–4)

Critics have justifiably seen this harmonic interaction of sun and soil in positive terms, as an emblem of the way the autumnal landscape "conspire[s]," that is, "breathes together" (*conspirare*), with the late-season sun "to load and bless" humankind with a harvest. But one should not ignore the possible darker breathings of landscape that this balance displaces, for medical topographers saw the combination of a rich landscape overloaded with vegetation and a hot sun as the primary cause of miasmas, the "misty pestilence" of the *Fall of Hyperion* (1. 205). James Annesley argues, for instance, that "when the action of the sun upon the rich moist soil takes place, exhalations are formed of a more noxious description, and malignant remittents, continued fevers of a bad type, yellow fevers, and dysenteries, usurp the place of the milder forms of disease, which the same place, when differently circumstanced, will produce" (22). Conspiring can become conspiracy, just as "close" is the antithesis of those healthy spaces "open to the currents of air" that Keats celebrates in his letter to Taylor (*Letters* 2: 155).[20] As William Babington and James Curry (who spent eight months in Bengal) noted in lectures similar to those Keats attended at Guy's Hospital, this dangerous combination of heat and decaying vegetation explained the greater incidence of fever during autumn: "Operation of heat shewn by the more noxious effects of marsh effluvia in warm, than in cold climates and seasons;—and especially in autumn, when heat is often greatest, and many vegetables spontaneously die and rot" (15). Under the influence of a less "mature" sun, such a "loading" of the earth, ripening fruit "to the core," would hardly be a blessing. Focusing on the conditions by which environmental pathogens were generated—the conspiracy of sun and soil that produces steams, mists, miasmas, effluvias, and "vegetable putrefactions"—Keats tempers the breath of autumn. There is a danger too in "continual summer" (qtd. in Kupperman 186), as life in the tropics (where "warm days . . . never cease") made abundantly clear. Too much honey makes the bees' hive uninhabitable: "For summer has o'er-brimm'd their clammy cells" (10–11). "Clammy" suggests "sticky," but it also conveys even more vividly the cold sweats, the "clammy perspirations" that accompany fever (Babington and Curry 54), as in Glaucus's declaration that "a clammy dew is beading on my brow" (*Endymion* 3.568).

In constructing this temperate landscape, Keats drew substantially on Leigh Hunt's 5 September 1819 *Examiner* column, "The Calendar of Nature," which I quote in part:

Autumn has now arrived. This is the month of the migration of birds, of the finished harvest, of nut-gathering, of cyder and perry-making, and, towards the conclusion, of the change of colour in trees. The swallows, and many other soft-billed birds that feed on insects, disappear for the warmer climates, leaving only a few stragglers behind, probably from weakness or sickness, who hide themselves in caverns and other sheltered places, and occasionally appear upon warm days. (574)

The three great themes of autumn—harvest, the coloring and defoliation of the landscape, and the southern migration—shape Hunt's naturalistic description. Despite his emphasis on the vitality of the season, he nevertheless notes that for the sick, and for the "few stragglers" who cannot migrate, it is a difficult time. Its "chill and foggy" mornings and evenings are "not wholesome to those who either do not or cannot guard against them." It is a season of abundance: "There is grain for men, birds, and horses, hay for the cattle, loads of fruit on the trees, and swarms of fish in the ocean." Nevertheless, for "the soft-billed birds which feed on insects," it is time for their departure to the "southern countries." For Hunt, England is structured not only by climatic, but also by dietary temperance: "Repasts apparently more harmless are alone offered to the creation upon our temperate soil."

Nicholas Roe has recently demonstrated that Hunt used his column to comment indirectly on recent political events and to call for political reform (257–63).[21] Roe's analysis recognizes how active a role constructions of nature played in the conceptualization of political life during this period.[22] This discourse drew much of its sustenance and vocabulary from a larger "politics of climate," grounded in the biomedical construction of national environments. In this regard the opening paragraph to Annesley's chapter "General View of the Causes Chiefly Productive of Disease in Warm Climates, Particularly in India" provides a useful counterpoint to the "Calendar of Nature." Annesley insists on the importance of medicine for any adequate "philosophical, civil, or political" view of societies. "When the obvious and intimate

relations subsisting between the earth's surface and the human species—
between man and the soil on which he moves, the productions of the earth
which surround and feed him, and the air which he is constantly inhaling into
his body are considered—the conditions of these agents, as far as they can be
recognized by sensible properties, or inferred from their manifest effects,
become matters of great interest in medical science, and of surpassing importance, in philosophical, civil, and political points of view." Conditions of the
atmosphere not only are "the chief and immediate sources . . . of the strength
and perfection of the mental and corporeal constitution of man . . . and . . . of
the diseases which harass him, stunting his physical and moral growth, or
sweeping him from amongst living animals, of which he is the head and
master," but are "also the most productive, although the more remote causes
of national character—of advancement in all the arts, sciences, and refine-
ments of life in some countries, and of moral and physical debasement in
others."

Following a logic similar to Keats's, Annesley argues that the differences
between the physical environments of temperate and tropical regions shape
their political institutions, "the freedom, prosperity, and greatness" of the
inhabitants of the former, and "the degenerate and debased condition of the
species" in the latter. Hunt's demand for a fairer and more balanced distribution of freedoms ("The poet still takes advantage of the exuberance of harvest
and the sign of the Zodiac in this month, to read us a lesson on justice" [574])
is thus based on the belief that a liberal politics should be the natural produce
of a temperate climate. As Annesley suggests:

The constitutions of the atmosphere derived from soil and situation, according to
their nature, are not only the productive sources of disease, but also the chief spring of
the perfection of the human frame, and of its degeneracy—the influential causes of the
various degrees of human science presented to us in the different kingdoms of the
world—of the freedom and greatness of nations, and of their enslaved and degraded
conditions—of the rise and downfall of empires. They should equally interest the
scientific physician, the philosopher, the enlightened legislator, and the arbiters of the
fates of nations. (8)

Read within the context of contemporary medical geography, the political,
philosophical, and medical symbolics of atmosphere, Keats's attempt to create
in "To Autumn" a poetic temperate space, which moderates the dangers of
more extreme world environments, is not "transhistorical" but expressive of a
larger geopolitics of environment that served as the ground of more specific
political arguments.

Keats's construction of the geography of Englishness through the active moderation of more extreme geographical environments, by cooling down and clearing away the tropical elements that enter the poem, can also be seen in the second stanza:

> Sometimes whoever seeks abroad may find
> Thee sitting careless on a granary floor,
> Thy hair soft-lifted by the winnowing wind;
> Or on a half-reap'd furrow sound asleep,
> Drows'd with the fume of poppies, while thy hook
> Spares the next swath and all its twined flowers.
>
> (13–18)

The phrase "whoever seeks abroad" has been reasonably glossed to mean "whoever seeks out of doors," especially since Autumn is portrayed in this stanza as an agricultural laborer. Yet more commonly, especially in medical literature, it refers to a journey outside one's own country, a "change of air." That Keats was considering going abroad at this point can hardly be doubted, yet the poem strives to produce conviction that a cure can be found at home. Recognizing this global positioning of Autumn helps explain Keats's extraordinary inclusion (oddly unremarked) of *opium*—"the fume of poppies"—in his catalog of the elements that compose an English autumn. Here Keats is recalling his letter to Taylor and his comments on the soporific and "enervating" effects of the fumes of the furrow, which are now a drug. The stanza's concluding image of Autumn at a "cyder-press, with a patient look," watching "the last oozings hours by hours" suggests that time has almost come to a standstill even as it extracts the essence of summer from the landscape to the very last drop. Ooze, however, also conveys darker meanings, as it refers to marshland and to the muddy decaying sediment that was largely blamed for tropical miasmas.[23] And "patient look" provides a wonderful condensation of meaning, for Keats could hardly use these words without reference to their obvious medical meaning or to the Latin root of "patient" meaning "to suffer." In a poem that seeks to achieve a calm acceptance of time, change, and mortality, the "patient" is indeed an exemplary figure. As the consumptive invalid Nathaniel Cheever II (1815–44) remarked when faced with the prospect of paying for a license to practice medicine when he was not sure he would even live long enough to recover this initial capital outlay, "We must act as though we expect to live, although we may be taken from this world at any moment" (qtd. in Rothman 55).[24]

In "To Autumn" Keats was as much intent on clearing his own poetic ground as on clearing physical space. In stanza 3, the formal features of this detropicalization are given their clearest expression. As others have noted, the opening question, "Where are the songs of spring?" recalls the feverish world of the odes, supplanted by English autumn. Here the floralism and "excess of greenth" of the earlier verse is replaced by "stubble-plains." Keatsian floralism nevertheless remains as a submerged element: the "*stubble*-plains" are more masculine, but they still have a "*rosy* hue" and the "barred clouds" still "*bloom.*" The "soft-dying day" voices the deeper elegiac tones of impending mortality, yet even here the sunset, as it "touch[es] the stubble-plains with rosy hue," echoes and contrasts with the angry diseased morning of *Hyperion:* Hyperion's palace "touch'd with shade of bronzed obelisks, / Glar'd a blood-red" (1.178–79). Insect life is at a minimum (only gnats and "hedge-crickets" remain), in contrast to the increasingly dominant idea of the tropics as dominated by insect life. Keats's reference to European willows, or "sallows," is another example of his extraordinary capacity to draw health out of a context of pathogenic meanings, for a "sallow" complexion, the sickly yellowish hue caused by liver complaints, was seen as a primary symptom of exposure to a tropical environment. Annesley remarks: "Not the least important of all the symptoms which ought to be viewed as premonitory of intertropical diseases, are, the states of the surface of the body, and the appearance of the counte-nance. . . . When the countenance is collapsed, sallow, and languid, then the powers of the system may be viewed as being deficient" (143).[25] Henry Marshall notes that women were not exempted "from the exhausting effects of a tropical climate. They in general soon lose the plumpness of health, the countenance becomes sallow, and the general complexion pale and colour-less" (75). The landscape of "To Autumn" presents an English face, yet it achieves this quality differentially, by rewriting the fever-ridden features of the tropics.

The landscape of the final stanza is still a breathing landscape, as the "win-nowing wind" of stanza 2 continues in the "light wind" of stanza 3, upon whose soft breath the dirgelike song of the gnats rises or falls, "lives or dies." Linda and Michael Hutcheon have noted the integral relation between breath, song, and disease in the European discourse on tuberculosis, most notably in the dramatic figure of the consumptive operatic heroine. "To Autumn" draws its song from similar sources as it rewrites dying in English terms: the tropical environment with its sudden enteric and hepatic fevers is rewritten in the tubercular language of a "soft-dying day."[26] Sallow, it is worth noting, was also used in regard to tubercular complexions. In the early stages of pulmonary consumption, James Clark notes, "the skin of such a patient will be found in an unhealthy condition: either harsh and dry, or moist, *clammy*, and relaxed. Its color, too, is often changed to a *sallow*, and, in some cases, to a dirty yellowish hue; and, except on the cheeks, there is always a deficiency of red vessels" (*Treatise on Pulmonary Consumption* 44, emphasis added). In the final image of the "gathering swallows" that "twitter in the skies," there is certainly an oblique reference to the sore throat that Keats had been suffering for more than a year—"each swallow a triumph" (P. Fry 218). Perhaps Keats was already considering leaving England, or maybe he was thinking of the "few stragglers" that Hunt mentioned as being left "behind, probably from weakness or sickness, who hide themselves in caverns and other sheltered places, and occasionally appear on warm days."

In a letter to J. H. Reynolds, Keats confirms the ideal of temperateness that shapes his view of autumn. Apparently sensing the strangeness of applying moral categories to weather, he writes: "How beautiful the season is now— How fine the air. A temperate sharpness about it. Really, without joking, chaste weather—Diane skies" (*Letters* 2: 166). The ideal of temperance also shapes his remarks on landscape. "I never lik'd stubble fields so much as now," he declares. "Somehow a stubble plain looks warm—in the same way that some pictures look warm." For the first time, he seems able to appreciate the stubble fields of England over their geographical alternatives. Keats makes "warm" into a heavily value-laden term: such fields look warm, and they produce within the viewer an equally moderated response. The reference to English landscape paintings emphasizes that the environment he is celebrating in "To Autumn" is itself a unique fiction, something he first saw in paintings and then read into the country environs of Winchester.

Just as "To Autumn" constructs the myth of a national environment, it also claims that English poetry should mirror the healthy temperate zone it comes from. Critics have correctly seen the poem as the celebration of a new kind of poetic voice. "I always associate Chatterton with autumn," Keats writes. "He is the purest writer in the English Language. He has no French idiom, or particles like Chaucer['s]—'tis genuine English idiom in English words" (*Letters* 2: 167). This emphasis on a pure, native language can be seen in the poem's verbal indebtedness to Thomson, Chatterton, and Coleridge and its avoidance of words with Latin roots. At the same time, Keats announced his decision to abandon *Hyperion* because "there were too many Miltonic inversions in it—Miltonic verse can not be written but in an artful or rather artist's humour. I wish to give myself up to other sensations. English ought to be kept up" (2: 167). In a related letter Keats expands on these comments, writing that "I shall never become attach'd to a foreign idiom so as to put it into my writings. The Paradise lost though so fine in itself is a curruption of our Language—it should be kept as it is unique—a curiosity. a beautiful and grand Curiosity. The most remarkable Production of the world—A northern dialect accommodating itself to greek and latin inversions and intonations" (2: 212). Milton is portrayed as a cultural monster, a hybrid, employing a "northern dialect" yet allowing too much of the south to enter his poetry. "The purest english I think—or what ought to be the purest—is Chatterton's," Keats goes on to say. "Chatterton's language is entirely northern— I prefer the native music of it to Milton's cut by feet." Having identified with Chatterton's pure "uncorrupted" language of autumnal England, Keats speaks of his recent recognition of the need to stand "on my guard against Milton." In words that have less to do with poetic influence than with a whole range of environmental and medical assumptions about the link between poetry, nationality, and climate, he asserts that "Life to [Milton] would be death to me." I doubt Keats intended this comment to be taken only metaphorically.

Following a chain of associations that link English landscapes and chaste skies to notions of linguistic purity, Keats concludes his letter to Reynolds with a reference to his sisters, now living in Devonshire. "Your sisters by this time must have got the Devonshire ees—short ees—you know 'em—they are the prettiest ees in the Language," he writes, punning on both the alphabetic letter and "ease" (2: 168). Where love—from *Endymion* to the "Ode on a Grecian Urn"—had produced fever, "A burning forehead, and a parching tongue" (30), Keats now seems to be seeking a less passionate, more "chaste" gendering of space. "O how I admire the middle siz'd delicate Devonshire girls of about 15," he declares. "There was one at an Inn door holding a quartern of brandy—the very thought of her kept me *warm* a whole stage— and a 16 miler too" (2: 168, emphasis added). Since *ease* is the root of "dis-ease," Keats's mythologizing of the "warmth" produced by Devonshire girls can be seen, like "To Autumn" itself, as a very personal expression of a desire for health. It is hardly surprising that Devonshire, during this period, was being promoted as a particularly equable climate, "a favorite resort of the invalid," a region particularly suitable for counteracting consumption because of its "atmosphere, soft, warm, and charged with aquaeous vapour" (Shapter, *Climate of the South of Devon* 122).[27] Keats admits that "To night I am all in a mist; I scarcely know what's what," and he points out that lately he has suffered from depression, the "blue-devils," yet he nevertheless hopes that the place has a prophylactic power; you "need not fear . . . while you remain in Devonshire" (2: 167–68).

In September 1819 Keats hoped he had finally found a poetic style that no longer depended on or produced fever, one that would allow him to "look / Upon his mortal days with temperate blood" ("On Fame," *Complete Poems* 1–2). He claimed he was no longer the person he once was. "From the time you left me, our friends say I have altered completely—am not the same person. Some think I have lost that poetic ardour and fire 'tis said I once had—the fact is perhaps I have." He echoes Wordsworth in seeking to "substitute a more thoughtful and quiet power. . . . Qui[e]ter in my pulse, improved in my digestion; exerting myself against vexing speculations—scarcely content to write the best verses for the fever they leave behind." He goes on to stress, "I want to compose without this fever. I hope I one day shall" (*Letters* 2: 208–9). Keats obviously hoped he had found a native poetry that would no longer make him ill, that having sojourned too long in a poetic tropics he had finally come home, gaining control over the fever that had become a regular part of his life. "I have got rid of my haunting sore throat—and conduct myself in a manner not to catch another" (*Letters* 2: 200).[28]

This hope was not fulfilled, and much of the pathos of "To Autumn" derives from the sad personal circumstances that motivated this extraordinary celebration of a nativist aesthetic. It is the only poem in which Keats was able to create an unfevered literary environment out of the fevered landscapes of his earlier poetry, an achievement based on the belief that a poetry modeled on the English countryside would be healthier than other literary spaces. Yet this ideal environment, drawn largely from English landscape paintings, was not a space Keats had much experience with. It was, indeed, largely a national fiction, which grew in importance as more and more people left Britain for the colonies.[29] Alongside Keats's claim that he had adopted a new self should be set his admission that London has itself become foreign. "I walk'd about the Streets," he writes, "as in a strange land" (*Letters* 2: 187). In March 1820, in one of many letters obsessed with the dangers of English weather, Keats remarks to Fanny Brawne, "What a horrid climate this is" (2: 278).

The Death of a "Young English Poet"

George H. Ford's remark that "if a Keats had not existed, the Victorians would have had to invent one" (180) is valid for several reasons, not least for epidemiological ones. His death in Rome in 1821, not from poetry but from consumption,[30] exerted a powerful hold on the imaginations of Victorians and occupies a central place in the history of nineteenth-century European representations of disease. Keats was not, of course, the first poet to die young. It was Chatterton and Burns that Wordsworth recalled in "Resolution and Independence" when he declared, "We Poets in our youth begin in gladness; / But thereof comes in the end despondency and madness" (*William Wordsworth* 48–49).[31] The replacement of these earlier poets by Keats (and sometimes by Shelley) suggests a corresponding shift of concern. By the 1820s Keats was a cultural myth, linking Western Romantic genius with poetry, passion, and consumption.

Given the epidemic rise of tuberculosis in industrialized nations during the nineteenth century (one of every four deaths in the United States in the 1830s, for instance, was caused by it), one would expect a large number of creative people to be affected, among them Percy Shelley, Emily Brontë, Frederic Chopin, Friedrich von Schiller, John Addington Symonds, and Robert Louis Stevenson.[32] Unique to nineteenth-century middle-class representations of the disease is its aestheticizing as a "romantic" sickness, a disease that both attacked and produced refined spirits. "There is a dread disease," writes Dickens in *Nicholas Nickleby*, "which so prepares its victim, as it were, for death; which so refines it of its grosser aspect, and throws around familiar looks, unearthly indications of the coming change; a dread disease, in which the struggle between soul and body is so gradual, quiet, and solemn, and the result so sure, that day by day, and grain by grain, the mortal part wastes and withers away, so that the spirit grows light and sanguine with its lightening load, and, feeling immortality at hand, deems it but a new term of mortal life; a disease in which death and life are so strangely blended, that death takes the glow and hue of life, and life the gaunt and grisly form of death" (637). Dickens describes a disease that spiritualizes the self, as the fever burns away the body to expose the spirit within. Consumptives occupied a threshold state between life and death and were often said to pass out of this world with such ease that neither the victim nor those looking on could discern when the boundary had been crossed.

For a modern reader, such representations may seem perverse. Sheila Rothman notes that "the death was anything but beautiful" (17). For most it was a painful and exhausting way to die, a gradual suffocation in which the mind usually retained full consciousness until the end. For René and Jean Dubos, "the romanticized portrait" of Keats's life and death, "of the fragile poet who fell victim to tuberculosis because his sensitive nature had been unable to withstand contact with a crude world," embodied everything that was wrong about the Romantic culture of tuberculosis (11). Susan Sontag draws a similar conclusion, asserting that "it is still difficult to imagine how the reality of such a dreadful disease could be transformed so preposterously"

(*Illness as Metaphor* 35). The aestheticizing of tuberculosis as a spirit-making disease was indeed a cultural construction whose place within the larger geographical understanding of diseases needs to be addressed. Yet one should not ignore its importance in giving meaning to an epidemic whose causes Europeans did not yet understand and that appeared (at least to them) to have singled out their young people for an early death. "Fully one half the deaths from consumption occur between the twentieth and fortieth years," remarks Clark. "Mortality is about its maximum at thirty" (*Treatise on Pulmonary Consumption* 137).[33] Consumption was "the great white plague," a disease of the temperate regions of the globe, particularly of the urban centers of Europe and North America. It is within this geographical context, in which Western peoples seemed to be set apart from others by their susceptibility to consumption, that the tragedy of Keats achieved such cultural importance, for it seemed to lie at the heart of what nineteenth-century Europeans saw as their biomedical identity. De Quincey went further, arguing that consumption was almost a defining national disease, "almost peculiar . . . to Britain, interlinked with the local accidents of the climate and its restless changes" (*Collected Writings* 3: 424). Keats's legacy was as much cultural and epidemiological as it was poetic. In framing the "death of Keats," Western middle-class disease experience was idealized and differentiated from its tropical and lower-class alternatives. It was also a gendered myth, adopted especially often by Victorian women, who saw in the poet's tragedy an image of their own epidemiological fortunes.

Yet such a role was not automatic. Before Keats could serve as an idealized cultural icon of the European consumptive, the social understanding of his illness had to be revised. In light of the conservative public perception of Keats as a "cockney" poet, his death might just as easily have served as a cautionary tale about the link between consumption, poverty, and sexual excess—the world of Cheapside and the East rather than of Hampstead or Rome. Consumption among the lower classes was hardly idealized, for it was associated with overcrowded housing, poor diet, unsatisfactory working conditions, and as Richard Cotton remarks, "the unnatural or unrestrained indulgence of the sensual passions" (70).[34] It is this dimension that the *Literary Gazette* emphasized when it portrayed Keats as "a radically presumptuous profligate," "a foolish young man, who, after writing some volumes of very weak, and, in the greater part, of very indecent poetry, died some time since of a consumption: the breaking down of an infirm constitution having, in all probability, been accelerated by the discarding his neckcloth, a practice of the cockney poets, who look upon it as essential to genius, inasmuch as neither

Michael Angelo, Raphael nor Tasso are supposed to have worn those anti-spiritual incumbrances" (Review of *Adonais* 772). Such animosity is rare in the 1820s, yet it suggests that the death of Keats need not have been understood in such idealized terms. Coleridge's encounter with Keats at Highgate illustrates how easily class shaped the framing of consumption. "A loose, not well dressed youth, met Mr Green and me in Manfield Lane—Green knew him and spoke. It was Keats—he was introduced to me, and stayed a minute or so—after he had gone a little, he came back, and said, 'Let me carry away the memory, Coleridge, of having pressed your hand.' There is death in *his* hand said I to Green when he was gone. Yet this was before the consumption showed itself" (*Table Talk* 1: 325). Much of the mythic power of this disease encounter derives from Coleridge's belief that he had palpably felt the disease in Keats's hand long before it was medically visible. What could be seen, however, and what must have contributed in no small degree to this diagnosis, was that Keats was "loose, not well dressed."[35]

Keats also believed that consumption was fundamentally linked to sexual activity and desire ("the pest / Of love" [*Endymion* 2.365–66]), for these anxieties are crystallized in "La Belle Dame sans Merci." "What can ail thee?" the narrator asks a sick knight at arms, whose wasted body and pallid face flushed with fever reveal that he is suffering from consumption:

> I see a lily on thy brow
>   With anguish moist and fever dew,
> And on thy cheeks a fading rose
>   Fast withereth too.   (9–12)

The knight's tale, as recent critics have noted, raises as many questions as it answers.[36] He recounts how he met a strange woman in the meads, that they fed on "roots of relish sweet, / And honey wild, and manna dew," and eventually went to her "elfin grot" (25–29). After a passionate encounter, he fell asleep and experienced a terrible nightmare in which he saw a long procession of victims, all pale like him:

> I saw pale kings, and princes too,
>   Pale warriors, death pale were they all;
> They cried—"La belle dame sans merci
>   Hath thee in thrall!"
>
> I saw their starv'd lips in the gloam
>   With horrid warning gaped wide . . .
>   (37–42)

"Starv'd lips" speak of a hunger that is both sexual and social, a striking contrast to previous images in the narrative. These "gaping" mouths hardly idealize consumption. In a dark reworking of Adam's dream, the knight awakes to find it true—that he is alone and sick ("palely loitering") on "the cold hill's side." With an ambiguity suggestive of the knight's belated attempt to understand a disease whose cause eluded early nineteenth-century medicine, it is ambiguous whether it is the "lady" or the "dream" that has the speaker in thrall. The poem is also about poetic creation, about the relation between the poet and the verbal spaces he sought to inhabit. For a poet who "look[ed] on fine Phrases like a Lover" (*Letters* 2: 139), poetic composition and sexual pleasure were not easily separated, so the transition from the exotic setting that allowed him to feed on "honey wild, and manna dew" to the barren northern landscape in which "no birds sing" (alluding to Goldsmith's America and to degeneration) is as much about postpoetic as postcoital depression.[37] Both poetic creation and excessive passion, it seems, summon up the thralling figure and landscape of consumption.[38] The word "thrall" would be taken up again by Keats in a late poem "I cry your mercy," where the title's reworking of "La Belle Dame sans Merci" should remind us that much of the anguish of these poems resides in the fact that both love and poetry are the cause and effect of disease.[39]

Shelley's *Adonais* represents an extraordinary reworking of the cultural meaning of the death of Keats because it shifted the understanding of his illness away from the themes of urban poverty and sexual passion toward a largely symbolic understanding of the relation between poetic genius and society. The poem was instrumental in popularizing the view that his illness did not derive from his own behavior and class affiliations but was brought on by his ill treatment at the hands of the Tory reviewers.[40] An important aspect of this strategy, Susan Wolfson persuasively argues, was that it feminized Keats. Shelley's preface speaks of the "genius" of Keats as "not less delicate and fragile than it was beautiful. . . . [W]hat wonder if its young flower was blighted in the bud? The savage criticism on his *Endymion,* which appeared in the *Quarterly Review,* produced the most violent effect on his susceptible mind; the agitation thus originated ended in the rupture of a blood-vessel in the lungs; a rapid consumption ensued, and the succeeding acknowledgments from more candid critics, of the true greatness of his powers, were ineffectual to heal the wound thus wantonly inflicted" ("Adonais," *Shelley's Poetry and Prose* 390–91). In the poem Keats is portrayed as a "broken lily," a "pale flower by some sad maiden cherished," the "extreme hope, the loveliest and the last, / The bloom, whose petals nipt before they blew" (48–54).

Susan Wolfson has examined in depth the cultural ramifications of Shelley's gendering of Keats as female ("Feminizing Keats"). On one hand, it produced more satire on his effeminacy. *Blackwood's,* for instance, in a mock apology, notes that if "we suspected that young author, of being so delicately nerved, we should have administered our reproof in a much more lenient shape and style" (Review of *Prometheus Unbound* 686). Byron's initial response, in a letter to Murray, was that "he who would die of an article in a review—would probably have died of something else equally trivial" (*Byron's Letters and Journals* 8: 163). More famous was his comment in *Don Juan:* " 'Tis strange the mind, that very fiery particle, / Should let itself be snuffed out by an Article" (*Byron* 11, st. 60). This feminization, however, made Keats a favorite of nineteenth-century middle-class women readers. In journals such as the *Ladies' Companion* and the *Victorian Magazine* and in the biographies and criticism of women such as F. M. Owen, Mrs. Oliphant, Amy Lowell, and Dorothy Hewlett, the tragic death of the delicate, fragile, and beautiful Keats at the hands of a violent set of reviewers was memorialized: "In poetry his was the woman's part" (Oliphant 3: 138).

A key factor in the feminization of Keats as "Adonais" was that during this period pulmonary consumption was itself a gendered disease: women suffered more often from the disease by a ratio of sixty to forty.[41] Physicians attributed this difference to several factors: women's more delicate frames and the impact of passions or sorrows on their constitutions; domestic or sedentary occupations; the use of corsets; the lack of appropriate physical exercise and fresh air; and weakened physical resistance to the disease because of pregnancy and menstruation. By feminizing Keats, Shelley was in many senses confirming this biomedical link and thus providing a general model of the relation between consumption, poetry, and femaleness. Through *Adonais,* the "death of Keats" was raised to the status of a gendered cultural myth, whose decided impact on nineteenth-century women arose partly because it explained in idealized terms their predisposition toward consumption. For nineteenth-century women, who had to make sense of the fact that they were significantly more susceptible to this disease than men, aestheticizing consumption helped them to deal with an epidemic.

Shelley describes the poet's words in "A Defence of Poetry" as being "instinct with spirit; each is as a spark, a burning atom of inextinguishable thought" (*Shelley's Poetry and Prose* 500). In an even more famous phrasing, he describes the mind of the poet in creation as "a fading coal which some invisible influence, like an inconstant wind, awakens to transitory brightness: this power arises from within, like the colour of a flower which fades and changes as it is developed" (504). A potent aspect of Shelley's mythologizing of Keats's death, which was taken up by others, is his adaptation of the notion of the burning coal that produces poetry to the etiology of a disease; he portrays consumption as the literal burning up of the poet's body, not by fever, but by the "power within." By the end of the poem he can thus argue that we need not weep for Keats because

> the pure spirit shall flow
> Back to the burning fountain whence it came,
> A portion of the Eternal, which must glow
> Through time and change, unquenchably the same,
> Whilst thy cold embers choke the sordid hearth of shame.
>
> (338–42)

Faced with an enigmatic disease ("Shall that alone which knows / Be as a sword consumed before the sheath / By sightless lightning?" [177–79]), Shelley represents Keats's consumption as a physiological expression of the poetics of creation, in which the dross of the body is burned away by the spiritualizing genius of the poet, the "burning fountain." This association leaves Shelley free to apply consumption not to Keats, but to those who are not poets:

> *We* decay
> Like corpses in a charnel; fear and grief
> Convulse us and consume us day by day.
>
> (348–50)

It is the public that suffers the "day by day," decline, whereas the poet becomes a "portion of the loveliness / Which once he made more lovely" (379–80). Keats was consumed not by disease, but instead by a poetic fire burning within, one that cannot be "extinguished" (389).

Adonais is an extraordinary mythologizing of disease, one that aestheticizes and spiritualizes it. By its conclusion Shelley, who felt that he too was consumptive, can identify fully with the disease, as he takes the poet's "consuming" "fire" and "breath" into himself, making it the source of his own poetic voice:

> The *fire* for which all thirst; *now beams on me,*
> *Consuming* the last clouds of cold mortality.
>
> The *breath* whose might I have invoked in song
> Descends on me; my spirit's bark is driven,
> Far from the shore, far from the trembling throng

> Whose sails were never to the tempest given;
> The massy earth and sphered skies are riven!
> (485–91, emphasis added)

Since consumptives normally died by suffocation, Shelley's invoking the breath of Keats suggests a fundamental revision of its meaning, one that links breath itself to the burning spirit of the poet. The contagion of the disease is now desired:

> I am borne darkly, fearfully, afar:
> Whilst burning through the inmost veil of Heaven,
> The soul of Adonais, like a star,
> Beacons from the abode where the Eternal are.
> (492–95)

Adonais played a major role in shaping how Victorians understood the relation between gender, poetry, and consumption. One might cite, for instance, James Russell Lowell's comparison of Keats and Wordsworth in his edition of Keats's poems, where he observes:

Poesy was [Wordsworth's] employment; it was Keats's very existence, and he felt the rough treatment of his verses as if it had been the wounding of a limb. To Wordsworth, composing was a healthy exercise; his slow pulse and unimpressible nature gave him assurance of a life so long that he could wait. . . . But every one of Keats's poems was a sacrifice of vitality; a virtue went away from him into every one of them; even yet, as we turn the leaves, they seem to warm and thrill our fingers with the flush of his fine senses, and the flutter of his electrical nerves, and we do not wonder he felt that what he did was to be done swiftly. (xxii)

Where for Wordsworth poetic composition was "healthy exercise," Keats's poetry was a "sacrifice of vitality," the heat of the senses, the "flush" of fever, and the "flutter" of a feminine sensibility still apparently capable of being felt by the fingers that turn the pages of his poetry. What a contrast to Coleridge's account of the diseased touch of Keats. Others found it necessary to reassert the masculinity of Keats's genius by distinguishing between the poet's "masculine" mind and his feminine body. George Gilfillan, for instance, argues that Keats's "great defect lay in the want, not of man-like soul or spirit, but of a man-like constitution. His genius lay in his body like sun-fire in a dewdrop, at once beautifying and burning it up" (1: 183).

One could explore further the way men and women during the nineteenth century used the death of Keats to frame an understanding of the relation between poetry, gender, and tuberculosis. I conclude this chapter by suggesting another way the public reception of Keats's poetry cannot be separated from the complex uses Europeans made of disease in differentiating themselves from colonial others. *Adonais* is a poem that relocates the Orient in the West. Not only does Shelley retain the traditional machinery of the pastoral elegy, but the poet's name derives from a combination of "Adonis" and the Hebrew name for God, "Adonai."[42] The movement from "Adonais" to "Keats" follows a westering course, yet it continues in a subtle manner to produce an extraordinary balance of East and West, as Keats is the genius of both Venus and Hesperus, the morning and evening stars. Through "consumption" he is portrayed as the most European of poets, yet equally important, his genius remains linked to its Eastern epiphanic sources.

Throughout the nineteenth century, consumption was consistently portrayed in the language memorialized by *Adonais* as a consuming fire that refined the body. In this regard one of the more remarkable negotiations of the complex geographical instabilities governing the contemporary representation of Keats is given in the personal recollections of Barry Cornwall. He follows what was fast becoming a convention in describing consumptives by observing the close connection between genius and consumption in the physiognomy of the poet: "There was a lustre in his look which gave you the idea of a mind of exquisite refinement, and high imagination; yet, to an observing eye, the seeds of early death were sown there; it was impossible to look at him, and think him long-lived" (392). Cornwall seeks to masculinize the poet by stressing that he did not have a feminine body type; instead, there was "a look of strength and durability about his chest and shoulders, which might have deceived a casual looker-on." The observer, however, "who could perceive the inner-workings, who could estimate the wear and wasting which an ardent, ambitious, and restless intellect makes in the 'human form divine,' must have felt persuaded that the flame burning within would shortly consume the outward shell."[43] Consumption is here portrayed almost as an expression of a masculine strength of intellect. Looking for an appropriate metaphor, Cornwall first suggests that Keats's "spirit was like burning oil in a vessel of some precious and costly wood, which when the flame has consumed its nutriment, will then burn that which contained it." Not fully satisfied, however, he recalls the Indian custom of *sati* or "widow burning": "Unlike the pyre that consumes the devoted widow of the Hindoo husband, where we may see the fire but not the victim, in him we saw the fire and the victim too. *He,* however, was a self-devoted martyr to intellect, and not to a senseless and brutal custom; and if literature had its army of martyrs, as Religion gloriously has, his name would not be forgotten in its calends"

(392). In a complicated negotiation of both culture and gender, Cornwall portrays Keats as a uniquely hybrid figure, whose disease constitutes a Western equivalent of *sati:* the poet's diseased body is the widow that is consumed by the fire within him.[44] The absent husband is, of course, most obviously the "Keats of literature," the idea of literary fame to whose service his body and these flames were devoted. Keats's poetry is thus seen as an ongoing performance of *sati,* the self being burned up in the very act of composition. Having established this relation, Cornwall is intent on differentiating Keats's sacrifice to poetry from the barbaric customs of the East. He expresses the European disgust for the "senseless and brutal custom" that authorizes the Eastern sacrifice of widows and suggests that Keats's self-sacrifice is the literary equivalent of religious martyrdom. Nevertheless, Cornwall's analogy just as easily suggests the cultural and gender ambiguities raised by Keats's poetry, the way the archetype of the English Romantic consumptive poet was built on a complex and unstable negotiation of a range of ideas about the geography and gender of disease.

FIVE

Joseph Ritchie and
"The Diseased Heart of Africa"

In a recent collection of essays, Gerald W. Hartwig and K. David Patterson stress the important role disease has played in African history even as they note that

historians of Africa have generally neglected the study of past health conditions—as well as the role of disease, health care, and medicine in history—despite the obvious importance of the disease burden on the African continent. Major epidemics, which have often accompanied ecological change, migration, or foreign contacts, have tested institutions and decimated populations. A host of endemic afflictions have restricted settlement of large areas, sapped the strength and shortened the lives of Africans, and limited their productivity. For centuries, the continent's disease environment contributed to its relative isolation from non-African civilizations. (3)

In recent years this subject has received more attention.[1] Studies of colonial Africa suggest that this burden was not lessened by European expansion into Africa but instead grew as a concomitant change in social structures, land-use practices, and diet added an array of new diseases to an already lengthy list. During the Romantic period, especially in the literature opposing the slave trade, the interior of Africa, largely unknown to Europeans, was often portrayed as a tropical idyll, violently ripped apart by the tribal trade in slaves. More often, however, Africa was seen as the worst of the world's pathogenic spaces, a plague-ridden climate that prevented its people from rising above nature and developing a culture equivalent to that of Europe. Since comparisons of the relative merits of places were implicitly comparisons of the merits of people and their social institutions, Europeans frequently saw in the "poor diseased heart of Africa" a sign of the backwardness or laziness of black people and their inability to control their disease environments. Later in the century, remarks Jean Comaroff, "savage natives were the very embodiment of dirt and disorder, their moral affliction all of a piece with their physical degradation and their 'pestiferous' surroundings" ("Diseased Heart of Africa" 306).[2] The sickness of Africa expressed the sickness of its people.

European ideas about the dangerous character of the African tropical environment, however, were not simply reflections of ethnocentrism, as they have often been understood; they also articulated in emphatic terms what had been the disease experience of Europeans on this continent for centuries. As an article in the second edition of the *Encyclopaedia Britannica* (1778) suggests, knowledge of Africa was structured by paradox. "Though the greatest part of this continent hath been in all ages unknown both to the Europeans and Asiatics, its situation is more favorable than either Europe or Asia for maintaining an intercourse with other nations." "In the centre of the three quarters of the globe," it nevertheless remained largely unknown to Europeans until the late eighteenth century. Henry Beaufoy, secretary of the African Association, observes that "the map of its interior is still but a wide extended blank, on which the geographer . . . has traced, with a hesitating hand, a few names of unexplored rivers and of uncertain nations" (Hallett, *Records* 44). The reviewer of Hugh Murray's *Historical Account of Discoveries and Travels in Africa* (1817) notes: "So imperfect, indeed, is our knowledge of this vast continent, that in what are deemed to be best charts, full two-thirds of it appear a blank; or, what is still worse, chains of mountains and trackless deserts, rivers, lakes and seas, are laid down *ad libitum;* their course and direction being determined by no other scale or dimensions than the mere whim of the mapmaker, and many of them having, in probability, no existence but on paper" (299). Read against the backdrop of European exploration and surveying, the absence of marks on the map of Africa, its "blank darkness," to cite the title of C. L. Miller's book, made Africa ideal for the projection of European racial fantasies about the relation between disease and darkness. Megan Vaughan declares: "In the post-Enlightenment European mind Africa, it seems, has been created as a unique space, as a repository of death, disease, and degeneration, inscribed through a set of recurring and simple dualisms—black and white, good and evil, light and dark" (2). As public health officials increasingly saw "ignorance" and "backwardness" as the breeding places of disease, these were also added to the list.

At the same time, these huge blank spaces in the European mapping of Africa spoke of innumerable tragedies. Since the existence of a map is a sign of the successful exploration of a region, the mark of failure is blankness. Swift notes:

> So geographers, in Afric maps,
> With savage pictures fill the gaps,
> And o'er uninhabitable downs
> Place elephants for want of towns.
> ("On Poetry," *Poetical Works* 2.177–80)

One cannot miss the way elephants (probably "Indian" elephants) quite literally stand for European ignorance of African geography, yet just as important, Swift's portrayal of the interior as "uninhabitable" voices a history of failed colonial efforts. He replaces the earlier geographers' elephants with "uninhabitable downs," but this new space is no longer a blank freely available to any inscription; its very silence speaks of its deadly pathogenic nature.[3] What Swift should have said was not that these spaces were "uninhabitable" for all human beings, but that they were so for foreigners. Europeans' accounts of Africa as a space of disease not only reflected their attitudes toward blacks but also their own experience in the region. For three centuries, attempts to explore and colonize tropical Africa had met with repeated failures as Europeans were decimated by malaria, yellow fever, and amoebic dysentery, to name only a few of the major diseases endemic to the region.

By the Romantic period, the West Coast of Africa, where British commercial interests were centered, was being referred to as "the white man's grave." This view was not an exaggeration. Among the subjects included in a Handbook of Useful Information for prospective settlers in the region is a section titled "How to Reach West Africa and How to Return." The second part of the handbook is typical of the kind of colonial humor normally reserved for Africa, since it begins: "If dead, this will not be needed" (qtd. in Scott 1: 69). Mary Kingsley, in *Travels in West Africa* (1897), provides a sober summary of the risks:

Remember, before you elect to cast your lot in with the West Coasters, that 85 per cent. of them die of fever or return home with their health permanently wrecked. Also remember that there is no getting acclimatised to the Coast. There are, it is true, a few men out there who, although they have been resident in West Africa for years, have never had fever, but you can count them up on the fingers of one hand. There is another class who have been out for twelve months at a time, and have not had a touch of fever; these you want the fingers of your two hands to count, but no more. By far the largest class is the third, which is made up of those who have a slight dose of fever once a fortnight, and some day, apparently for no extra reason, get a heavy dose and die of it. A very considerable class is the fourth—those who die within a fortnight to a month of going ashore. (690)[4]

With her characteristic unwillingness to pull punches, Kingsley notes that "other parts of the world have more sensational outbreaks of death from epidemics of yellow fever and cholera, but there is no other region in the world that can match West Africa for the steady kill, kill, kill that its malaria works on the white men who come under its influence" (681).

Throughout most of the eighteenth century, British commercial enterprise in West Africa was primarily restricted to the slave trade. The end of the century, however, saw an increase in colonialism, linked ironically to the rising movement against the slave trade. In 1787, under the direction of Granville Sharp, Granville Town was established in Sierra Leone. Composed of 456 settlers—poor blacks from England and a motley mixture of white settlers, some of them prostitutes who had been inveigled into joining them—the settlement struggled on for two years. However, poor planning, poor soil, but most of all epidemic disease led to the failure of the settlement, as 46 percent of the Europeans and 39 percent of the blacks died in the first year, leaving fewer than 130 by the summer of 1788.[5] Then in December 1789 the settlement was burned to the ground by a local chief. Maria Falconbridge describes the outcast state of some of the remaining women, whom she met in 1791:

I never did, and God grant I never may again witness so much misery as I was forced to be a spectator of here: Among the outcasts were seven of our country women, decrepid with disease, and so disguised with filth and dirt, that I should never have supposed they were born white; add to this, almost naked from head to foot; in short, their appearance was such as I think would extort compassion from the most callous heart; but I declare they seemed insensible to shame, or the wretchedness of their situation themselves; I begged they would get washed, and gave them what cloaths I could conveniently spare. (64)

In January 1792, 1,200 free blacks set sail from Nova Scotia and joined 119 white Europeans to establish a new settlement, Freetown. Maria Falconbridge, who was among this latter group, speaks of the tremendous natural beauty of the region: "Those mountains appear to rise gradually from the sea to a stupendous height, richly wooded and beautifully ornamented by the hand of nature, with a variety of delightful prospects" (18–19). She admits that she would be quite willing to spend many years in Africa if she could be guaranteed "a little agreeable society, a few comforts, and could ensure the same good health I have hitherto enjoyed." Yet this optimism is continually tempered by the awareness of the risk, caused by an "unhealthy putrid vapour that almost constantly hovers about these mountains; the poisonous effects of which carries off numbers of foreigners" (73). Her fears were justified. In the first year of the new settlement, at least 17 percent of the Nova Scotia blacks died of fever. European losses were even greater, totaling 49 percent. Falconbridge describes Freetown at the height of the epidemic in July 1792:

There is about twelve hundred souls, including all ranks of people, in the Colony, seven hundred, or upwards, of whom, are at this moment suffering under the affliction of burning fevers, I suppose two hundred scarce able to crawl about, and am certain not more, if so many, able to nurse the sick or attend to domestic and Colonial concerns; five, six, and seven are dying daily, and buried with as little ceremony as so many dogs or cats.

It is quite customary of a morning to ask "how many died last night?" Death is viewed with the same indifference as if people were only taking a short journey, to return in a few days; those who are well, hourly expect to be laid up, and the sick look momentarily for the surly Tyrant to finish their afflictions, nay seem not to care for life! (148)

As the wife of the agent responsible for the new settlement, Falconbridge insists that the high rates of disease and death are not primarily caused by the "baseness" of the climate of Sierra Leone. Instead, she argues that lack of adequate medical assistance, inadequate preparation for the rainy season, and unsanitary living conditions are the main reasons.[6] Walking amid "so much sickness and so many deaths," she wonders "what kind of stuff I am made of," for she feels "much better than when in England" (149). Less than a month later, however, Falconbridge almost died: "Confined three weeks with a violent fever, stoneblind four days, and expecting every moment to be my last; indeed I most miraculously escaped the jaws of death." She credits her recovery to the arrival of "a Physician" (Thomas Winterbottom). Her narrative provides a unique perspective on how a middle-class woman responded to colonial disease. Pathetic or absurd, depending on one's point of view, her primary regret is that she lost her hair: "I am yet a poor object, and being under the necessity of having my head shaved, tends to increase my ghastly figure. You will readily guess it was very humbling and provoking for me to lose my fine head of hair, which I always took so much pride in, but I cannot help it, and thank God my life is preserved" (154–55).

At the same time as plans for colonizing Sierra Leone were under way, the Association for Promoting the Discovery of the Interior Parts of Africa, formed on 9 June 1788 and headed by Joseph Banks, was committed to exploring the Niger River, which promised European access to the western interior. After several failed attempts by Simon Lucas, John Ledyard, and Daniel Houghton, the African Association finally achieved a notable success with Mungo Park's 1795–97 expedition. With the publication of his *Travels* (1799), the African Association was euphoric. Banks's address at its 1799 General Meeting indicates the close relation between geography and British imperial ambitions in the region:

We have already by Mr. Park's means opened a Gate into the Interior of Africa, into which it is easy for every Nation to enter and to extend its commerce and Discovery from the West to the Eastern side of that Immense continent. The passage by Land, from the Navigable waters of the Gambia to those of the Joliba is not more than — days march. A Detachment of 500 chosen Troops would soon make that Road easy, and would build Embarkations upon the Joliba—if 200 of these were to embark with Field pieces they would be able to overcome the whole Forces which Africa could bring against them. (Hallett, *Records* 168)

In 1798, on the recommendation of J. F. Blumenbach, another expedition was undertaken by Frederick Hornemann, which ended with his death from dysentery. Another was sponsored in 1805, but Henry Nicholls died of fever in Calabar, on the Guinea coast, at its outset. At this point, the African Society turned to Park for another expedition. Reservations were expressed about the obvious risks, but Banks responded, "I am aware that Mr Park's expedition is one of the most hazardous a man can undertake; but I cannot agree with those who think it too hazardous to be attempted: it is by similar hazards of human life alone that we can hope to penetrate the obscurity of the internal face of Africa" (qtd. in Gascoigne 19). In 1805, just as the rainy season was beginning, Park set out again from the coast of Guinea with forty-four men to seek the mouth of the river. His last letter, written to Lord Camden, speaks of a tragic loss of men through fever on the march from the Gambia to the Niger:

Your Lordship will recollect that I always spoke of the rainy season with horror, as being extremely fatal to Europeans; and our journey from the Gambia to the Niger will furnish a melancholy proof of it.

We had no contest whatever with the natives, nor was any one of us killed by wild animals or any other accidents; and yet I am sorry to say that of forty-four Europeans who left the Gambia in perfect health, five only are at present alive, viz. three soldiers (one deranged in his mind), Lieutenant Martyn and myself. (2: 80)

After losing another man a few days later, Park disappeared in a desperate effort to reach the mouth of the river. In 1809 another expedition was attempted, this time by the Swiss Johann Ludwig Burckhardt, but he too died of dysentery before leaving Cairo for the Fezzan. It was not until 1815 that two other expeditions were undertaken. Both of these, however, achieved very little in the way of new geographical knowledge, though they did succeed in losing more Europeans through disease. By 1817 the Colonial Office had concluded that any expeditions that attempted to reach the Niger via the coast of Guinea were doomed to failure. The alternative northern route, proceeding along the old Garamatian way, across the Sahara from north to south, from Tripoli, through Murzuk (the capital of the Fezzan), to Bornu on Lake Chad, seemed more likely to be successful. W. H. Smyth, a young naval officer, assessed the prospects in a letter to his admiral, Sir Charles Penrose:

I am becoming still more convinced that here—through this place, and by means of these people—is an open gate into the interior of Africa. By striking due south of Tripoli, a traveller will reach Bornu before he is out of [the Bashaw of Tripoli] Yusuf's influence; and wherever his power reaches, the protecting virtues of the British flag are well known. In fact, looking to the unavoidable causes of death along the malarious banks of the rivers on the western coast, I think this ought to be the chosen route, because practicable into the very heart of the most benighted quarter of the globe. (487)

All that was needed now was someone to lead the expedition.

Joseph Ritchie's Travels

"Have you seen Lalla Rookh? I never met with anything that carried me so completely away into the midst of Roses and Bulbuls and Perfumes and Hummingbirds and Jewels and all manner of Precious Stones. How rich English Poetry is by the additions it has received ever since we last talked about it" (qtd. in Garnett). The author of this letter, written in 1818, is not Keats, though he sounds a good deal like him, but instead is Joseph Ritchie, a young English surgeon, naturalist, and occasional poet.[7] Born in 1788, Ritchie received his surgeon's certificate in 1811 and accepted a position at the Lock Hospital, London, in 1813. In a letter written to his Yorkshire countryman Richard Garnett, Ritchie provides a lengthy critical commentary on contemporary poetry: on the third canto of Byron's Childe Harold as his best; on Coleridge's "Christabel"; and especially on the poetry of Wordsworth. "I have read a good deal of Wordsworth lately and have become completely a convert to the heretical doctrines promulgated by him and his school. I think I have met with finer poetry in his two vols. of Minor Poems than anything I have read except the best passages of Milton and Akenside."

At this point he turns to Keats. "If you have not seen the Poems of Keats, a lad of nineteen or twenty, they are well worth your reading," he writes. "If I am not mistaken he is to be the great poetical Luminary of the Age to come."

At the conclusion of the Napoleonic Wars Ritchie visited Paris, where he took courses in natural history, astronomy, and chemistry and came to the notice of Alexander Von Humboldt. The latter must have been impressed with the young man's knowledge of science and natural history, for when the opportunity presented itself he recommended Ritchie to Joseph Banks (and through him to the Colonial Office) as the ideal person to lead the expedition then being planned to explore the Niger River and to discover Timbuktu, while "collecting and preparing objects of natural history" (Lyon 1).[8] Ritchie's education and career thus exemplify the fusion of natural history and exploration that shaped European colonial expansion during the eighteenth and nineteenth centuries.[9] An article in *Blackwood's* in January 1818, for instance, extols the benefits of linking voyages of discovery with scientific expeditions: "Voyages of discovery, and expeditions by land, have been lately undertaken at the command of the King, and in all these enterprizes, the examining and collecting of natural productions has been considered as a principal object" ("Notices in Natural History" 380). In tropical regions, medical training was of additional importance, for not only were physicians trained in botany, but in regions where epidemics could quickly decimate an expedition, a knowledge of medicine was often a key to success.

Ritchie met Keats at the famous party held by Benjamin Haydon in December 1817, which also included Wordsworth, Lamb, Thomas Monkhouse, John Landseer, and the redoubtable comptroller of the Stamp Office, John Kingston. His brief entrance into literary history, largely forgotten by literary critics, provides a useful insight into how African exploration was perceived during the Romantic period. When Ritchie was introduced as "a gentleman going to Africa," Charles Lamb is said to have shouted, "And pray, who is the Gentleman we are going *to lose?*" (Haydon, *Diary* 2: 174). It is typical of Lamb's humor that it simultaneously disarms anxiety and draws attention to it. Given the history of African exploration and colonization, it was an incredibly insensitive remark, especially from an employee of the East India Company. Yet it makes explicit what everyone in the room must have known—that Ritchie's chances of surviving this expedition were minimal. As Haydon notes in his diary, the comment alluded "to the dangers of penetrating into the interior of Africa." He adds that the remark produced "a roar of laughter, the *victim* Ritchie joining with us" (2: 174). In his *Autobiography,* Haydon adds a further irony: "We then drank the victim's *health,* in which

Ritchie joined" (2: 269). Nineteenth-century colonialism, especially in Africa, produced its own special brand of gallows humor, a style whose most eminent practitioner was Ryder Haggard.

Haydon does not indicate what Keats thought of Lamb's joke. A year later Keats was considering whether he too might have better opportunities as a surgeon on an East Indiaman. During the party, however, Keats did make a significant gesture: perhaps recalling the Ptolemaic idea that the Nile had its source in the Mountains of the Moon, he asked Ritchie to take a copy of *Endymion* with him on the expedition and fling it into the Sahara Desert (Haydon, *Autobiography* 2: 271).[10] Ritchie appears to have joined in the revelry, perhaps from embarrassment. In the poem "A Farewell to England," published in 1820, he suggests that silence was indeed an accepted way of dealing with such anxieties. Adopting the valedictory tone that Keats used in "To Autumn," Ritchie makes sense of the danger he faces by putting his life at the service of a nationalist ideal. After evoking the "chalky cliffs" of Dover, he speaks of the "beauty" of England's "daughters," the valor of its "haughty chivalry," its wisdom, and its poets, "who fill the spacious earth with their and thy renown" (1–18). Britain's imperial destiny functions as a consolatory myth. May peace continue at home, "When I am gone," Ritchie writes, and may England

> be a mark to guide the natives on,
> Like a tall watch-tow'r flashing o'er the deep.
> Long may'st thou bid the sorrowers cease to weep,
> And dart the beams of truth athwart the night
> That wraps a slumbering world—till from their sleep
> Starting—remotest nations see the light,
> And Earth be blest beneath the buckler of thy might.
>   (28–36)

Faced with the prospect of his own death, Ritchie sets it within the context of a global imperial destiny. Instead of appealing to nature, as in the traditional pastoral elegy, he asks England in her imperial authority to "bid the sorrowers cease to weep," making his own possible sacrifice a worthy one:

> Strong in thy strength I go—and, wheresoe'er
> My steps may wander, may I ne'er forget
> All that I owe to thee,—and O! may ne'er
> My frailties tempt me to abjure that debt.
> And what if far from thee my star must set!
> Hast thou not hearts that shall with sadness hear

The tale—and some fair cheeks that shall be wet,
And some bright eye in which the swelling tear
Shall start for him who sleeps in Afric's deserts drear?
(37—45)

"Melancholy bodings" are here presented as a kind of irreverence, as "pro-phan[ing] a charge like mine," so the poem concludes by rejecting the fears that have authorized it, thus insisting on a self-imposed silence as the appropriate etiquette for responding to this anxiety. If there are to be tears, they will be cast by the "fair" sex of England.

Late in 1818, in a letter written to his brother George shortly after Tom died, Keats declared that "one of the grandeurs of immortality" is that "there will be no space" (*Letters* 2: 5). After asking George, then living in Louisville, Kentucky, "Have you shot a Buffalo? Have you met with any Pheasants?" Keats adds that "my Thoughts are very frequently in a foreign Country—I live more out of England than in it—the Mountains of Tartary are a favourite lounge, if I happen to miss the Allegany ridge, or have no whim for Savoy" (2: 9). The hope that one might use the imagination to escape the limitations and isolation imposed by geography led him to recollect Ritchie and how strangely his poetry was making its way through what must have seemed to him two of the most extreme environments of the globe. "Haydon show'd me a letter he had received from Tripoli—Ritchey was well and in good Spirits, among Camels, Turbans, Palm Trees and sands—You may remember I promised to send him an Endymion which I did not—however he has one—you have one—One is in the Wilds of america—the other is on a Camel's back in the plains of Egypt" (2: 16). Ritchie writes to Haydon, "Pray tell Keats that *Endymion* has arrived thus far on his way to the Desert, and when you are sitting over your Christmas fire will be jogging (in all probability) on a Camel's back 'over those Afran Sands immeasurable'" (2: 16, n. 4).

As it turned out, Ritchie was far too optimistic: it was not until the end of March that the expedition was finally under way, by which time the party, made up of Ritchie, a shipwright named John Belford, and George F. Lyon, who eventually published *A Narrative of Travels in Northern Africa, in the Years 1818, 19, and 20* (1821), barely had enough money left for hiring camels to take them to Murzuk. Ritchie was partly to blame. Although given an initial disbursement of £2,000, he spent over £400 in Paris on scientific instruments, and another £1,000 for trading goods, so that, with incidental expenses, the expedition had only somewhere between £65 and £225 when they left Tripoli, and further funds from London would not arrive for months

(Bohen 51–53).[11] With barely enough money to survive, with inadequate goods for trade, living on dates and grain, the three men quickly came down with dysentery and malaria. As Lyon notes, "From that time it rarely happened that one or two of us were not confined to our beds" (100). Over the next six months, despite brief periods of health, Ritchie grew progressively worse and increasingly reclusive. On 8 November he suffered another relapse, and Lyon fell ill the next day; both were attended by Belford, now deaf and "an invalid" (189). On 20 November Ritchie died, quietly entering Kingsley's third epidemiological category of those Europeans "who have a slight dose of fever once a fortnight, and some day, apparently for no extra reason, get a heavy dose and die of it." Shortly thereafter funds arrived from England. When Lyon was sufficiently recovered to open Ritchie's sitting room, he found no "mementos of the scientific mind with which he certainly was gifted . . . only a few scattered papers, an unfinished journal, and some letters." These he burned, so we will never know what Ritchie thought during his months of sickness. When he opened the chests Ritchie had packed in Tripoli, which had accounted for the load of eight of the twenty-two camels on the expedition, Lyon found six hundred pounds of lead, "a camel load of corks for preserving insects on, and two loads of brown paper for preparing plants," two "large chests of Arsenic bottles" for killing insects, two chests of instruments, and five hundredweight of books—one of which must have been *Endymion* (195–96).

Rereading his diary in 1823, Haydon recollected the famous party of 1817 and added a short note: "Since writing this, poor Ritchie is dead! He died on this route. 1819. Lamb's feeling was prophetic.

Keats too is gone! How one ought to treasure such evenings, when life gives us so few off them" (2: 176n). In January 1837 Haydon once again took up his pencil, noting that "Lamb is gone too! Monkhouse, the other Friend, is gone. Wordsworth & I alone remain of the party." Perhaps as an afterthought, he added, "If the Comptroller lives I know not."

Percy Bysshe Shelley and Revolutionary Climatology

In *Queen Mab,* Shelley makes a claim for the practical benefits of vegetarianism that would have been hardly conceivable before the Romantic period. "There is no disease, bodily or mental, which adoption of vegetable diet and pure water has not infallibly mitigated," he writes, "wherever the experiment has been fairly tried" (*Poetical Works* 830). Debility becomes strength, disease is converted into health, and life expectancy is extended even as the ability to enjoy bodily pleasure is heightened: "Old age would be our last and our only malady" (830). Arresting here is the idea that for the first time perfect health might be within the grasp of human beings. In the light of human history this belief in a total conquest of disease might seem impossibly idealistic, but it is also very modern. A chorus of similar declarations have been made over the past two hundred years, if not for all then certainly for many diseases, and these constitute one of the revolutionary and enduring social claims of modern medicine. Edwin Chadwick, the famous Victorian sanitation engineer, can hardly be called an idealist, yet he too voiced the hope that "if sanitation were carried out in its completeness, disease, which was the cause of all death before the appointed time, would itself die" ("Obituary"). With the emergence of germ theory during the last quarter of the nineteenth century, optimism reappeared, especially in the field of tropical medicine. "Get rid of or avoid these disease germs," one article argued, "and we get rid of a principal obstacle to the colonization of the tropics by Europeans" ("Europeans in the Tropics" 94).[1] The 1950s and 1960s, as Laurie Garrett observes, were also years of immense medical optimism:

Nearly every week the medical establishment declared another "miracle breakthrough" in humanity's war with infectious disease. Antibiotics, first discovered in the early 1940s, were now growing in number and potency. So much so that clinicians and scientists shrugged off bacterial diseases, and in the industrialized world former scourges such as *Staphylococcus* and tuberculosis had been deftly moved from the "extremely dangerous" column to that of "easily managed minor infections." Medicine was viewed as a huge chart depicting disease incidences over time: by the twenty-first century every infectious disease on the chart would have hit zero. Few scientists or physicians of the day doubted that humanity would continue on its linear course of triumphs over the microbes. (30)

From our present vantage point, which has seen the appearance of an increasing array of new diseases or formidable new strains of old diseases, declarations like these may seem utopian. Medicine nowadays is ambiguously both more and less confident about its ability to control disease, especially as health costs rise and many nations, especially the poorer ones, become less able to afford newer treatments. Yet drug companies, not without reasonable justification, repeat their promises. Charles Rosenberg observes that most Americans continue to believe "in the laboratory and its products; they see AIDS as a time-bound artifact of that unfortunate but essentially transitional period between the discovery of this new ill and the announcement of its cure" (*Explaining Epidemics* 288). Shelley's idea of a future world in which "Health floats amid the gentle atmosphere" (*Queen Mab* 8.114) therefore should be seen as an early articulation of a profoundly modern stance toward the body and overall human health, one that has shaped the course of medicine. The cure has changed—from vegetarianism, to Beddoes's "pneumatics," to sanitation, to bacteriology, to antibiotics, to the mapping of genes—but the belief that disease can be completely controlled remains a deep, if frequently troubled, modern faith.

Shelley was not alone among his contemporaries in believing that human beings might attain perfect health. His immediate medical debts, Timothy Morton notes, were to the dietary writings of vegetarians, books such as William Lambe's *Reports of the Effects of a Peculiar Regimen on Scirrhous Tumours and Cancerous Ulcers* (1809) and *A Medical and Experimental Inquiry into the Origin, Symptoms, and Cure of Constitutional Diseases* (1805), George Cheyne's *Essay of Health and Long Life* (1724), Joseph Ritson's *Essay on Abstinence from Animal Food* (1802), and John Newton's *The Return to Nature, or A Defence of the Vegetable Regimen* (1811) (*Shelley and the Revolution in Taste* 13–56). Nora Crook and Derek Guiton have shown that Shelley was knowledgeable about contemporary medicine. In 1811 he briefly considered becoming a surgeon, duly enrolling in a course of anatomical lectures and visiting Saint Bartholomew's with his cousin Charles Grove (1). Over the next two years he read a wide range of medical texts: Hippocrates; Celsus's *De Medicina;* Darwin's *Zoönomia* (1794–96); Thomas Trotter's *View of the Nervous Temperament* (1807) and his *Essay . . . on Drunkenness* (1804); and Robert Thornton's *Medical Extracts on the Nature of Health* (1796–97).[2] His second cousin Thomas Medwin remarks: "If Shelley was at that time a believer in alchymy he was even more so in the Panacea" (*Life of Percy Bysshe Shelley* 50).

Shelley's focus, as a "physiological critic" (*Poetical Works* 833), was less on the practice of medicine than on its philosophy and politics, an approach that links him strongly with the Enlightenment, an intellectual milieu dominated by physicians. For writers such as Godwin, Condorcet, and Cabanis, the philosopher is a social physician who uses knowledge and inquiry to cure social and bodily ills.[3] Disease is less a product of nature than a *social problem*. Political reform is thus metaphorized as a movement from sickness to health, an undertaking that perfects both the social and the physical body. Godwin remarks in *Of Population* that "there is no evil under which the human species can labour, that man is not competent to cure" (615). Earlier, in the *Enquiry concerning Political Justice,* he argued that "we are sick and we die . . . because we consent to suffer these accidents" (1793 ed. 869). Reason and technology are necessarily progressive, so Godwin envisions a time when human life will see "a total extirpation of the infirmities of our nature" and an indefinite prolongation of life (1985 ed. 775). "In all instances," he declares, disease is "the concomitant of confusion" (772). Godwin is every bit a spokesman for the Enlightenment and for a mainstream position of modern public health policy in his insistence that disease and *ignorance* are fundamentally linked. In *Queen Mab,* Shelley also asserts: "It is certain that wisdom is not compatible with disease" (*Poetical Works* 808). Both writers provide a powerful crystallization of what I will call "ideopathology," the notion that the real causes of the emergence and transmission of disease are to be found not in climate or nature but in the sphere of ideas, in human ignorance. When Shelley writes in a letter of 10 September 1815 that "the human beings which surround us infect us with their opinions" (*Letters* 1: 292), he is not speaking metaphorically. Because diseases live in the dark breeding spaces produced by confusion, misunderstanding, and ignorance, truth is sanitary: the advance of knowledge, embodied in public education, technology, medicine, and social reform, not only enfranchises but cures.

The ideopathogenic link between ignorance and disease is a two-way street: wisdom is a precondition of health, but just as important, health is necessary for true knowledge. "Whenever the cause of disease shall be discovered," Shelley writes, "the root, from which all vice and misery have so long overshadowed the globe, will lie bare to the axe" (829). His promotion of the vegetarian diet seeks to make possible healthy thinking, and thus social reform; a change of diet would cleanse the mind of the antisocial and aggressive heating of the blood produced by meat, thus ensuring "a calm and considerate evenness of temper, that alone might offer a certain pledge of the future moral reformation of society" (830). Unnatural diets are the source of "all putrid humours," "all evil passions, and all vain belief" (*Queen Mab* 8.215–16). A carnivorous society cannot escape bloody thoughts. In one of Shelley's most striking formulations, a vegetarian Napoleon Bonaparte would not have had "either the inclination or the power to ascend the throne of the Bourbons" (*Poetical Works* 830). Empire, one might conclude, is essentially an eating disorder: "On a natural system of diet we should require no spices from India; no wines from Portugal, Spain, France, or Madeira; none of those multitudinous articles of luxury, for which every corner of the globe is rifled, and which are the causes of so much individual rivalship, such calamitous and sanguinary national disputes" (832). Without entering into the merits of vegetarianism, one can recognize that throughout his work Shelley refuses to separate reason from the biological and social preconditions of a healthy physical body. A social revolution that is not intrinsically guided by medicine is not a real revolution at all.

Anticipating one of the central aspects of modern medicine, Shelley insists that disease is a *social phenomenon:* "Man, and the animals whom he has infected with his society, or depraved by his dominion, are alone diseased" (827). He goes on to argue, employing an early form of comparative medicine, that "the domestic hog, the sheep, the cow, and the dog, are subject to an incredible variety of distempers; and, like the corrupters of their nature, have physicians who thrive upon their miseries" (827). Not only is Shelley here reflecting critically on the newly developing field of veterinary medicine, but he is unique in recognizing that human disease cannot be adequately understood in isolation from our relationships with domestic animals, which share and transmit many of our diseases. Although he does not use the word "ecology," which emerged in the latter half of the nineteenth century, he is nevertheless unwilling to think of disease outside the nexus of human interaction with nature. The geography of disease, which thus extends beyond human life to incorporate the entire biota affected by human beings, is not a reflection of any physical factors or limits inherent in nature but expresses the social interactions—the "dominion"—of human beings over each other and over animals. Shelley is not averse to setting contemporary disease ecologies against more traditional pastoral notions of a pristine nature that preceded the fall into the sicknesses of social life. Nevertheless his primary thrust is not toward a nostalgic recovery of a pristine state of nature, when there was no disease, but toward the development of a social theory of disease and disease ecologies that might lead to their transformation through science and reform. The struggle is preeminently a social and ideational war that aims at the sociophilosophical conquest of diseased space. All utopias must be biosocial ones, spaces of health, because health is itself a precondition of utopia.

In this chapter I explore the important ways Shelley's geographies are shaped by his medicalizing of social life. He shares with medical meteorologists and topographers the view that it is not people but places that are sick, yet whereas most saw disease as primarily a symptom of the physical environment, as climatological factors combine with specific aspects of a rural or urban landscape (marshes, forests, narrow streets, dockyards, etc.) to produce harmful poisons or miasmas, Shelley sees the physical environment itself as a social product. It is "kings, and priests, and statesmen" who produce the "venomed exhalations" that "spread / Ruin, and death, and woe" (*Queen Mab* 4.80–85). Geography is thoroughly a social construction. To "socialize the natural," to take up such seemingly "natural" aspects of the environment as "soil" and "climate" and rewrite them as expressions of social relations, is thus a central aspect of Shelley's medical thought that has not received the attention it deserves. In confronting disease, the poet believed he was confronting not a physical organism but social spaces fundamentally shaped by power and ideas. Shelley's social theory is profoundly influenced by medical geography, but rather than seeing the physical environment as a given, he understands it as a product of social relations. This is why he refuses to separate ideopathology from the analysis of power. "Power" is a "desolating pestilence" that "Pollutes whate'er it touches" (3.176–77). Literature has often employed epidemics as metaphors for social ills, but the environmental and demographic aspects of "desolating" go beyond metaphor to suggest that power *is* disease; it is the force that creates pathogenic spaces in the world. Pathology *is* the study of power. Ignorance, vice, misery, and disease are not just useful metaphors for describing its effects but are part of its being. Alluding to the upas tree of tropical Asia, Shelley argues that "commerce" is a "poison-breathing shade" beneath which "no solitary virtue dares to spring" (5.44–45). This link between power, disease, and the environment can be seen again in his description of the world that meets the eyes of the human soul:

> Ah! to the stranger-soul, when first it peeps
> From its new tenement, and looks abroad
> For happiness and sympathy, how stern
> And desolate a tract is this wide world!
> How withered all the buds of natural good!
> No shade, no shelter from the sweeping storms
> Of pitiless power.   (4.121–27)

Anticipating the "living storm" (466) of the *Triumph of Life,* Shelley describes power in meteorological terms as the "sweeping storms" that "desolate" the earth, withering "the buds of natural good." In confronting disease, Shelley was therefore confronting social spaces that he believed derived their pathogenic character from the desolating power of "evil, the immedicable plague" (*Prometheus Unbound* 2.4.101). Medicine provided him with a vocabulary for reading social geographies as disease environments. As he suggests in the conclusion to "The Sensitive Plant," one of the primary tasks of the poet is to provide a visionary alternative to such landscapes, the vision of a healthy world:

> That garden sweet, that lady fair
> And all sweet shapes and odours there
> In truth have never past away—
> 'Tis we, 'tis ours, are changed—not they.
>   (4.17–20)

Shelley's social therapeutics are constituted as a recovery of a nature that preceded the fall into sickness, but this recovery proceeds through a radical critique of contemporary disease geographies as preeminently social formations.

Shelley's writings constitute an extended reflection on the intertwining of social power and disease. The understanding of this relation, however, was not fixed but underwent significant changes of emphasis. After the utopian optimism of the early writings, in which he celebrated people's power to control and transform their environments through social reason, an increasing pessimism dominates his work. In *Mont Blanc* this pessimism derives from his recognition of the limits of our control of nature. In the *Triumph of Life* a far deeper pessimism emerges as he recognizes the depths of social power and disease. In this poem social evils have become pandemic. Shelley's comprehension of the ideopathology of space was not removed from the colonial world but frequently advanced through a reflection on colonial spaces, for it was there that the dynamic interaction of social and natural forces was writ large. As the embodiment of a pathogenic space that had come into being through the misuse of power, colonial space thus provided Shelley with a means and vocabulary for understanding European society. His increasing pessimism about the world's human environments can be said, then, to express anxiety about the direction British society was heading and fear that its imperial contact with other nations was becoming as great a plague to them as the East had originally seemed to be for England.

The Social Environment

With the exception of *Prometheus Unbound, Queen Mab* represents Shelley's greatest articulation of a biosocial utopia. In book 8 he envisions a total conquest and transformation of the world's diseased environments, a global ecological revolution made possible by science and love:

> All things are recreated, and the flame
> Of consentaneous love inspires all life:
> The fertile bosom of the earth gives suck
> To myriads, who still grow beneath her care,
> Rewarding her with their pure perfectness:
> The balmy breathings of the wind inhale
> Her virtues, and diffuse them all abroad:
> Health floats amid the gentle atmosphere,
> Glows in the fruits, and mantles on the stream.
> (8.107–15)

As in much of Shelley's writing, social revolution is here registered by a change in the physical environment. Countering the miasmas, those "terrestrial emanations . . . [or] causes of disease which float in the atmosphere" (Annesley 45), Shelley presents a world in which love, health, and reason are diffused everywhere. Man, with "taintless body" (8.199), rules and guides the changes taking place on earth: "his being notes / The gradual renovation, and defines / Each movement of its progress on his mind" (8.142–44). Shelley's biosocial utopia remains centered in human beings as he describes how reason and passion, no longer at war with each other, extend over the entire earth "Their all-subduing energies, and wield / The sceptre of a vast dominion there" (8.233–34).

Although criticism has generally been satisfied with seeing *Queen Mab* as simply visionary, Shelley's optimism concerning humans' power to extend their "all-subduing energies" over nature must have received confirmation and impetus from his active involvement, while writing a major portion of the poem, in a massive land reclamation project in Wales. The Tremadoc Embankment project, named after its initiator William Alexander Madocks, involved "nearly a hundred workmen, who were reinforcing a massive embankment across the mouth of the estuary to the little port of Portmadoc, and draining and clearing the land behind it" (Holmes 163). It may pale in comparison with the imperial engineering megaprojects of the later nineteenth century, yet it shares with them a fundamental belief that human beings can use technology to make physical environments suit their needs. When Shelley arrived the project was in serious trouble, since the Grand Cob embankment had been breached by flooding the previous spring. Shelley promised financial assistance to the almost bankrupt Madocks and also helped raise funds. The *North Wales Gazette's* report of one of Shelley's speeches suggests how adaptable his social utopianism was to large-scale capital projects:

The Embankment at Tremadoc, is one of the noblest works of human power—it is an exhibition of human nature as it appears in its noblest and most natural state—benevolence—it saves, it does not destroy. Yes! the unfruitful sea once rolled where human beings now live and earn their honest livelihood. Cast a look round these islands, through the perspective of these times,—behold famine driving millions even to madness; and own how excellent, how glorious, is the work which will give no less than three thousand souls the means of competence. How can anyone look upon that work and hesitate to join me, when I here publicly pledge myself to spend the last shilling of my fortune, and devote the last breath of my life to this great, this glorious cause. (qtd. in Holmes 166)

Shelley's social concerns are obvious; at a time when "famine" is driving "millions to madness" ("disease" may have been omitted by the reporter), the project is giving employment to three thousand people. Here physical nature is fully subservient to human needs and purposes, while "human nature" "in its noblest and most natural state" is expressed in those actions that increase the productivity of an otherwise "unfruitful" earth.

Shelley's geographical ideas are similar to those of Comte Georges-Louis Leclerc de Buffon, whom he first read in 1811. Like the French naturalist, he believes that large areas of the earth need improvement if they are to be adequate human habitats. Thomas Hogg notes the scientific culture shaping Shelley's geography. "What is the cause of the remarkable fertility of some lands, and of the hopeless sterility of others?" Shelley asked. "A spadeful of the most productive soil, does not to the eye differ much from the same quantity taken from the most barren. The real difference is probably very slight; by chemical agency the philosopher may work a total change, and may transmute an unfruitful region into a land of exuberant plenty" (48–49). Shelley's belief that chemical fertilizers can make an "unfruitful region" produce "exuberant plenty" was not, as Hogg believed, fanciful but instead shows the influence of Sir Humphry Davy's lectures on behalf of the Board of Agriculture early in 1802. There Davy argued that agriculture is "an art intimately connected with chemical science" (2: 315).[4] Having already suffered ridicule for his enthusiasm over the medical benefits of nitrous oxide, Davy was careful to avoid looking "to distant ages . . . [to] amuse ourselves with brilliant, though delusive dreams concerning the infinite improveability of man, the annihilation of labour, disease, and even death. . . . We consider only a state of human progression arising out of its present condition" (323). The infertility of the soil, however, was not the only factor standing in the way of agricultural improvement. Finding adequate water supplies was just as important. Shelley believed that chemistry would ultimately discover "a simple and sure method of manufacturing the useful fluid, in every situation and in any quantity," a knowledge that would produce a total ecological transformation of North Africa. "The arid deserts of Africa may then be refreshed by a copious supply," he declared, "and may be transformed at once into rich meadows, and vast fields of maize and rice." Nor would the coldness of some climates constitute an insurmountable obstacle to human ingenuity; it might be possible "perhaps at no very distant period . . . to produce heat at will, and to warm the most ungenial climates as readily as we now raise the temperature of our apartments to whatever degree we may deem agreeable or salutary." Shelley's science provides the means for making the entire earth serve human needs. We make a serious mistake if we treat his notions about ecological revolution as simply visionary. They also express many of the ideas that led to the radical transformation of the landscapes of England and that informed the engineering megaprojects of later nineteenth-century colonialism.[5] An anti-imperialist on one level, Shelley nevertheless shares with the promoters of empire the "technotopian" belief that European science should contribute to the transformation of global environments.[6]

In *Queen Mab,* Shelley follows Hippocrates in drawing a parallel between different climates and the health of the people who inhabit them. He divides the world into three primary environmental zones—the polar, the tropical, and the temperate. The first two are extreme pathogenic spaces. Whatever might be said about the extreme environment of those who dwell in "the gloom of the long polar night," a much harsher world awaits them in the poem. Shelley speaks of people who are biologically degenerate. Man "shrank with the plants, and darkened with the night," he writes:

> His chilled and narrow energies, his heart,
> Insensible to courage, truth, or love,
> His stunted stature and imbecile frame,
> Marked him for some abortion of the earth,
> Fit compeer of the bears that roamed around,
> Whose habits and enjoyments were his own:
> His life a feverish dream of stagnant woe.
> (8.149—56)

Drawing on Buffon's description of the disastrous impact of the cold American climate on its indigenous people, Shelley produces an even more negative picture of environmental and reproductive degeneration as he repeatedly speaks of the narrowing of moral and biological energies, of shrinking, stunting, imbecility, and abortiveness, and the absence of the Shelleyan virtues of "courage, truth, and love." Disease has often been understood as a punishment for moral offenses. Shelley applies this idea to entire regions, as if the world's pathogenic spaces were a punishment upon their inhabitants: "All was inflicted here that Earth's revenge / Could wreak on the infringers of her law" (8.163—64).

Since Shelley associates sickness and fever with social stasis—the word "stagnant" deriving from *stagnum* ("swamp")—the people who inhabit the tropics are little different:

> Nor where the tropics bound the realms of day
> With a broad belt of mingling cloud and flame,
> Where blue mists through the unmoving atmosphere
> Scattered the seeds of pestilence, and fed
> Unnatural vegetation, where the land
> Teemed with all earthquake, tempest and disease,
> Was man a nobler being . . .   (8.166—72)

Again disease is understood as a deviation from nature, as the "blue mists" of miasma, their color suggesting death, are born from "*unnatural* vegetation" and an "unmoving" atmosphere. One popular explanation for the unhealthy character of tropical environments during the dry season was "the want of the free ventilation afforded by the trade-winds during the rest of the year" (Tulloch and Marshall 102).[7] Shelley draws on this idea, but for him the "unmoving" state of the atmosphere or of the swamp—both productive of miasmas—is a *symptom* of social stagnancy, not its *cause*. Shelley goes on to argue that disease combines with slavery and constant warfare to make the tropics a bane to human existence.

Given the analogy drawn in medical geography between the moral and intellectual qualities of a people and the qualities of the environments they inhabit, Shelley's contemporaries would not have been surprised by his turn from these extreme environments to the "milder zone" (8.187), the "favoured clime" (8.193) of England, where "truth" has finally arisen to combat disease. Yet Shelley describes it as also being diseased:

> Even where the milder zone afforded man
> A seeming shelter, yet contagion there,
> Blighting his being with unnumbered ills,
> Spread like a quenchless fire; nor truth till late
> Availed to arrest its progress.   (8.187–91)

Shelley does not celebrate the enviromedical superiority of Europe as a physical space, although he does place it higher in the scale of world regions. Instead, he values its role in bringing truth to light. For Shelley, disease environments are not "essentialized" but are symptoms of the absence of truth, which is the only force needed to "arrest" their development.

Michael Scrivener argues that Shelley's "'nature' not only presents no insuperable obstacles to reason, but is itself rational" (68). From such a viewpoint, disease-bearing environments are unnatural because they deviate from reason. Their cure is seen as a "recovery" both of reason and of their "nature." Shelley supports this idea through an interesting revision of the extensive "ruins of empire" literature. Where the contemplation of the ruins of ancient cities frequently gave rise to a melancholy sense of historical change and to the moral that all empires must eventually fall victim to time, Shelley focuses on the destruction of habitable environments indicated by such ruins. Take Palmyra, for instance, where "the aspect of a great city deserted, the memory of times past, compared with its present state" ushers in the political reverie of Volney (3–4). Shelley follows the French ideologue in using these ruins to reflect on the course of empires and on social and political decay. "Monarchs and conquerors there / Proud o'er prostrate millions trod— / The earthquakes of the human race" (2.121–23). Yet his association of the rulers with destructive geological forces suggests that the poet is more fascinated by the clear evidence these ruins provide of a physical environment that no longer exists. To the obvious question raised by such ruins—Why would a people build a great city in the middle of a desert?—Shelley drew the obvious conclusion that Palmyra had not always been in the desert, that some massive change had radically altered its character. His explanation is political: a change in moral and political institutions, notably the advent of an increasingly despotic government, caused depopulation and with it a progressive decline in the people's capacity to maintain the fertility and moderate climate of the region. The emergence of the desert, as both a demographic and a physical process, is thus a political development, concomitant with the emergence of despotism.[8]

The contemporary condition of Jerusalem evokes a similar sense of the link between politics and environmental degradation:

> Behold yon sterile spot;
> Where now the wandering Arab's tent
> Flaps in the desart-blast.
> There once old Salem's haughty fane
> Reared high to heaven its thousand golden domes,
> And in the blushing face of day
> Exposed its shameful glory.   (2.134–40)

After noting that "where Athens, Rome, and Sparta stood / There is a moral desert now" (2.162–63), Shelley turns to the ancient Mayan civilization. Where once "arose a stately city / Metropolis of the western continent," there is now only a wilderness (2.187–88). States that deviate from the virtues of independence, labor, and equality produce wildernesses. Shelley takes his republican environmentalism further to reach the extraordinary visionary conclusion that there is no spot on earth, no matter how wild, that was not once a populous city. "There's not one atom of yon earth," he writes:

> But once was living man;
> Nor the minutest drop of rain,
> That hangeth in its thinnest cloud,
> But flowed in human veins:
> And from the burning plains
> Where Libyan monsters yell,
> From the most gloomy glens
> Of Greenland's sunless clime,
> To where the golden fields
> Of fertile England spread
> Their harvest to the day,
> Thou canst not find one spot
> Whereon no city stood.
>
>   (2.211–24)

Here Shelley articulates a social ecology more radical than anything currently claimed by contemporary social constructionists, arguing that all nature "once was living man." He thus inverts the traditional understanding of the relation between the city and the wilderness by claiming that *cities come first.* In *Queen Mab* the wilderness and the depopulated desert—emblems of environments that have proved uninhabitable to humankind—are not viewed as an "essential" nature that precedes social life but instead are seen as the vestiges of cities in ruin. Diseased environments are not the cause of social and political disorder but are their result, the effects of a power that is truly a "desolating pestilence" (3.176). Shelley denies that nature is conceivable apart from human life. The wilderness is always the signature of a population decline produced by social inequity, resulting in the collapse of the habitable environments produced by rational, social labor: it is always the city gone wild. Whereas Wordsworth argues for the need to humanize nature, Shelley understands revolution as the recovery of the human face of nature, the cities that once existed everywhere on earth.

Shelley's belief that the wilderness is a "depopulated nature" contributes to a century-old demographic debate, begun by the *Persian Letters* (1721), in which Montesquieu argued that the modern world was suffering from depopulation. "After a calculation as exact as is possible in such matters," Rhedi writes to Uzbek, "I have found that hardly one-tenth as many people are now on the earth as there were in ancient times." Even "more astonishing," he goes on to argue, "is that this depopulation goes on daily, and if it continues, the earth will be a desert in a thousand years" (188). He concludes that there must be "a secret and hidden poison, a corrupting disease afflicting human nature itself" (188). Uzbek responds that the problem lies not in nature, but in the sphere of morals and government, as the small, densely populated Greek city-states were replaced by large, ineffective empires shaped by antirepublican values. Shelley is a population pessimist who employs the idea of depopulation to argue against vice and bad government. Cities become deserts through changes in the moral and civil nature of human beings.[9] In *Hellas,* both the desert and paradise are politically determined: "Let the tyrants rule the desert they have made; / Let the free possess the paradise they claim" (1008–9).

As Shelley and his contemporaries looked at various parts of the globe, they saw ample evidence that some regions had undergone substantial climatic changes. They were quite aware that North Africa and the Middle East had once been immensely fertile, with sufficient rainfall to allow them to serve as the granary of the Roman Empire. Seeing deserts where there once were major croplands, they reached the not unwarranted conclusion that these environmental changes were linked to changes in social and political institutions. Colonial regions, associated with poverty, disease, and depopulation, far from being "naturally" this way, were seen as having undergone ecological degradation. Early on, as Richard Grove notes, Europeans had seen in the Canary Islands and Madeira how quickly deforestation can produce a radical decline in rainfall and consequent desiccation (*Ecology, Climate, and Empire* 6). Shelley shares the anxieties that shaped early conservationist thinking as he sees in tropical colonial regions the forces that produce social ruin. "Ozymandias" is probably Shelley's most powerful depiction of the relation between poor government and a degraded physical environment. A traveler recounts his encounter with the "colossal Wreck" of a monument to Ramses II in the desert of an "antique land." The poem has long been read as a classic example of dramatic irony. The words on the pedestal of the broken statue read, "My name is Ozymandias, King of Kings, / Look on my Works, ye Mighty, and despair!" Kelvin Everest sees them as conveying "a simple moral. The tyrant's affirmation of his omnipotence, sneeringly arrogant and contemptuous of its human cost, has been ironised by time. . . . It is simply true that tyranny does not last" (26–27). Such a view, though correct on one level, does not recognize how far-reaching is the desolating power of Ozymandias, so that his true works are still everywhere present in the "lone and level sands" that "stretch far away." The tyrant's words should be taken literally, though in a manner the speaker did not intend. Shelley looked at depopulated nature—the *desert*—as a far more ominous monument than the broken sculpture, showing not tyranny's susceptibility to time, but its continuing presence not only *in,* but *as* physical space. Tyranny *is* ruin, and Shelley intended his readers to recognize that "those passions . . . *yet survive* stamped on these lifeless things." "Ozymandias" is thus very much a poem about colonial space, which sees the ecologically degraded and depopulated character of such regions as a sign of the continuing survival of desolating power. Ecology and politics are inseparably allied.

Because Shelley denies that climate is "natural" because he sees all climates as "climates of power," addressing climate in his poetry is always a political gesture. As I argued in chapter 1, colonial regions were seen not only as sites of social ruin, but also as places whose environments were undergoing radical renewal. Rather than seeing it as an "immovable barrier to the political improvement of the species" (Godwin, *Enquiry,* 1985 ed. 146), many writers thought that climate itself could be radically transformed, as appeared to be the case in America. Climate change was indeed seen as one of the chief benefits of the introduction of European technologies, knowledge, and polit-ical institutions. In the concluding utopian vision of *Queen Mab,* the fairy describes a world in which a total ecological transformation has taken place: "The habitable earth is full of bliss" (8.58). Social revolution engenders a world in which the polar wastes and tropical deserts no longer exist and the climatic differences that once characterized the globe have been eliminated:

> Those wastes of frozen billows that were hurled
> By everlasting snow-storms round the poles,
> Where matter dared not vegetate or live,
> But ceaseless frost round the vast solitude
> Bound its broad zone of stillness, are unloosed;
> And fragrant zephyrs there from spicy isles
> Ruffle the placid ocean-deep
>
> . . . .
>
> Those desarts of immeasurable sand,
> Whose age-collected fervors scarce allowed
> A bird to live, a blade of grass to spring,
> Where the shrill chirp of the green lizard's love
> Broke on the sultry silentness alone
> Now teem with countless rills and shady woods,
> Corn-fields and pastures and white cottages.
>
> (8.59–76)

The centrality of "Corn-fields, pastures, white cottages" in this renovated earth shows how difficult it is, even for the most radical of English anti-imperial poets, to avoid using English landscapes as the measure of utopia. Yet Shelley criticized English society not for its utopian self-representation as an "island garden" but because it did not live up to this ideal.[10] Having provided Ianthe with a vision of what the earth can become, the fairy brings her back to reality. "The present now recurs. / Ah me! a pathless wilderness remains / Yet unsubdued by man's reclaiming hand" (9.143–45). Revolution is ecolog-ical reclamation, the recovery of a nature produced by human labor and love that has been destroyed by social degradation.

Shelley's belief that climate is social might seem impossibly idealistic, but it voices a central strand in nineteenth-century scientific thought. For instance, his prophecy of a time when the deserts will "teem with countless rills and shady woods" almost became a reality in the 1870s. As early as 1738, Thomas Shaw had suggested, in his *Travels, or Observations relating to Several Parts of Barbary and the Levant,* that the Sahara had once sustained a huge inland sea or lake. He speculated that three large saline depressions, or "chotts," were the last remnants of the Sea of Triton, once connected to the Mediterranean. James Rennell returned to this idea in 1800, in his *Geographical System of Herodotus, Examined*. In the 1870s, during the excitement created by the building of the Suez Canal, French engineers considered the possibility of increasing "the commercial and environmental potential of North Africa by creating a vast, inland 'sea' deep within the arid wastes of the Sahara" (Heffernan 95). The project of constructing a series of canals that would connect the Saharan chotts to the Gulf of Gabès was first proposed by the surveyor François Élie Roudaire. Reintroducing water to the region, he believed, would moderate the climate and return it to its original temperate condition. Agriculture would regain its rightful place in the area, and the health of the people would be improved. As Roudaire observed, "The inland sea will be for Algeria what the Mediterranean is for France" (qtd. in Heffernan 103). Victor Hugo's support for the project—its rhetoric reminiscent of the language of Shelley at Tremadoc seventy years earlier—provides one measure of how greatly such a project appealed to a nineteenth-century European imperial audience: "The people [of North Africa] are disinherited, their world is a desert. . . . Must we conquer this world by force of arms? No! Let us astonish the universe by great achievements which do not involve warfare. It is up to us, it is the duty of civilization. Algeria requires a sea: let us create it there. A sea brings with it ships, ships create towns, and towns create civilization" (qtd. in Heffernan 105). In Hugo's panegyric, imperialism has two forms, military and environmental, and only the latter expresses the values of civilization. Imperial engineering is presented as a means of ecological recovery; through knowledge, the "disinherited" of North Africa will be given back the climate and the world they have lost. Roudaire could not gain enough state and private financial support to set the project in motion, especially when a later geological survey suggested that the chotts were the remnants of a lake rather than being connected to the sea. Nevertheless the idea continued to influence French policy in Africa, and its feasibility continues to be debated among contemporary climatologists.

In light of later imperial developments, Shelley's celebration of the "greening the desert," in Timothy Morton's phrasing, his belief that geography is only the naturalized embodiment of political life, is at once less visionary than one might assume and more closely affiliated with the Promethean projects of imperial landscape transformation so characteristic of the nineteenth century.[11] Although Shelley was critical of aristocratic privilege, he shares with the landed gentry and the more commercial entrepreneurs of the nineteenth century the belief that science can produce a nature adapted to human needs.

Mont Blanc *and "the Winter of the World"*

Against Shelley's faith that human environments, and with them human bodies, might be made healthy through science and love, must be set his own experience, which confirmed his remark that "in the present state of the climates of the earth, health, in the true and comprehensive sense of the word, is out of the reach of civilized man" (*Poetical Works* 808). Shelley's list of health complaints was long and ongoing, from his early bout with "brain fever," for which his father is said to have considered sending him to an asylum, through an assortment of nervous and possibly hypochondriac ailments and stomach spasms, to ophthalmia, premature aging, possible venereal infection, severe pulmonary attacks, and fears of consumption. Nora Crook and Derek Guiton note that "for most of the last four years of his life, Shelley was living either at a watering place, the seaside or a centre of medicine. . . . [O]ne cannot ignore the constant pressure of illness. Shelley's principal pursuit was health" (112). Even during the composition of *Queen Mab*, Mary Shelley notes, "ill-health made [Shelley] believe that . . . a year or two was all he had of life" (*Poetical Works* 837). The celebration of the world-transforming powers of science and technology in the poem therefore should be set against a personal history of ill health and its attendant anxiety. Since Shelley could not conceive of health apart from the diagnosis of social power, it would not be difficult to read his continuing complaints as a fundamental kind of social criticism, as expressions of a fluctuating sense of the prospect of social reform.

In this regard, one of the stranger episodes in Shelley's life took place during late 1813, when he feared he had contracted elephantiasis. Hogg writes that the poet, shortly after reading "a formidable description in some medical work," believed he had come into contact with the disease by sitting across from "an old woman with very thick legs."[12] Fearful that an epidemic was about to occur in England, he obsessively examined himself and others for signs of the disease:

One evening, during the access of his fancied disorder, when many young ladies were standing up for a country dance, he caused wonderful consternation amongst these charming creatures by walking slowly along the row of girls and curiously surveying them, placing his eyes close to their necks and bosoms, and feeling their breasts and bare arms, in order to ascertain whether any of the fair ones had taken the horrible disease. He proceeded with so much gravity and seriousness, and his looks were so woebegone, that they did not resist, or resent, the extraordinary liberties, but looked terrified and as if they were about to undergo some severe surgical operation at his hands. (457–58)

During these years, and increasingly in the later poetry, Shelley's biosocial utopianism must be read against a deeper anxiety that England, by virtue of its increasingly despotic social policies, was becoming another "East," the first signs being epidemiological. Indeed, for Shelley the East is not a geographical entity restricted to a specific climate or people but instead is a political condition. The "East" therefore occupies an important place in the language of the ideopathologist, *not* as the cause or source of diseases, but as the exemplum of a pathology of power that can take root anywhere. Shelley thus consistently portrays the confrontation with autocratic government as a confrontation with the primary diseases of the East—with leprosy, plague, and elephantiasis. In a letter written in June 1811 he remarks about Southey's *Curse of Kehama*, "Is not the chapter where Kailyal despises the leprosy grand" (1: 126). Probably the most powerful of these encounters is described in "Ozymandias." Crook and Guiton perceptively suggest that the swollen limbs of the monument convey the telltale symptoms of elephantiasis: "The stone legs stand obstinately, hypostasizing the horror, like an inveterate disease or memory of disease which embeds itself in the boundless and bare sand of consciousness" (99).

Because social and environmental ruin mirror one another, the difference between the traveler's encounter with the monumental wreck of Ozymandias in the desert and the stony dialogue of the poet with the depopulated Mont Blanc is not as great as one might think.[13] Despite the apparent oddity of speaking of the Alpine regions of the highest mountain in the European subcontinent as a colonial landscape, *Mont Blanc* should be read as a European "wilderness poem" that reflects on the boundaries between society and nature and on the limits of the human transformation of nature. Originally placed as the coda to the travel narrative *A History of a Six Weeks' Tour*, it describes Shelley's response to a wilderness landscape, where nature operates on a sublime scale. In a note added to the preface of the narrative, Shelley writes that he sought "to imitate the untameable wildness and inaccessible solemnity from which [his] feelings sprang" (vi). In his letters to Peacock, he adopts the language of a naturalist describing the flora and fauna of a foreign region: he talks about wolves ("A wolf is more powerful than the fiercest & strongest dog"), notes that there are "no bears in these regions," and describes "an exceedingly rare animal called the *Bouctin.*" He mentions a visit to a "Cabinet d'Histoire Naturelle" at Chamonix and notes that he has purchased "some specimens of minerals & plants & two or three chrystal seals at Mont Blanc." His best purchase, he declares, "is a large collection of the seeds of rare Alpine plants, with their names written upon the outside of the papers which contain them. These I mean to colonise in my garden in England; & to permit you to make what choice you please from them." Although the people of Chamonix are noticeably absent from the poem, figured only by their incapacity in the face of the destructive power of nature, Shelley's attitude toward them is explicit in the letters to Peacock. Immediately after citing Buffon's "gloomy theory" that the earth "will at some future period be changed into a mass of frost," he turns his attention to the Chamoniards. "Add to this the degradation of the human species, who in these regions are half deformed or idiotic & all of whom are deprived of anything that can excite interest & admiration. This is a part of the subject more mournful & less sublime;—but such as neither the poet nor the philosopher should disdain," Shelley writes, as he reserves the "development" of his "views" on the topic for later conversation (*Letters* 1: 496–99).[14]

The poem's indebtedness to colonial exploration narratives, most obviously to the great African narratives detailing the search for the origins of the Nile or the Niger River, may not be as obvious as it is in *Alastor,* yet *Mont Blanc* is nevertheless shaped by the same concern to map the limits of human control over nature.[15] It too recounts a journey, mostly by the imagination, to discover the source of a "majestic River" (123). From a bridge over the River Arve, on the frontiers of civilized life, the poet ascends upward to the deserted summit of the mountain whence "Power in likeness of the Arve comes down / From the ice gulphs that gird his secret throne" (16–17). Like *Queen Mab,* the poem examines the relation between social power and the environments through which it is expressed; yet unlike the earlier poem, *Mont Blanc* is much more skeptical about humans' power to control nature and adapt it to their needs.

It is not difficult to recognize that *Mont Blanc* is a poem about the power of glaciers. What has not been recognized is that it is also a poem about *climate change* and about how human beings can transform physical environments. It would not have been difficult during the early part of the nineteenth century to convince the people of Chamonix that climate changes. From the sixteenth century, when the glaciers first began a destructive descent on the valley settlements, through the seventeenth and eighteenth centuries, which were periods of minor glacial advances and retreats, to the middle of the nineteenth century, when a major advance of ice was once more under way, the Chamoniards lived in constant apprehension of what climatologists now call "the Little Ice Age."[16] In the 1690s, for instance, they sent a deputation to Jean d'Arenthon, bishop of Geneva, asking him to "exorcise and bless these mountains of ice. . . . [T]hey said that since his last visit the glaciers had retired more than eighty paces." Their delegation was successful, for he returned to

Chamonix, with the happy result, his hagiographer states, that "the glaciers have withdrawn an eighth of a league from where they were before, and . . . have ceased to cause the havoc they used to do" (qtd. in Le Roy Ladurie, *Times of Feast* 180–81). Because the augmentation or decrease of glaciers directly reflected changing climatic conditions and could easily be measured, and because their expansion and movement were of such consequence to those who lived near them, the study of glacier expansion and contraction played a central role in the early development of the science of climatology. Le Roy Ladurie thus remarks that "to talk about glaciers is the same thing as talking about climate" (99). As early as 1821, Ignace Venetz, an engineer from Visperterminen, saw glacier augmentation and diminution as evidence that temperature "rises and falls periodically but in an irregular manner." In 1817, a year after its members began to study glaciers, the Société Helvétique des Sciences concluded that the climate of Switzerland was becoming colder.[17] In talking about the descent of the glaciers of Mont Blanc, therefore, Shelley was contributing to debates about climate change and humans' relation to it.

During the summer of 1816, when the poem was written, the weather was terrible. Mary Shelley notes in the *History of a Six Weeks' Tour* that "the spring, as the inhabitants informed us, was unusually late, and indeed the cold was excessive" (90). Recalling this period, Mary notes that "it proved a wet, ungenial summer, and incessant rain often confined us for days to the house" (*Frankenstein* 224). The cold weather was not unique to Switzerland but was part of global cooling caused by the eruption of the Tambora volcano in Indonesia on 11 April 1815. It produced one of the coldest summers in history, comparable to those of 1316 and 1675, and 1816 was popularly known as "the year there was no summer."[18] In many regions of the world, especially India, Canada, and Europe, there were famines and large-scale food shortages, and the weather also probably played a role in the outbreak of cholera in 1817. John D. Post observes: "The catastrophe of 1816 may have had only one comparable antecedent in the history of Europe—the monumental medieval ecological disaster of 1315–17" (730). For a poet who used climatology as a political gauge, the summer of 1816 could only be interpreted pessimistically. In *The Revolt of Islam*, Cythna describes the nadir of revolutionary hopes in language that aptly characterizes the climatic politics of *Mont Blanc:* "This is the winter of the world" (*Poetical Works* 3685).

Shelley describes a world in which the human power to create temperate environments seems impotent in the face of a power that dwells apart from human control. "I never knew I never imagined what mountains were before," he writes to Peacock. "The verge of a glacier presents the most vivid image of desolation that it is possible to conceive. No one dares approach it, for the enormous pinnacles of ice perpetually fall, & are perpetually reproduced." Noting the geologist H.-B. de Saussure's comment that the glaciers "have their periods of increase & decay," Shelley disagrees, arguing along with the Chamoniards that they "perpetually augment" and that they will eventually overflow the vale. In one year, he remarks, "these glaciers have advanced three hundred feet into the valley. . . . "[T]hese glaciers flow perpetually into the valley ravaging in their slow but irresistible progress the pastures & the forests which surround them, & performing a work of desolation in ages which a river of lava might accomplish in an hour, but far more irretrievably—for where the ice has once been the hardiest plant refuses to grow—if even, as in some extraordinary instances, it should recede after its progression has once commenced" (*Letters* 1: 497–99). In the glaciers of Mont Blanc, Shelley saw a vision of the end of the world. Against the utopian ideal of a temperate universe under total human control, he adopts the "gloomy theory" of Buffon, seeing these glaciers as the "first essays" of the power or god that is "throned among these desolating snows" (1: 499), a force that could lead to a state of perpetual winter.

In the wilderness world of *Mont Blanc*, there are limits to humans' power to create social habitats, yet it remains unclear whether these limits have been established by nature or by the failure of social institutions. Shelley's assertion that "the wilderness has a mysterious tongue / Which teaches awful doubt, or faith" and "a voice . . . to repeal / Large codes of fraud and woe" (76–81) is less a statement of confidence than a means of leaving the question open.[19] As in *Queen Mab*, the wilderness is depicted as a depopulated space, a world of "frozen floods" and "unfathomable deeps," a "desert peopled by the storms alone" (64–67). Yet here Shelley appears less willing to assert the primacy of the social over the natural. He rewrites *Queen Mab* from a more pessimistic viewpoint, describing a "city of death" that has been built up "in scorn of mortal power":

> there, many a precipice,
> Frost and Sun in scorn of mortal power
> Have piled: dome, pyramid, and pinnacle,
> A city of death, distinct with many a tower
> And wall impregnable of beaming ice.
>
> (102–6)

Shelley presents a city that is actually a desert, and he almost reverses the argument of *Queen Mab* that all wildernesses are the relics of unpeopled cities.

Here nature parodies and thus ridicules the cities of the humanly constructed
or "daedal earth" (86). Instead of expressing the rational laws of nature,
mirrored by human reason, this city is actually a ruin:

> Yet not a city, but a flood of ruin
> Is there, that from the boundaries of the sky
> Rolls it perpetual stream; vast pines are strewing
> Its destined path, or in the mangled soil
> Branchless and shattered stand: the rocks, drawn down
> From yon remotest waste, have overthrown
> The limits of the dead and living world,
> Never to be reclaimed.   (107–14)

The admission that these glaciers represent an incursion of the "dead" or
frozen world into the "living world" that is "never to be reclaimed" reflects
Shelley's increased skepticism in 1816. In the face of this destruction, human
beings are powerless: their "work and dwelling / Vanish, like smoke before
the tempest's stream, / And their place is not known" (118–20).

Shelley partially resolves the contradiction between the power of nature
and that of human beings by reading it across the axis of colonial geography.
Although the descending Alpine glaciers contribute to the misery of the
disease-ridden and deformed Chamoniards, they also are the source of "one
majestic River, / The breath and blood of distant lands" (123–24). The fertile
"distant lands" referred to here, odd as it may seem, are of course Europe,
where the power of the glaciers and the river has been harnessed to serve human needs. Early in 1818, searching for a theme on the Nile River that could
be developed quickly in a sonnet competition with Leigh Hunt and Keats,
Shelley rewrote Mont Blanc. In "To the Nile," the colonial geography that
shaped his understanding of the European socialization of nature is quite clear:

> Month after month the gathered rains descend
> Drenching yon secret Aethiopian dells,
> And from the desert's ice-girt pinnacles
> Where Frost and Heat in strange embraces blend
> On Atlas, fields of moist snow half depend.
> Girt there with blasts and meteors Tempest dwells
> By Nile's aërial urn, with rapid spells
> Urging those waters to their mighty end.   (1–8)

Like Mont Blanc, Atlas produces a river that, as it flows "O'er Egypt's land of
Memory" (9), becomes the ambiguous source of agricultural renewal and
epidemic disease—"soul-sustaining airs and blasts of evil," "fruits and poi-

sons" (11–12). As Shelley reflected on the depths of empire, the dangers of the natural limits placed upon human life by nature seemed less threatening than the reach of empire. Just as in *Mont Blanc*, where the power of nature is mirrored in the power of the mind that imagines this scene, Shelley shifts his attention from the contradictory power that is embodied in the likeness of the Nile to the contradictory power of knowledge. The world-historical sources of disease seemed much closer to home: "Beware, O Man—for knowledge must to thee, / Like the great flood to Egypt, ever be" (13–14).[20]

Empire and Pathogenic Space in The Triumph of Life

In *The Triumph of Life* Rousseau, now disfigured beyond recognition, describes how life triumphed over him:

> "I among the multitude
> Was swept; me sweetest flowers delayed not long,
> Me not the shadow nor the solitude,
>
> Me not the falling stream's Lethean song,
> Me, not the phantom of that early form
> Which moved upon its motion,—but among
>
> The thickest billows of the living storm
> I plunged, and bared my bosom to the clime
> Of that cold light, whose airs too soon deform."
> (460–68)

This is an extraordinary moment in an extraordinary poem. Like one of Dante's damned, Rousseau describes how he "plunged" into "the thickest billows of the living storm." Nowhere in Shelley's poetry is the relation between power and the creation of the world's pathogenic environments more powerfully expressed, for the "clime" and "storm" that ultimately disfigure Rousseau are both "living," produced by human beings. As in *Mont Blanc*, Shelley's focus is on the agency of power in history, and the *nature* it produces. Whereas the earlier poem left unanswered the question whether the extreme environments of colonial spaces were attributable to the power of nature or to the failure of government in these regions, the *Triumph* explores the pathogenic reach of empire. Its central organizing metaphor, the imperial "triumphs" or public pageants that were staged in ancient Rome to celebrate the return of victorious generals and their armies, emphasizes that Shelley's explicit topic is *imperial* power:

> Imperial Rome poured forth her living sea
> From senatehouse and prison and theatre
> When Freedom left those who upon the free
>
> Had bound a yoke which soon they stooped to bear.
>
> (113–16)

The poem is about the ideology, produced by a combination of politics, law, and art, that sponsored this "living sea" of colonists. The Roman pageant provided Shelley with an allegorical structure for an anatomy of empire and of the imprisoning links forged between those who enslave and those enslaved. As Demogorgon declares, "All spirits are enslaved who serve things evil" (*Prometheus Unbound* 2.4.110).

In examining the fundamental link between disease and empire, Shelley drew extensively on Petrarch's *Trionfi*, a poem portraying life as a medieval progress, a series of "triumphs," summarized by A. C. Bradley as "in turn the triumph of Love over man, especially in his youth; the triumph of Chastity over Love; that of Death over all mortality; that of Fame over Death; that of Time over Fame; and that of Divinity over Time" (441). Like Shelley's poem, the *Trionfi* is explicitly a disease narrative, an attempt to make sense of the first bubonic plague pandemic that ravaged Asia, the Middle East, North Africa, and Europe during the middle of the fourteenth century. As a cultural document, it powerfully conveys how medieval Europeans sought to make sense of an epidemic that destroyed between a third and a half of their people. The poem is also a personal response to the Black Death, for *The Triumph of Death,* written in 1348, includes Petrarch's account of Laura's death by plague:

> Not like a flame that forcibly is quenched,
> But like to one that doth itself consume,
> Her soul, contented, went its way in peace,
>
> Like to a light that is both clear and sweet
> And loses slowly its own nutriment,
> Keeping its dearness to the very end.
>
> (59–60)

Shelley's Rousseau draws an explicit parallel between himself and Laura, noting that had he burned with a brighter light, "if the spark with which Heaven lit my spirit / Earth had with purer nutriment supplied" (201–2), he would not now be so disfigured. Like the others who people the pageant, Rousseau is a plague victim, a point Hazlitt made when he suggested that the *Triumph* was "a new and terrific Dance of Death" (16: 273). The "wild dance" (138) of those chained to the car mimes popular descriptions of plague victims, yet the cause of this sickness is not *Yersinia pestis* but imperial power— "Evil, the immedicable plague." By the end of his career, Shelley sees empire as a pandemic "pour[ing] forth" *from Europe!* That Shelley would see Petrarch's disease narrative, which he first read in 1819, as an appropriate structure for analyzing imperial power is not surprising, for he used the word "triumph" for similar purposes in *Queen Mab.* "The pestilence that stalks / In gloomy triumph through some eastern land," he argues, "Is less destroying" (4.188–90) than the actions of European statesman, "those royal murderers, whose mean thrones / Are bought by crimes of treachery and gore" (4.170–71). In the *Mask of Anarchy,* the *Trionfi* also served as the allegorical structure for a political anatomy of England. Through the lens provided by medieval dream narrative, nineteenth-century imperialism was a terrible *danse macabre,* a "ghastly dance" (540). The epidemiological consequences of this expansion were no less frightening than the original expansion of *Yersinia pestis* into Europe. As will become clear, however, the cause of this somber reflection on disease and empire was not plague but the outbreak in 1817 of pandemic cholera.

Whereas the limits of human power in the face of colonial nature structure *Mont Blanc,* the *Triumph* focuses on the devastating reach of empire. Shelley shows how the world-shaping and mind-transforming power of empire has become as deep as life itself. As in *Mont Blanc,* the universe is not separate from the mind that perceives it, so the difficulty of recovering a world unaffected by the deformations of imperialism lies in the fact that the pageant transforms not only the universe but also the minds of those who participate in it. Empire and its ideologies shape human perceptions along with human bodies, "Temper[ing] its own contagion to the vein / Of those who are infected with it" (277–78). As in Wordsworth's "Intimations Ode," where language itself is a barrier to recovering childhood nature, the poet-dreamer of the *Triumph* is not removed from the imperial culture and ideology that he wants to see beyond. The essay "On Life" suggests that the pageant threatening to enslave him takes place as much in his mind as anywhere else, in the ideological sphere of language and ideas: "All familiar objects are signs, standing not for themselves but for others, in their capacity of suggesting one thought, which shall lead to a train of thoughts.—Our whole life is thus an education of error" (*Shelley's Poetry and Prose* 477).

In both the narrator's and Rousseau's accounts of the appearance and progress of the pageant, the idea of a "habitable earth" "full of bliss" is presented as something that continues to exist in human experience, though its presence has been all but obliterated from thought. The poem opens with a utopian image of the morning of a world in which all things share in equitable labor:

> Swift as a spirit hastening to his task
> Of glory and of good, the Sun sprang forth
> Rejoicing in his splendour, and the mask
>
> Of darkness fell from the awakened Earth.
>
> (1–4)

The earth responds in kind, the birds "temper[ing] their matin lay," and "Continent, / Isle, Ocean, and all things" bear "their portion" (8–19) of the toil. The ontological status of this temperate world, however, is one of the central problems of the poem. The opening frame seems to be a record of an immediate perception of the world, yet Shelley refuses to separate the world one perceives from the linguistic measures (poetic or otherwise) that mark its movement; as in a Turner painting, which draws attention to its medium, this world is perceived through a "transparent" shadow, the product of a "strange trance," that brightens all it touches:

> for the shade it spread
>
> Was so transparent that the scene came through
> As clear as when a veil of light is drawn
> O'er evening hills, they glimmer.   (30–33)

An already complex fiction, a waking dream, becomes more complex when Shelley insists that this scene is not only the product of heightened perception, literally achieved through poetry, but also a recovery of an earlier state of the world and of the mind that once perceived it: "I knew / That I had felt the freshness of that dawn. . . . And sate as thus upon that slope of lawn" (33–36).

Social space, like the mind, is layered and thus supplies equivocal access to what has been lost. Just as the geographies of the poem appear as transparencies or veils, each blotting out or shading others, so too perception is layered. Each new world displaces those that preceded it, but not without leaving traces, which can be recovered as déjà vu. Rousseau's experience parallels that of the dreamer-poet as he too recollects a time when he discerned "a gentle trace / Of light diviner than the common Sun / Sheds on the common Earth" (337–39). Language has the power to heighten perception, and Rousseau's account of his encounter with "a shape all light" (352) suggests the way a naive perception of the world is increasingly displaced by "words and signs, the instruments of its own creation" (*Shelley's Poetry and Prose* 477). The light's "fierce splendour" "displaces the darkness of the previous night and his previous thoughts. The three metaphors Shelley uses to describe this vision emphasize the close connection between perception and language. Like poetry, "her feet, no less than the sweet tune / To which they moved," "blot[s] / The thoughts of him who gazed on them, and soon / All that was seemed as if it had been not" (382–85). Poetry is inextricably bound up with perception, for the vision here is either a stain that blots out all other thoughts or something that obliterates them by soaking them into itself. The second metaphor is that the "gazer's mind" is "strewn beneath" these "feet like embers, and she, thought by thought, / Trampled its fires into the dust of death" (386–88). Here the link between power and perception is obvious. Each vision, like each author who draws "new figures" on the world's "false and fragile glass / As the old faded" (247–48), comes into being by triumphing over and annihilating all that preceded it. The third metaphor, which I consider here, is that of light supplanting light. "Like day she came," Rousseau declares, treading out "the lamps of night," "making the night a dream" (390–93). The stars continue to shine during the day, but they can no longer be seen.

The *Triumph*, like many of the poems written in Italy, is structured by a "semantics of light." Just as the "shape all light" displaced the stars, it too is supplanted by the burst of "a new Vision never seen before" (411). The philosophical meaning of this continual process of enlightenment—light displacing light—need not concern us here. I want to concentrate on the way Shelley's emphasis on light is influenced by colonial medical discourse. A nineteenth-century colonial physician may not have noticed that in describing how the sun "radiantly intense / Burned on the waters" (345–46) Shelley was alluding to Coleridge's portrayal of the tropical moon in the "Ancient Mariner," "where the ship's huge shadow lay, / The charmèd water burnt alway / A Still and awful red" (269–71). Nevertheless, he would have had no difficulty recognizing that in speaking of this "light's severe excess" (424) Shelley was introducing a language normally reserved for the tropics, for over this period an extensive discourse had developed on the danger the "tropical sun" held for Europeans. By the end of the nineteenth century, as Dane Kennedy notes, the danger was believed to be so great that a new disease— "tropical neurasthenia"—entered medical terminology.[21] Foremost among those providing a theoretical description of the disease was Charles Edward Woodruff in his *The Effects of Tropical Light on White Men* (1905). Lacking adequate skin pigmentation to protect themselves from the effects of actinic (or ultraviolet) radiation, white Europeans, he believed, inevitably became neurasthenic within a year of their arrival in the tropics. The condition produced a wide range of symptoms, among them "fatigue, irritability, loss of concentration, loss of memory, hypochondria, loss of appetite, diarrhoea and digestive disorders, insomnia, headaches, depression, palpitations, ulcers, alcoholism, anemia, sexual profligacy, sexual debility, premature and prolonged menstruation, insanity, and suicide" (Kennedy, "Perils of the Midday Sun" 123). On this basis Woodruff concluded that Europeans could never become *acclimatized* to tropical climates.

During the first half of the nineteenth century exposure to tropical light was considered just as dangerous, only now it was the combined impact of heat and light on the skin and nervous system, which was believed to be the cause of fevers and debility. As in Rousseau's description of the changing effect of light on him in the *Triumph,* tropical light was deceiving. Initially it was a physiological *stimulant,* as an increase in skin secretions gave rise to a corresponding increase in liver function. "Exhilarated in mind" and in a state of "nervous excitability," James Martin suggests, the newcomer initially feels a heightened pleasure, one enhanced by the light and tropical scenery (37–38). "An elevated range of temperature" felt on "the surface of the body," he adds, "tends, along with the increased excitability of the nervous and vascular systems, to raise the animal spirits, and impart a feeling of invigoration and health delightful to the senses" (451). But such a state is only temporary, a prelude to the most dangerous of tropical illnesses: "The lengthened application of these operations of climate, which at first appeared beneficial, are sure to impair the health, and that, too often, with a termination so suddenly dangerous or fatal, as at once to shock and terrify all who behold it" (451). As an example of how quickly such changes can take place, Martin cites a report on Ensign F. in the Bengal army: "'Has been in India only three years and a few months, and has already had four separate attacks of hepatitis, two of dysentery, one of continued fever, and two severe tertian intermittent fevers, besides numerous other illnesses.'" Although this man ultimately recovered his health, Martin notes that "this officer bore the marks of his stormy career of disease" (451).

Shelley's depiction of Rousseau draws on several sources. Through one of its most famous philosophes, Shelley places the Enlightenment under critical scrutiny. Dante's technique of punishing the damned by making them allegories of their sins is also important, as is his use of Virgil as a guide through the Underworld. Of central importance here, however, is that Rousseau is also portrayed as a "colonial invalid," as someone who lost his health serving the imperial car, the "living storm." In the *Triumph,* Dante's Hell serves as a master trope for European colonial experience, and Rousseau, like any number of colonial servicemen, administrators, and settlers, is marked by the experience of having "bared my bosom to the clime / Of that cold light, whose airs too soon deform" (467–68). Rousseau's retrospective account of his participation in the "triumph" therefore has much in common with other texts recounting the experience of colonial service. Our last image of him is of a "cripple," who looks on as the car he has dedicated his life to serving disappears in the distance, leaving him behind as little more than refuse:

> the cripple cast
> His eye upon the car which now had rolled
> Onward, as if that look must be his last.
>   (544–46)

Shelley does not sentimentalize Rousseau. P. M. S. Dawson notes that Rousseau, though he was an active participant in the pageant, "loathes his own condition, and describes the fate of his erstwhile companions with no more generous feeling than fascinated horror" (265). The *Triumph* can be said, then, to be a profound study of the "psychopathology of empire," as it analyzes the combination of guilt, horror, ambition, and the devotion to an ideal that increasingly defined British colonial psychology. Rousseau does not fully understand how he has been brought "to this dread pass" (302). Having at first advised the poet-dreamer to "forbear / To join the dance" (189–90), he then urges him to join it, so that perhaps he may himself learn what has motivated him:

> But follow thou, and from spectator turn
> Actor or victim in this wretchedness,
>
> And what thou wouldst be taught I then may learn
> From thee.   (305–8)

Since in Shelley's view human beings inhabit the worlds they create, in contrast to many colonial physicians, he does not understand "the clime" that has destroyed Rousseau as being separate from his participation in the pageant. The *Triumph* not only describes *the climates of empire* it seeks to show how these unhealthy environments, characterized by extremes—of light and dark, heat and ice—came into being, replacing the healthy temperate world, the "native noon" (131), that Shelley believed existed before contemporary societies. The splitting of space into mimetic extremes, which we saw at work in Wordsworth's "The Brothers" and in De Quincey, is made the focus of the poem's critique of empire. Whereas "Ozymandias" reflects on colonial space after the fact, the *Triumph* explores its emergence. "What a world we make," declares Beatrice in the *Cenci*, "The oppressor and the oppressed" (5.3.74–75). Consider, for instance, the first simile that Rousseau uses to describe the effects of drinking the nepenthe:

> And suddenly my brain became as sand
>
> > Where the first wave had more than half erased
> > The track of deer on desert Labrador,
> > Whilst the fierce wolf from which they fled amazed
>
> > Leaves his stamp visibly upon the shore
> > Until the second bursts—so on my sight
> > Burst a new Vision never seen before.   (405–11)

Rousseau is describing more than the emergence of a new vision: a new kind of space comes into being as his mind becomes the sands of "desert Labrador." A more extreme environment—or perhaps state of mind—can hardly be imagined, especially since Shelley rids it of all signs of life.

In contrast to *Queen Mab*, where the fairy envisions a time when the climatic extremes of the colonial world will give way to a climate in which "Health floats amid the gentle atmosphere" and "No storms deform the beaming brow of heaven" (8.114–16), the *Triumph* examines the opposite process—the pathogenic fracturing of the temperate clime into colonial extremes. This explains why, as the poem progresses, the climate gets progressively colder and hotter, darker and more intensely light, *at the same time*—a climatic hybridity of an extraordinary sort. A striking example of this contradictory fracturing is the emergence of a "cold tropic sun." Early in the poem, the approaching chariot, sounding like "the South wind," is described in this manner:

> And a cold glare, intenser than the noon
> But icy cold, obscured with [ ] light
> The Sun as he the stars.   (77–79)

The chariot produces a light that blots out the sun, because it is "intenser than the noon," yet it is at the same time "icy cold." Rousseau is enslaved by the same "cold bright car," and in the passage with which I began this section, he describes how into "The thickest billows of the living storm / I plunged" (466–67). Rousseau's journey behind the triumphant car eventually takes him to a place that is a phantasmic double of the West Indies. Following the "savage music" and the dancers that evoke the link between sensuality and death so characteristic of the colonial discourse on disease, he describes how the grove

> Grew dense with shadows to its inmost covers,
>   The earth was grey with phantoms, and the air
> Was peopled with dim forms, as when there hovers
>
> A flock of vampire-bats before the glare
> Of the tropic sun, bringing ere evening
> Strange night upon some Indian isle,—thus were
>
> Phantoms diffused around, and some did fling
>   Shadows of shadows, yet unlike themselves,
> Behind them, some like eaglets on the wing
>
>   Were lost in the white blaze . . .   (481–90)

By the end the journey the morning grove has become a tropical jungle, the earth "grey with phantoms," the air "peopled with dim forms" that look like a "flock of vampire-bats," emblems of those life-denying signs or "shadows" continually thrown off by human beings in their triumph, amidst the "white blaze" of a "tropic sun": "Each, like himself and like each other were, / At first, but soon distorted, seemed to be" (530–31). Shelley represents the West Indies in gothic terms, as a horrific space of death, a cemetery haunted by ghosts. Its inhabitants are "restless apes," "vultures," and "gnats and flies, as thick as mist / On evening marshes" (493–509). In a dramatic fracturing of light, this environment suffers at once both the "glare" of a "tropic" noon and the darkness of evening beside a miasmatic swamp.

In constructing this complex literary dialogue between a colonial invalid and the dreamer who is tempted to join the progress of the car, Shelley drew on several literary sources in addition to Dante. "The Rime of the Ancient Mariner" obviously shapes this colonial encounter, as do the ambivalent dialogue between Victor Frankenstein and Robert Walton and the encounter with the pathogenic ruin of the tyrant in "Ozymandias." Another literary source, which has not been remarked, came from Shelley's close personal and intellectual relationship with Thomas Medwin. Nigel Leask has recently drawn attention to the importance of Medwin's work in establishing "a hitherto neglected link between Shelley and India" (70).[22] Shelley met Medwin in 1820, shortly after he returned from India, having served there since 1813 as a cavalry officer in the Twenty-fourth Light Dragoons. Although Medwin saw little military action in India, his health was permanently impaired. Ernest J. Lovell Jr. notes that he was listed as "'sick present' during eleven different months between June, 1814, and April, 1818" (54–55). Like many, he returned to Europe, on officer's half pay, suffering from an abscessed liver. In *The Angler in Wales* (1834), Julian (Medwin's fictional persona) is described as having arrived "from Bengal, with the brevet rank of Captain, and half a liver, to pay his devotions to Hygeia" at Bath (1: 4). Through Medwin, the Shelleys were also introduced to another retired Indian officer, Edward Ellerker Williams, whose father had served most of his life as an officer with the East India Company. His companion, Jane Cleveland Johnson (Jane Williams), whom he met in India, was the sister of General John Wheeler Cleveland of the Madras army. The Shelley circle at Pisa, during the final two years of the poet's life, was thus dominated by Anglo-Indians. In view of Shelley's close association with both Medwin and Edward Williams, there can be little doubt that he was well informed about imperial politics in India. Just as important, Shelley would have been acquainted with the medical hazards Europeans faced there, both in theory and in practice, for on 23 November 1820 Medwin suffered a recurrence of what was probably amoebic dysentery, and Shelley nursed him. Through contact with this circle, Shelley was able to recognize in a far more immediate fashion the impact of colonial power not only on the colonized, but on the minds and bodies of colonists.

Shelley's active role in revising Medwin's work and in helping him publish it is well documented. In his introduction to the collection *Oswald and Edwin,* Donald Reiman observes that "it appears that almost every poem in Medwin's volume *Sketches in Hindoostan, with Other Poems* had been criticized and corrected by Shelley" (vii). Over the course of two months, from April to May 1820, Shelley read, corrected, and commented on *Sketches,* paying special attention to "The Pindarees," a semifictional allegory of Medwin's stay in India. While reading the poem, Shelley must have experienced a feeling of déjà vu, not unlike that of the narrator of the *Triumph,* for Medwin's Indian poems, as Leask has noted, are profoundly indebted to Shelley's orientalist poetry, especially as "they adapt the male and female protagonists of *Alastor, The Revolt,* and *Prometheus Unbound* to their author's own experience of India" (160). "The Pindarees" reworks *Alastor,* representing colonial India by the Indian woman Seta, who has relinquished her community for the protagonist Oswald. "Home—parents—caste—oh deem not I repine," she declares to him, for India is now "A world of love and life to me, / A paradise while shared by thee" (64, 68). Oswald, for his part, has also given up his cultural ties, having converted to Brahmanism. Whereas others guess that his conversion is simply a means of cheating the Brahmans of their lore or a political strategy, Medwin suggests that love underlies this renunciation. Medwin's is a poetry of colonial nostalgia. Critical of both British and Indian culture, he celebrates what he perceives as the precarious ideal of colonial India, embodied in the love of Oswald and Seta. "The Pindarees" recounts the destruction of this fragile paradise through violence and disease. When the predatory Pindarees destroy Seta's village, Oswald leaves her to seek retaliation. The description of the village, where the soldiers can hardly walk for fear of slipping "on corses weltering in their crimson tide" (73), and of Oswald's march against the Pindarees constitute the poem's traumatic core. "That day of horrors ne'er shall I forget!" the narrator writes: "Though years have passed, it haunts my memory yet" (74). The march against the Pindarees produces a horrific waste of lives as some "fell by plague," others "by the sword." With a glance to his own physical condition, Medwin remarks that most "in the unequal strife / With nature lingered out the dregs of life" (76).

"The Pindarees" is an important cultural document because it is the first poem in British literature to describe the appearance of modern cholera. Medwin and Edward Williams were both serving in the Grand Army of the Marquis of Hastings when on 14 November 1817 cholera broke out among the ten thousand soldiers of his division. At least three thousand men died, among them two officers in Medwin's Twenty-fourth Light Dragoons. Hastings, in his diary, describes the horror of the march to healthier environs: "15 November. We crossed the Pohooj this morning, and encamped on its eastern bank. The march was terrible, for the number of poor creatures falling under the sudden attacks of this dreadful infliction, and from the quantities of bodies of those who died in the waggons, and were necessarily put out to make room for such as might be saved by the conveyance. It is ascertained that above 500 have died since sunset yesterday." On 22 November, when the epidemic finally showed signs of letting up, Hastings writes: "No one who has witnessed the dismay and melancholy which have lately visited our people, can comprehend my sensations on hearing laughter in the camp this morning" (qtd. in Macnamara 50–51). In 1863 Samuel Dickson, the medical officer in charge of the regiment, wrote: "Never before had I seen anything so awful as this disorder" (23).

In a note to a later version of "The Pindarees," Medwin explains that the poem is essentially an allegorical response to these events. "One march I shall never forget, it has haunted me to-day," he writes: "I was in the rear-guard, and did not get to my new ground till night, and then left eight hundred men, at least, dead and dying, on the road. Such a scene of horror was perhaps never witnessed. The disease first made its appearance among the coolies, next our servants were affected, afterwards the Sp'hees, then the European soldiers, and last the officers. . . . We lost a whole troop" (*Angler* 2: 346). Since "The Pindarees" is to some extent veiled autobiography, the impact of the march on Medwin must have been enormous. Oswald returns home to find Seta dead—all that is left of the colonial idyll is an empty urn: her dust "is all that fills his arms!" (80). The final image of Oswald essentially reworks the description of the poet of *Alastor:*

> And moon by moon slow lingering, waned away;
> And Oswald's hair turned prematurely grey;
> Grief has a hand more furrowing far than time's:
> Effects more fatal than the worst of climes;
> 'Twas this, like wax before the taper's ray,
> Made all that cheer'd existence melt away;
> Then grew his form attenuate . . . (82)

Grief is more wasting than the fevers of "the worst of climes." Oswald is portrayed as one of the walking dead, a "corpse in open day," estranged from others, knowing that the world "contains not ought beside, / A blank" (80–81). In the *Angler in Wales,* the disillusionment is clear: "The spell is broken— it was a protracted dream. . . . Call it exile—call it what you will, India was *my* country. There I had friends, a home, congenial employments—pursuits to rouse the mind to energy: here all is torpor—stagnation—death!" (1: 265).

After reading "The Pindarees" in May 1820, Shelley wrote Medwin that he found "the conclusion rather morbid; that a man should kill himself is one thing, but that he should live on in the dismal way that poor Oswald does, is too much. But it is the spirit of the age & we are all infected with it" (*Letters* 2: 189). Self-recognition must have shaped Shelley's reading of the poem, for Oswald is a Shelleyan pastiche. The *Triumph* constitutes Shelley's poetic response to Medwin's colonial nostalgia. The Rousseau of the *Triumph* is not simply a foil for Medwin, but the experience he articulates, of an ideal that has been eclipsed by a power to which he is nevertheless chained, is deeply expressive of Medwin's own colonial despair. Medwin was himself a Rousseauist, and this may have influenced his decision, while in Geneva, to rent the Maison Petit, where Rousseau was said to have lived in 1754. "If I have been extinguished," declares Rousseau, "yet there rise / A thousand beacons from the spark I bore" (206–7). Although, as I have already pointed out, the description of the imperial pageant derives from many sources, certainly one source is Medwin's description of the Hoolee festival, an orgiastic Saturnalia in which all "dance, vault wildly from the ground; / Or wheel in dizzying mazes round and round" (60). The *Triumph* describes how

> Swift, fierce and obscene
> The wild dance maddens in the van, and those
> Who lead it, fleet as shadows on the green,
>
> Outspeed the chariot and without repose
> Mix with each other in tempestuous measure
> To savage music. . . . Wilder as it grows,
>
> They, tortured by the agonizing pleasure
> Convulsed and on the rapid whirlwinds spun
> Of that fierce spirit . . .   (137–45)

Shelley also probably had in mind the festival of the Juggernaut, in which the car of Vishnu was pulled by pilgrims and was said to crush those who threw themselves in its way. In *The Curse of Kehama,* a poem Shelley knew well, Southey describes its progress:

> The ponderous Car rolls on, and crushes all.
> Through flesh and bones it ploughs its dreadful path.
> Groans rise unheard: the dying cry,
> And death and agony
> Are trodden under foot by yon mad throng,
> Who follow close, and thrust the deadly wheels along.
>   (*Poetical Works* 598)

The hybrid aspects of the pageant, as it combines Eastern festivals with the celebrations of an imperial Rome, also reads medieval descriptions of the plague across its modern, imperial equivalent—the Asiatic cholera. It owes much to Medwin's description of the march of Hastings's Grand Army. Shelley would have learned of this march not only through reading "The Pindarees" but also in conversation with Medwin and Williams. Claire Clairmont, for instance, notes laconically that the topic of conversation on 7 December 1820 was "1st Toast at the Indian Mess. A bloody war, a sickly season and a field officer's Corpse" (192). Medwin also read parts of his Indian journal to the Shelleys in November. The conventional reading of the *Triumph* as a *danse macabre* based on Shelley's knowledge of the history of the Black Death needs to be revised, therefore, to recognize how the poem responds to the first pandemic of cholera and Hastings's march through the interior of India:

> One falls and then another in the path
> Senseless, nor is the desolation single,
>
> Yet ere I can say *where* the chariot hath
> Past over them.   (159–62)

A journal entry for 16 November 1817, when the epidemic was at its height, provides a remark applicable to Shelley's *Triumph:* "Thus may it well be said of us, that 'In the midst of life we are in death'" ("Journal of the Central Division of the Army" 7).

The *Triumph* does not offer many answers. It insists, however, that Europeans need to understand their role in creating the pathogenic environments that victimize them. For Shelley despondency was not enough. One had to maintain faith in the possibility of recovering a healthful world:

> So knew I in that light's severe excess
> The presence of that shape which on the stream
> Moved, as I moved along the wilderness,
>
> More dimly than a day appearing dream,
> The ghost of a forgotten form of sleep,
> A light from Heaven whose half extinguished beam
>
> Through the sick day in which we wake to weep
> Glimmers, forever sought, forever lost.   (424–31)

Conclusion

In pointing out the close connection between Shelley's medical geography and European imperialism, I have sought to avoid the misleading idea that Shelley's writing promotes what has loosely been called "cultural imperialism." The term has been far too vaguely defined to be of much critical use. Shelley *does* speak in global terms, but to avoid such a perspective in light of the world created by colonialism would be myopic. Writing after Malthus, who claimed that disease was inescapable, a necessary consequence of the fact that population always exceeds the physical constraints placed on it by the environment, Shelley recognized that the relation between disease and the environment was of fundamental importance to any theory of reform. By understanding diseases and the physical surroundings that produce them entirely in social terms, by denying that there is anything natural about disease, Shelley shifted the focus of therapy away from the relation between medicine and the environment, away from the scientific attempt to cure these settings, toward a recognition that the primary reason one people may suffer diseases from which others are largely exempt has less to do with climate or geography than with social relationships, human behavior, and economics. Shelley shared with many nineteenth-century imperialists the idea that the world's geographies were epiphenomena that could be radically transformed through education, technology, and political change. Unlike them, however, he also recognized that such changes would be ineffectual if they increased, rather than decreased, social inequalities. As we look on the world from our modern vantage point, when the medical promise of the global elimination of many diseases has been replaced by recognition that the cost of medical technology has actually widened the gap between those who can be said to be healthy and those who are not, Shelley's attempt to go beyond a local understanding of disease, his recognition that its cause is "the root, from which all vice and misery have so long overshadowed the globe," remains one of the most important social theories of disease articulated in the nineteenth century.

Cholera, Sanitation, and the
Colonial Representation of India

On 19 November 1831 the *Lancet* published an article on "the history of the disease which has recently so deeply engaged the attention of the public and of the medical profession." "The History of the Rise, Progress, Ravages, etc. of the Blue Cholera of India" appeared at an opportune moment, for the first cases of cholera were being reported in Sunderland, in County Durham. Aimed at providing a comprehensive "geographical history" (252) of the cholera epidemic, it documents how the disease was understood when it finally reached the shores of England. The British first learned about "the outbreak of a new and terrible disorder in our Indian possessions" (241) early in 1818. They anxiously watched as it spread from the Ganges Delta across India, through Persia and Turkestan into Russia, Poland, and Austria, then on to Hamburg, whence it crossed the North Sea. William Sproat, a keelman, had the dubious honor of being its first diagnosed victim on English soil. Significantly, the *Lancet* insists that epidemic cholera is a *new disease.* By the "hurried and almost *popular* imposition" of the name "cholera" to this epidemic, "*a name* most injudiciously . . . applied to the disease," the mistaken impression was produced that it is "identical with the disease of that title familiar to the English practitioner" (241), the endemic or sporadic diarrheal disease cholera morbus or cholera nostras. A familiar name suggests a familiar disease, and the *Lancet* emphasizes that this new cholera is unlike anything the British have seen before. Even as the article acquiesces to accepted linguistic usage, referring to "the cholera" or "the blue cholera," it is far more comfortable with terms such as "the distemper," "the epidemic," or most explicitly, "*the disease,* whatever it be denominated, which has travelled from India to Europe since the year 1817" (259).

Just as significant, the article also argues that the disease is new to India. Ancient Hindu medical literature was not very helpful in clarifying the origin of the disease, though in Lower Bengal natives worshiped the goddess of cholera as Oola Beebee. Local outbreaks of a similar disease had occurred sporadically throughout India's history, at Goa in 1589, at Calcutta in 1781–82, and then two years later, at the holy city of Hurdwar, where twenty thousand pilgrims died in less than eight days. The first description of a cholera epidemic by an English physician had also been given at Madras by J. Paisley as early as 1774.[1] Duly noting these signs that cholera was endemic to India, the *Lancet* nevertheless stresses that before 1817 cholera had never *traveled* like this disease: "If cholera, identical with the present disease, did previously exist in Hindostan, it did not spread as in the present instance" (259). In *The History of the Contagious Cholera* (1831) James Kennedy agreed, arguing that though "the species of cholera to which this variety belongs" had long existed in India, in 1817 "the disease assumed a contagious property, which there is no evidence to prove it ever before possessed; and a name was then wanting to distinguish the new variety" (x). The need to deal with new maladies was not unusual during the colonial period; both colonizers and colonized regularly confronted new diseases and parasites. Epidemic cholera was significantly different, however, in that it was a new disease (or perhaps a new "variety" of an older one) for *both* colonizers and colonized. The conservative *Quarterly Review* declares: "We have witnessed in our days the birth of a new pestilence, which, in the short space of fourteen years, has desolated the fairest portions of the globe, and swept off at least FIFTY MILLIONS of our race. It has mastered every variety of climate, surmounted every natural barrier, conquered every people." An imperial age produced an imperial disease: "It has not, like the simoom, blasted life, and then passed away; the cholera, like the small-pox or plague, takes root in the soil which it has once possessed" (Macmichael 170).[2]

In light of the recent outbreak of AIDS, we are in a better position to understand the confusion and uncertainty produced by the appearance of a new disease. Epidemic cholera questioned the traditional distinction between endemic and epidemic diseases. Especially during its first fifteen years of existence, between 1817 and 1832, it was not clear how far it would spread or whether it might become permanently rooted in England. Kennedy pessimistically remarks: "Cholera may exist in every habitable part of the globe" (217). Michael Durey argues that cholera "tested received attitudes and mentalities, probed society's resources and resourcefulness, and exploited its weaknesses and shortcomings, structural, political, social and moral. Cholera accordingly offers a unique opportunity to study contextually a society under stress, struggling to comprehend and control a new factor in the environment" (2). Yet the British understanding of and response to cholera cannot be explained without reference to its global context. Cholera crossed many of the boundaries—cultural, geographical, and climatic—that were thought to exist between Britain and its colonial possessions, and by so doing it challenged those boundaries and led to their reconceptualization. It changed how the British saw themselves and their place in the colonial world. Significantly, this new understanding emerged in tandem with a new conception of India, which now was perceived as the cause, the geographical locus, and the primary exporter of a modern plague. Throughout the nineteenth century, "Asiatic" or "India" cholera competed with malaria as the "tropical disease" par excellence, and in framing an understanding of this "oriental scourge" (Rosenberg, "Cause of Cholera" 257) Europe renegotiated its relation to the "tropical world." After 1817, modern cholera was distinguished from the cholera morbus that had been common to both England and India. Framed differently, cholera was now seen as having an Indian origin. Contact with India had always had its dangers, but now they were magnified tenfold. For troops stationed there, such contact was immediate, so the dangers of cholera were paramount. Yet where did contact with India begin or end? Spread along the main transportation and commercial arteries of the nineteenth century—by river, sea, road, and later by railway—cholera mapped the many lines of communication between Britain and its colonial possessions. Its spread thus demarcated the reach of empire, demonstrating that there were no longer any boundaries.

The *Lancet* follows other contemporary accounts in placing the beginnings of modern cholera at Jessore, a city on the Ganges Delta that conformed to the assumptions of colonial medical topography: "All infectious epidemics . . . have ever emanated from tropical climates, and from the alluvial districts bounding the mouths of mighty rivers" (252). It is described as "a crowded, filthy place, surrounded by impenetrable and marshy jungles, and consequently exposed to all the horrors of a malarious and ill-ventilated atmosphere" (242). Dirty and overcrowded, situated in a marshland whose malarial qualities are exacerbated by water tanks, irrigation ponds, and the heat of the tropical sun, Jessore is portrayed as a pathogenic time bomb requiring only two years of irregular weather to "transmute" decaying vegetation into "pestilence." "Never perhaps was there, in the history of the world," the *Lancet* declares, "a more close and abundant concatenation of the causes, which transmute the decay of vegetable life into the pestilence of the living animal; and never perhaps was a malady thus produced which swept the world with more destructive virulence" (242). The *Lancet's* account of the spread of the disease from the Ganges Delta to encompass all of India proceeds in tandem with a theoretical generalizing that associates *all* of India with the pathogenic environment of Jessore. As it recounts how cholera changed from being a sporadic, *local* disease endemic to the delta and the Sunderbunds to being one of *national* dimensions, destroying over twenty million people, the *Lancet* engages in a radical epidemiological remapping of India as a human habitat: "In every soil over which it travels, it deposits the source of successive genera-tions of calamity . . . in whatever part of India it broke forth, there it seems to have deposited the seeds of new irruptions of the distemper, of which not less than two hundred instances have occurred up to 1831, in the chief cities already named" (241, 244). The history of the spread of cholera over the Indian subcontinent is thus more than the history of a disease; it also repre-sents a revision of the European understanding of the biomedical identity of modern India, the emergence of the idea that *all* of India is cholera-ridden. In this new frame, epidemic cholera is now seen as a permanent part of the Indian landscape. James Martin is typical: "The cholera epidemics which have ravaged various parts of Hindustan since 1817, have always originated *in* and issued forth *from* India, but not, to my knowledge, been imported into India by ships from infected countries. . . . It may therefore be inferred, that the cause of the disease, however latent or submerged for a time, *is never actually absent from the soil of India, or from some of its localities"* (297, emphasis added).

Although it is unnecessary to examine the *Lancet's* detailed account of the spread of cholera over the Indian subcontinent, the article does suggest that during this period India underwent an enormous epidemiological crisis.Like other colonial regions, in the nineteenth century India was a far more deadly disease environment than it had been before. Reginald Orton, surgeon to the Thirty-fourth Regiment of Foot in Madras, notes this change in the 1820 preface to *An Essay on the Epidemic Cholera of India:* "CHOLERA is well known as a disease of tropical climates and warm seasons, but, as far as our informa-tion extends, it has rarely prevailed to any great degree in this country, until the autumn of the year 1817; when it appeared in Bengal, in the form of a very peculiar and malignant epidemic, which has since extended its ravages, apparently over the whole of the immense territories under the authority and influence of the British in India. This disease has swept off a very considerable proportion of the population of India" (v). The historical factors underlying this change are not difficult to discern. R. J. Morris suggests they had to do with the rise of British colonial influence in India, notably the rise of trade and of troop movements across the whole subcontinent (21). The *Lancet* confirms this view as it draws attention to "the coincidence between the irruption of the disease in previously-uninfected places, with the arrival of ships, of caravans of fugitives or pilgrims, of individuals, and with the progress of armies" (261). For instance, the rise of British naval commerce with Bombay after 1815 is credited for the city's emergence as "a centre and point of departure for the itinerary lines, by which the cholera has advanced to the Persian Gulf, to the Mediterranean, the Caspian and the Baltic; and we may now, unfortunately, add, to the German ocean and the river Wear [i.e., Sunderland]" (246). In the East, British control of the harbors of Calcutta and Madras produced similar results.

The *Lancet* devotes considerable attention to demonstrating the close link between British troop movements and the spread of cholera across the subcontinent:

Fact 1.—When cholera appeared in the 34th regiment, on the route from Bellary to Bangalore, all the villages through which the 34th passed suffered the disease immediately afterwards, and a native soldier travelling from Bangalore to Nundedroog, at neither of which stations cholera had appeared, on passing through the camp of the 34th while the disease prevailed, was attacked and died. (261)

In another instance,

The 15th native regiment of infantry, while affected with cholera, were marched on Gooty; the villages through which it passed were immediately after desolated by this scourge, from which the inhabitants had ever before been exempt. (262)

The movement of troops provides a key to understanding not only the epidemiological unification of India, but also the spread of cholera across the globe. In 1823, for instance, "coincident with the Burmese war, and the march of our troops from sick districts in British India, the Birman empire became affected" (245). In 1831 a Cossack detachment from Koursk and the Ukraine was ordered to march on Poland: "Wherever these troops went, as they marched through the vast districts of Podolia and Volhynia, the towns and villages were infected in their order of succession from the east to Warsaw" (251). It is hardly by accident that the *Lancet* uses military metaphors to describe "this disease in its marchings and countermarchings in every direction of the compass" (244–45). Even "the great wall of China was traversed, and the inhabitants of Cocu-Coton, a town in the great desert of Cobi, were attacked" (246).

Although the *Lancet* considers cholera to be a poison produced and exported by tropical India, it follows a contagionist model in arguing that "mankind [is] the chief agent for its dissemination" (261). In delineating the "geographical history" of the pandemic, therefore, it is also mapping the contact lines of empire. This leads to an extraordinary conclusion: that nature or climate is no longer the determining factor in establishing the geographical range of the disease:

We have seen, as we followed it from clime to clime, how contemptuously it braved the opposing power of every atmospheric condition; how the burning heat of a Bengal or Molucca sun influenced its violence not more than the cold of a Moscow winter. We have found that extreme moisture, and excessive dryness, were alike unconnected with its maintenance, and still less essential to its existence, for we watched it desolating the dry and calcareous plains of Persia and the parched sands of Arabia, with the same fury that it manifested in the isles of the Indian ocean and the swampy Deltas of the Ganges, Euphrates, the Volga, and the Dnieper. Again, the preceding itinerary has more than once pointed out the remarkable fact of elevation of region affording no immunity against its rage; great chains of mountains, the Gauts, the Caucasus, Mount Ararat, and the Himalayas, having been traversed with the same violence that the malady swept the low jungle and the morass. Again, the route has shown the independence of the pestilence on any geological formation or terrestrial peculiarity, as it has traversed with equal ease the sandy plains of the Yemen, the basaltic declivities of the Mauritius and Bourbon, the steppes of Tartary, and the banks of the Euphrates, the Tigris, and Burrampooter. (252)

The spread of epidemic cholera demonstrated that colonial disease maps, based on notions of "climate" and "soil," were no longer secure, since the movements of disease were defined less by nature than by the lines of military and commercial power. In the new disease map produced by the *Lancet*, the British had little cause to feel secure:

We have traced the pestilence through 700 irruptions, and shown it ravaging nearly 2000 towns. We have seen it cutting off in Hindostan one-sixth of the whole population, in the cities of Arabia a third, in Persia a sixth, in Mesopotamia a fourth, in Armenia a fifth, in Syria a tenth, and in Russia, Poland, and Germany, a number not yet estimated with sufficient accuracy. Lastly, in the geographical route we have described we have been able to contemplate the enormous area of the disease, from the Mauritius 20°S. lat., to Archangel, 68 N.; and again from the Yellow Sea to the meridian of Greenwich. (252)

The *Lancet* displays in powerful terms the anxiety raised by the presence of "the meridian of Greenwich" in the modern disease map that the British had been instrumental in creating.

Romanticism and the New Disease Geography of India

In the opening pages of *The History of the Contagious Cholera*, James Kennedy speaks of the disappointment a newcomer feels on approaching Calcutta. "The stranger who visits Bengal, alive to the 'splendour of the East,' discovers little to gratify his expectation." Instead of the luxury, pleasure, and exoticism of a "romantic" India, a flat and monotonous region greets the eye. Kennedy nevertheless knows that this unremarkable landscape is also the cradle of epidemic cholera, and he strains to read this recent history in its silence. "Weighing anchor at day-break," the stranger "leaves the treacherous 'Sand Heads' behind him, and enters the estuary of the River Hooghly. . . . The Sun is now gathering strength, and the malarious vapours are seen coiling themselves up from the surface of the land, which presents the unbroken aspect of an endless swamp, covered with low, black, impenetrable jungle." Having reached the Diamond Harbour, thirty-five miles from Calcutta, Kennedy describes it as "the place where thousands of our countrymen have been sacrificed to marsh fever. The Company's ships, in delivering their cargoes here, send ashore many a gallant tar never to return. The malignant cholera, also, soon after its ravages were begun, travelled through the shipping at the anchorage, and carried off many victims." The "dead and dying" of recent history are nowhere to be seen in this now silent landscape, but Kennedy knows that the conditions for recurrence are still present: "These remarks, in passing, fill the stranger with a tide of mournful emotions, and evil anticipations: his home, and the expectant faces of parents, brothers, and sisters, on the one hand; his own untimely death, and their unutterable sorrow, on the other" (1–3). Anxiety now shapes the European colonist's dealings with the Indian subcontinent. "In this unhealthy region," he "discovers, sooner or later, that the source of his best enjoyment must ultimately repose on the hope of returning in independent circumstances to his native land," a desideratum that requires him to "avoid, as far as possible, the physical causes of disease" (5). In other words, get out as quickly and safely as you can.

Kennedy's somber depiction of the landscape of India is typical of the literature of the 1820s and 1830s and suggests that a substantial change took place in how India was imagined by Europeans. Compare it, for instance, with a passage from Thomas Moore's *Lalla Rookh*, published only a few months before the first outbreak of cholera:

The day of LALLA ROOKH's departure from Delhi was as splendid as sunshine and pageantry could make it. The bazaars and baths were all covered with the richest tapestry; hundreds of gilded barges upon the Jumna floated with their banners shining in the water; while through the streets groups of beautiful children went strewing the most delicious flowers around, as in that Persian festival called the Scattering of the Roses; till every part of that city was as fragrant as if a caravan of musk from Khoten had passed through it. . . . Seldom had the Eastern world seen a cavalcade so superb. From the gardens in the suburbs to the Imperial palace, it was one unbroken line of splendour. (*Poetical Works* 340)

Moore is not concerned with portraying modern India. Instead he draws on the traditional idea of India as an earthly paradise, the rich and luxurious land of spices and perfumes. In light of postcholeric representations, his mention of a city redolent with "fragrant" scents seems almost ironic, for the India that came into being during this period is not one of poetic beauty but a country of dirt, disease, and poverty. As the nineteenth century progressed, fewer writers celebrated a "romantic" India, leaving the region to be represented instead by colonial physicians, mostly Sanitarians, who saw it as an excremental space where filth, inadequate public sanitation, poverty, and overcrowding produced virulent forms of disease. In the eyes of colonial physicians, the sacred sites of Hindu pilgrimages, and most emphatically the sacred Ganges, were centers of pollution. Hindu religion was itself the problem, as James Johnson stresses in his description of a pilgrimage site: "The banks of this river present, particularly about the rising and setting of the sun, a motley group of all classes, and sometimes both sexes, sacrificing to the Goddess Cloacina, in colloquial association; not, indeed, offering their gifts in temples, but committing them freely to the passing current" (49).

By the middle of the century, when sewerage was seen as the great panacea, India provided the prototype of the colonial world. John Strachey, for instance, argues in 1864 that "the most important streets and thoroughfares of the northern division of Calcutta form to all intents and purposes a series of huge public latrines, the abominable condition of which cannot adequately be described" (qtd. in Goode 169). Major William Clemesha, in *Sewage Disposal in the Tropics* (1910), notes:

In India things are different. It must be understood that there is a certain percentage of the population in this country, who, when they are thirsty, will drink practically any water they come across. . . . The people themselves are extremely careless about the pollution of water; bathing, washing of clothes, not to mention other still more objectionable practices, are very common in village tanks, from which the people draw their daily supply. . . . An inspection of the bank in the morning shows very clearly that the foreshore is used as a latrine by the very people who rely on the river for a drinking supply. (203–5)[3]

From 1820 onward, medical representations of cholera-ridden India were increasingly structured by a single equation: people who suffer from endemic cholera live in filth. By the 1850s the meaning of filth had undergone further modification. Now cholera preyed on people who had not found the means to separate themselves from their own excrement. Cholera was a boundary issue, a sign of a people's inability to ensure that what they take into themselves is not the same as what they excrete.

Mary Douglas notes that the recognition of dirt "is never a unique, isolated event. Where there is dirt there is system" (35). Her argument that the body frequently serves as the symbolic nexus for understanding social and cultural relationships is aptly applied to representations of cholera, because the geographical difference between Europe and the tropical world was articulated in terms of the geography of the body. Take, for instance, the following description:

The climate of India tends powerfully to the production of disease within the abdominal cavity, while that of Europe tends as powerfully to production of disease within the thoracic cavity. As the two hemispheres are divided, the eastern from the western, by the meridional line so the diaphragm separates the two great cavities of the body, in one of which, the thoracic, is manifested very generally the morbid results of the Western, while in the other, the abdominal, are generally manifested the morbid results of Eastern climates. (qtd. in Scott 1: 5)

Here the diaphragm is equivalent to the "meridional line" separating the East and the West; the axis, however, is now horizontal, separating the diseases of the upper body from those of the lower stratum. Western diseases (for instance, tuberculosis) occupy the thoracic cavity while those of India inhabit the bowels (dysentery and cholera). To move from West to East is to move from the lungs to the bowels, from the soul to the body, from diseases of respiration to those of excretion, from breath to dirt. The place of the third body cavity, the cranium, in this model is clarified by James Martin when he asserts that tropical climates exacerbate both mental and abdominal disorders:

In the instance of Europeans desiring to proceed to India, or in those of officers wishing to return to their duties there, I always rest the question of their fitness to encounter the climate on the existence or otherwise of organic disease in any of the three cavities. Where, on careful examination, none such is discoverable, I determine at once that such person may proceed to a tropical climate with an average probability of enjoying health. When any considerable degree of functional disturbance is apparent, within the cerebral or abdominal cavities especially, I call for delay, and await their removal.

On the other hand, where there exists a hereditary or other disposition to morbid affections of the chest, I recommend such persons to proceed to India, as offering the best prospect of escape from a condition of disease which, in England, terminates too frequently in hopeless pulmonary consumption. (454–55)

Linked to insanity on one hand and excremental disorders on the other, tropical regions were hardly attractive, except for Europeans suffering from pulmonary complaints.

Attitudes toward cholera helped to produce and confirm this model. Tuberculosis might be seen as a "romantic" disease, which aestheticized and spiritualized its victims, even making them more sexually attractive. The Brothers Goncourt, in *Madame Gervaisais,* describe it as a disease in which the body does not get in the way: "In contrast to the diseases of the crude, baser organs of the body, which clog and soil the mind, the imagination, and the very humors of the sick as though with corrupt matter, phthisis [consumption], this illness of the lofty and noble parts of the human being, calls forth in the patient a state of elevation, tenderness and love, a new urge to see the good, the beautiful and the ideal in everything, a state of human sublimity which seems almost not to be of this earth" (qtd. in Dubos and Dubos 53). There was nothing beautiful or transcendent about cholera. Europeans were not only terrified by the speed with which it killed, but also disgusted by it. Body mass shrinks as the victim, suffering from vomiting and massive diarrhea, dies of dehydration; the skin of palms and soles becomes corrugated; victims of lighter complexions turn a blackish or bluish color, so dark, in fact, that their fingernails stand out against their skin; cramps and muscle spasms occur throughout the sickness and even after death (thus giving rise to the name "spasmodic cholera" and to stories among the working class of people's being buried or anatomized alive). Richard Evans notes: "The massive loss of body fluids, the constant vomiting and defecating of vast quantities of liquid excreta, were horrifying and deeply disgusting in an age which, more than any other, sought to conceal bodily functions from itself. . . . Cholera broke through the precarious barriers erected against physicality in the name of civilization" (*Death in Hamburg* 229).

It may be that much of the nineteenth-century emphasis on linking "civilization" to the advancement of hygiene and the spread of toilets and sewerage throughout the world was itself a response to the growing threat of diseases associated with filth—cholera, typhoid, typhus, and later polio. The intensity with which the word "civilization" is repeated almost as a prophylactic talisman against disease registers the anxiety with which nineteenth-century Europeans looked on the world they inhabited. Writers such as Mary Douglas and Julia Kristeva have suggested that feelings of disgust are not simply a response to what transgresses boundaries but also play a role in their creation. Douglas notes that "all margins are dangerous. . . . We should expect the orifices of the body to symbolise its specially vulnerable points. Matter issuing from them is marginal stuff of the most obvious kind. Spittle, blood, milk, urine, faeces or tears by simply issuing forth have traversed the boundary of the body. So also have bodily parings, skin, nail, hair clippings and sweat. The mistake is to treat bodily margins in isolation from all other margins" (121). Julia Kristeva uses the term "abjection" to describe the action by which an autonomous self is constructed as separate from the physical world that threatens it: "Loathing an item of food, a piece of filth, waste, or dung. The spasms and vomiting that protect me. The repugnance, the retching that thrusts me to the side and turns me away from defilement, sewage, and muck. The shame of compromise, of being in the middle of treachery. The fascinated start that leads me toward and separates me from them" (2). "Abjection" provides a valuable model for understanding European culture's response to the cholera pandemics. Disgust was the assertion of a boundary, both by individuals and by the state, a means by which Europeans separated themselves from the larger world of disease. The boundary was permeable, so much of the Victorian obsession with avoiding contact with dirty spaces, dirty people, and bodily dirt is an attempt to guard against incursions across this boundary. On the other side stood the world created and rejected by abjection operating on a global scale, the excremental colonial world, whose prototype was India.

Whereas the cultural construction of India as an abject other of Europe shapes much of nineteenth-century colonial literature, the primary focus of middle-class disgust and disease anxiety was directed not toward the East, but toward the British working class—the "Great Unwashed." A good deal of excellent work has been done on the impact of the 1831–32 cholera outbreak on British class relations and on the emergence of the Public Health movement.[4] Social historians such as R. J. Morris, Durey, and Evans have examined the way cholera exposed the dreadful living conditions of the nineteenth-century working class. Since this population was also believed to be the means by which epidemic cholera spread its tentacles from India into the very heart of the imperial metropolis, class relations were also refracted across colonial lines. The framing of "tropical disease" is not easily separated from the framing of the diseases of the English poor, especially since the latter were seen as the purveyors of sickness. The concept of abjection allows a more dynamic view of how cholera provided an impetus for social reform, for it implies that we need to read the "exposure" of the filthy living conditions of the poor as itself a product of middle-class anxiety and the attempt to set up boundaries against a population now considered a health threat. Disgust provided a map of middle-class disease anxieties in which the immediate danger posed by the working class and their "fever-nests" was a simulacrum of the dangers of the East.

Coleridge, Abjection, and the "Dirty Business of Laudanum"

Like the current AIDS epidemic, cholera in 1831–32 produced an epidemic of signs, as the disease intensified class anxieties that were already high in the period leading up to the passage of the Reform Bill on 4 June 1832. The framing of cholera was a public debate, much of it taking place, R. J. Morris notes, "by handbill as well as by press report and letter," where cholera produced "appeals, denials and derision" (116). Henry Gaulter went so far as to claim that the flood of handbills posted to local hoardings itself played a major role in aggravating the epidemic: "Without any adequate counterbalance of benefit, these systems committed the capital offence of setting and keeping at work, through a whole community, that agitation and fear which, as we have seen, render the human frame most capable of being acted upon by the cause of cholera. The perpetual appearance of fresh placards headed by this dreadful word—the daily parade of reports . . . all this ostentation of pestilence was most pernicious" (137). William Cobbett saw the epidemic as a fiction disseminated by health authorities, a "hobgoblin" (515) that gave them "powers wholly unknown to *English law!*" (513). He cites approvingly a placard recently posted in Lambeth:

CHOLERA HUMBUG!—Inhabitants of Lambeth, be not imposed upon by the villainously false report that the Asiatic Cholera has reached London. A set of half-starved doctors, apothecaries' clerks, and jobbers in the parish funds, have endeavoured to frighten the nation into a lavish expenditure; with the Government they have succeeded in carrying a bill which will afford fine pickings. A ruinous system of taxation, starvation, and intemperance, has been long carried on; it has now arrived at its acme, and disease is the natural result. (523)

Cobbett's view was not unjustified, for the conditions of the urban poor were so bad that this new disease, if it really existed, was the least of their worries.[5] He shrewdly recognized that fear of cholera was primarily a middle-class emotion, and that current efforts to assist the poor might stem from self-interest: "The *danger to themselves* has now awakened their compassion" (514). Nevertheless, even if the disease existed only in the *"alarming paragraphs"* (516) produced by the Board of Health, "an imaginary may be just as effectual as real pestilence" (517) if it encouraged efforts to improve conditions. Middle-class reformers, especially those of the Sanitarian movement, also hoped the epidemic might prove socially beneficial. James Kay (later Kay-Shuttleworth), in *The Moral and Physical Conditions of the Working Classes* (1832), suggests that "the ingression of a disease, which threatens, with a stealthy step, to invade the sanctity of the domestic circle; which may be unconsciously conveyed from those haunts of beggary where it is rife, into the most still and secluded retreat of refinement . . . ensures that the anxious attention of every order of society shall be directed to that, in which social ills abound" (12). Until the mid-1840s, Kay's was a minority position. Nevertheless, the consequences of the medical framing of the laboring classes as a *health threat* not only to themselves but to others were enormous. Class anxieties were now very much structured along epidemiological lines. Working-class districts—"the precincts of vice and disease" (4)—were seen as a source of continuing infection, the portals through which foreign diseases entered British society. For middle-class conservatives such as Rev. Newton Smart, not only cholera but aspirations toward democratic rights were contagious: even "pestilence" was to be preferred to "the horrors of revolution and anarchy" (382). Robert Southey thought that cholera might assist the anti-reform movement, as "a more effectual ally in aid of the Constitution" (*Selections from the Letters* 4: 230). Working-class radicals thus joined middle-class reformers in seeing the numerous proclamations of the Board of Health as part of a larger conspiracy "to frighten people out of their wits, and thus set up Cholera as the rival of Reform" ("Cholera in the Gazette").

The contemporary engraving *John Bull Catching the Cholera* (fig. 18) encapsulates the middle-class association of the politics of reform with the cholera epidemic. The broadsheet turns the anxiety of "catching" the disease into an assertion of the superiority of the British nation. Cholera, depicted as an emaciated Indian, blue from the disease, has been caught sneaking through a break in "The Wooden Walls of Old England," a conventional metaphor for the ships that linked a commercial England to the colonial world (again the source of the anxiety, maritime commerce, is transformed into a barrier). He should have known better, for two signs, one inscribed "Beware of the Bull," the other, "Board of Health," mark this territory as being guarded by nationalism and medicine. With one hand holding a club inscribed "Heart of

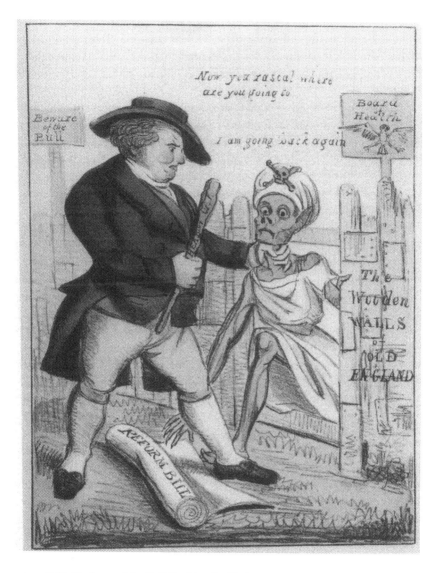

FIG. 18. D. Hodgson, *John Bull Catching the Cholera* (ca. 1832). The Wellcome Institute Library, London.

Oak" while the other grabs this outsider by the throat, John Bull asks, "Now you rascal where are you going to?" Cholera answers, "I am going back again." Meanwhile the disease reaches for the broadside titled "Reform Bill," which he apparently has brought along with him to assist in his invasion of England.

In July 1832 Coleridge entered this political fray with a poem titled "Cholera Cured Before Hand."[6] His attitude toward the Reform Bill was unambiguously conservative. Even as he believed in the need for social reform, and was critical of the degrading commercialism of the age, he feared the consequences of extending political power beyond its traditional limits. To the American H. B. McLellan he remarked that "care like a foul hag sits on us all . . . things have come to a dreadful pass with us, we need most deeply a reform, but I fear not the horrid reform which we shall have; things must alter, the upper classes of England have made the lower persons, *things;* the people in breaking from this unnatural state will break from their duties also" (*Table Talk* 1: 281–82n). In the letter to J. H. Green in which he included "Cholera Cured Before Hand," Coleridge draws out the analogy between the cholera epidemic and the politics of reform, writing: "I am jealous of the Glory of this new-imported Nabob, from the Indian Jungles, his Serene Blueness, Prince of the Air—lest he should have the presumption—for there is no bounds to the arrogance of these Oriental Imports—to set himself up in Hell against Lords Grey, Durham, & the Reform-Bill." Cholera, it appears, is likely to win more hellish followers than the reform movement, though Coleridge doubts whether "filling the Church-yard [can] be reckoned an equal service with stripping and emptying the Church!" (*Collected Letters* 6: 916).

"Cholera Cured Before Hand" is an unusual text for Coleridge because it appears to be addressed to the working class. In 1816 he had planned to write three lay sermons, addressed respectively to the upper class, the higher and middle classes, and the working class, but the last of these was never written. The poem can be seen, therefore, as a belated gesture in this direction. It is not, however, written in Coleridge's voice but instead appears under the pseudonym of a working-class reformer. The first version, signed "Demophilus Mudlarkiades" (917), suggests that the poet is both a democrat or "lover-of-the-people" and a "mudlark," a Dunciadic singer in or of dirt. "Mudlark" was slang for a hog, but also referred to people who scavenged in rivers, bays, and harbors at low water for old ropes, iron, and so on. Describing himself as "the People's, loyal Subject," he ends the poem by shouting the populist slogans:

Vivat Rex Popellus!
Vivat Regina Plebs!
Hurra! 3 times 3 thrice
repeated.—Hurra!—

The two other versions also emphasize the poet's affiliation with Catholicism
and the sovereignty of the "Plebs," but now he signs himself

Philodemus Coprophilus,
Physician prophylactic to their
Majesties, the He and She People.[7]

Here the "lover-of-the-people" is a "lover-of-dung": the poet-physician
who would claim to treat the poor also reduces them to filth and to the Yahoo
"He and She People."

As with Swift's satires, it is difficult to establish Coleridge's attitude toward
this fictional "doctor of the people." Clearly, however, the parody is directed
less toward the working class than toward its democratic pamphleteers, intimating that these people degrade those they claim to help. In a notebook
entry of 1816 he writes: "The Cobbetts & Hunts address you (= the lower
Ranks) as Beasts who have no future Selves—as if by a natural necessity you
must *all* forever remain poor & slaving. But what is the *fact?* How many scores
might each of you point out in your own neighborhood of men raised to
wealth or comfort from your own ranks?" (*Notebooks* 3: 4311). "Cholera
Cured Before Hand" undercuts working-class democratic discourse by arguing that it is itself the disease, since it produces and feeds on the degradation of
the poor, turning them into "He and She People" to justify the need for a
political cure. As Carl Woodring notes, the poem invents "a contemptible
persona as author of a transparently ironic set of verses" (229). The poem is
not patterned on literary texts, but instead parodies the deluge of "handbills"
that were produced by local health authorities as they sought to control
cholera by giving the working class information about the new disease and
how to avoid it. The title draws attention to its status as a pastiche: "CHOL-
ERA CURED BEFORE HAND: Premonitory promulgated *gratis* for the use of
the useful Classes, specially those resident in St Giles's, Saffron Hill, Bethnal
Green, &c—and likewise, inasmuch as the good man is merciful even to the
Beasts, for the benefits of the Bulls and Bears of the Stock Exchange." Coleridge provides instructions that this "premonitory" should be "so printed as
to secure a facile legibility to a current eye." He even suggests that "a number

of Copies [might be] struck off, pasted to parallelograms of Deal, and sent abroad as Placards Ambulant." By way of "attracting notice and giving authority to the thing, I would have each superscribed in red Capitals, THE BOARD OF HEALTH." To the epidemic of signs produced by cholera and the Reform Bill, Coleridge added his own politicomedical broadside.

That Coleridge did not actually publish the poem in the newspapers or as a handbill, but instead distributed it to three physicians, suggests that its real audience was not the working class or its spokespersons but the "clerisy," whom he believed should play a key role in governing the nation. With so many "ligneous" ("woody" or "mad") doctors using hoardings to give advice, "a few additional Doctor Lignums cannot fairly be complained [of]," he writes. In the letter to J. H. B. Williams, he argues that one sign of the "malignity" of cholera is that it "called into notoriety so many ligneous Doctors." He further writes that the poem was "as much activated by indignation as by philanthropy . . . at the presumptuous folly of sundry cholerophobists" (in the letter to H. N. Coleridge, they are a "herd of Cholerophilists"). Coleridge thus uses the cholera epidemic to highlight the failure of political authority that has given rise to both cholera and Reform. The poem is a tour de force pastiche, a rough parodic satire, not only of the deluge of cholera literature produced during the 1820s and 1830s but also of the "woody" authorities (both cholerophobes and cholerophiles) who were producing it.[8] In "Cholera Cured Before Hand" another ligneous doctor enters the political arena offering advice to the poor. Through him and his "iatro-gnomonic prophylactic Anthro[po]philous Doggrel," Coleridge mocks the contemporary political framing of cholera.

Coleridge was well positioned to write such a parody, for he had a substantial knowledge of contemporary medical theory and was well read in the cholera literature.[9] Accepting the consensus of contemporary physicians in the 1830s, he understands cholera to be a poison produced by the physical environment that under certain conditions can become virulent. In a letter of 24 February 1832, he suggests that the English ague, malaria, and cholera differ only as "Grades of intensity":

I think, however, that I could give the theory with an important completing adjunct, and so fill up the whole line of transit and connection from an Essex Ague thro' a Pontine Marsh-fever to the present Malignant Cholera—and explain the super-induction of the *Epidemic* on the two latter—the reason, I mean, why they are likely to be modified by aerial influences in unlucky states of the atmosphere—tho' of the three Factors of the Disease, viz. the Predisposition of the Patient, the unknown Virus, and the predisposing Circumstances, in which word I include quaecunque stant circum circa, state of atmosphere, soil, air, temperature & condition of the Habitat, &c—it is on the *first* that the *third principally* acts. (*Collected Letters* 6: 887–88)

Disease depends on the "Predisposition of the Patient" (general health, diet, age, behavior, etc.) as it is acted upon by "predisposing Circumstances" (factors such as filth, overcrowding, and lack of ventilation). During the early history of cholera, British and colonial physicians, especially those connected with the Sanitarian movement, drew many of their ideas about cholera from what was already known about the behavior of "fevers," especially epidemic typhus. Pelling notes, for instance, that under the direction of Chadwick, the Board of Health in 1848 left in doubt "whether typhus, plague, scarlatina, influenza, yellow fever, and cholera depended on peculiar and specific causes or on one common agent modified by circumstances; and then stated that, regardless of the answer to this, these diseases were all fevers, all dependent upon certain atmospheric conditions, all obedient to similar laws of diffusion, all infesting the same sorts of localities, all attacking the same classes and age groups, and all increased in severity by the same sanitary and social conditions" (64–65).[10] Referring to "virus" in its contemporary meaning as "poison," Coleridge asserts that one need not suppose "a specific *Virus* for the different diseases" (*Collected Letters* 6: 887).

Since epidemics are produced by "predisposing circumstances" acting on "predisposed populations," the premonitory is addressed to the population generally believed most likely to fall victim to it, the poor living in the "Cholera districts"—"St Giles's, Bethnal Green, Saffron Hill, &c." The hand-bill provides a typical list of dietary and behavioral recommendations:

> Pains ventral, subventral,
> In stomach or entrail
> Think no longer mere prefaces
> For Damns, Grins and Wry Faces;
> But off to the Doctor, fast as ye can crawl:
> Yet far better 'twould be not to have them at all.
>
> Now to 'scape inward aches
> Eat no plums nor plum-cakes;
> Cry, Avaunt, New Potato!
> And don't drink, like old Cato.
> Ah beware of Dis Pipsy,
> And therefore don't get tipsy!
> For tho' Gin and Whisky
> May make you feel frisky,

> They're but Crimps to D i s P i p s y:
> And nose to tail with this Gypsy
> Comes, black as a Porpus,
> The D i a b o l u s ipse
> Call'd Cholery Morpus:
> Who with Horns, Hoofs and Tale croaks for Carrion to feed him,
> Tho' being a Devil, nobody never has see'd him.

Since stomach ills (dyspepsia) were believed to predispose one to cholera, the poem recommends that the working class "Eat no plums nor plum-cakes," avoid the "New Potato," and later, beware of "Hot drams and cold Sallads." Dietary recommendations, however, express moral attitudes. Like the *Wesleyan Methodist Magazine,* which emphasized that cholera seeks out "the dissipated, dissolute, profane, and intemperate," this pseudo public health notice warns of the dangers of drink.[11] "Gin and Whisky" are "Crimps" to dyspepsia, the means by which the dissolute among the working class are forced against their will to serve "this Gypsy." Wherever she goes, cholera, described as a "black porpus" (the "hog-fish"), follows her "nose to tail."

The representation of cholera as a companion of Gypsies suggests the attitudes toward gender, sexuality, vagrancy, and colonial otherness conveyed by British ideas of this new disease. England is here shown to be threatened not by the India over there, but the "E-gyptians" who live within it, a threatening nomadic population associated with sexuality, poverty, and disease. The gypsy "Dis Pipsy" (her name, punning on "dyspepsia," "hell," and the colloquial word for a minor ailment, "pip") serves a similar purpose, since she embodies heightened middle- and lower-class anxiety about the new populations produced by colonialism—immigrants. Dr. Samuel Busey expresses the dominant nineteenth-century viewpoint: "In the cities, those direful and pestilential diseases, ship fever, yellow fever, and small pox, are almost exclusively confined to the filthy alleys, lanes, and streets, and low, damp, filthy and ill-ventilated haunts, which are exclusively tenanted by *foreigners*" (125). On 23 July 1832 the New York *Evening Post* described the local red-light district, the Five Points, as being "inhabited by a race of beings of all colours, ages, sexes, and nations, though generally of but one condition, and that . . . almost of the vilest brute. With such a crew, inhabiting the most populous and central portion of the city, when may we be considered secure from pestilence. Be the air pure from Heaven, their breath would contaminate it, and infect it with disease" (qtd. in Rosenberg, *Cholera Years* 33–34). Cholera was a disease especially associated with harbors and dockyards, places where foreign populations promiscuously associated with one another. It was here too that the "mudlarks" carried on their business, sometimes being accused of robbing ships as they unloaded their goods.

The British middle-class emphasis on women's propriety was profoundly shaped by colonial experience. Female colonists' "temperate" behavior and their greater concern for hygiene were seen as making them less susceptible than men to tropical disease. In an England increasingly worried about epidemics introduced from elsewhere, female propriety took on a new importance: it was now considered a primary means of safeguarding the health of the nation. By the 1850s, as Florence Nightingale became a cultural icon, women came to be seen as having a social responsibility to employ their virtue to defend against "foreign" disease. The first major health act to deal with contagious diseases, the Contagious Disease Act (1864), focused on prostitutes, whose "improper" behavior was now deemed not only immoral but a threat to society. Judith R. Walkowitz observes that pollution assumes a "heightened scatological significance in a society where the poor seemed to be living in their own excrement. . . . Literally and figuratively, the prostitute was the conduit of infection to respectable society" (4).[12] During the first cholera outbreak much was made of the fact that cholera seemed to have a special liking for prostitutes. Rosenberg notes that newspapers in the United States reported that "of 'fourteen hundred lewd women' in one street in Paris . . . thirteen hundred had died of cholera" (*Cholera Years* 41). The next stanza of "Cholera Cured Before Hand" draws on these concerns as it targets working-class women, the "She people" associated with the "gas-light[ed]" world of the urban metropolis and with prostitution:

> Ah! then, my dear Honeys!
> There's no Cure for you
> For Loves, nor for Moneys—
> You'll find it too true!
> Och! the halloballoo!
> Och! och! how ye'll wail
> When the offal-fed Vagrant
> Shall turn you as blue
> As the gas-light unfragrant
> That gushes in jets from beneath his own Tail:
> Till, swift as the Mail,
> He at last brings the Cramps on,
> That will twist you, like Sampson.

Mention of Samson suggests that a lower-class woman is a Delilah, the harlot ("For Loves . . . for Moneys") hired by the Philistines to betray Samson. The disgust that abjects an other is intense in this stanza, as working-class women's sexuality is seen as a threat to the integrity of the male body. "Bring the Cramps on," the speaker seems to say, as if the physical sign of a woman's sexuality—menstruation—also links her to disease and pollution; the punishment, the spasms of cholera, suits the crime. Kristeva notes that "menstrual blood . . . stands for the danger issuing from within the identity (social or sexual); it threatens the relationship between the sexes within a social aggregate and, through internalization, the identity of each sex in the face of sexual difference" (71). Sex is abjected as a sickness. "There is no Cure for you," the premonitory declares, as it takes a grotesque pleasure in the traditional language of the incurability of the prostitute. Abjection, the elimination by the self of all that threatens its autonomy, produces its own pleasures, especially as sexual anxiety is expelled violently by the speaker, "swift as the Mail" [male]. He describes how "the offal-fed Vagrant" will turn these "dear Honeys" as "blue" as "the gas-light unfragrant / That gushes in jets from beneath his own Tail." The disgust created by cholera, sexuality, and working-class women is heightened as the handbill, seeking to see into the bottom of cholera, describes the very fundament of evil. The poetics of cholera is, indeed, a poetics of filthy doggerel.

Evans has observed that in Europe the high incidence of cholera among working-class women was frequently blamed on their failure to keep their homes clean (ironically, it was through cleaning that they frequently became sick) (*Death in Hamburg* 450–65). The "premonitory" affirms this domestic ideology as it employs cholera as a demon to punish women who ignore their place in the home to seek the pleasure of the streets. Cholera is gendered as a male demon, a Samson or "Son of Sam" who "twists" his female victims, and a "Vagrant" who feeds on "offal." In this late poem of the Romantic period, the link between colonialism and vagrancy is given its darkest interpretation. Vagrants were commonly viewed as spreading cholera (among other diseases), and urban health authorities established policies to control their movement. The personification of cholera as an "offal-fed Vagrant" powerfully condenses contemporary knowledge of the link between this disease and filth, yet it also heightens readers' disgust by collapsing the distinction between food and excrement. Cholera is a dirty business that confuses the two, breaking down the boundaries that preserve the body. Yet disgust is also the means by which boundaries are reestablished. The premonitory spits out what *is not* "me" in an anxious effort to establish what *is* "me."

The final stanza turns from lower-class women to their male partners:

So without further Blethring,
Dear Mudlarks! my Brethren!
Of all scents and degrees
(Yourselves with your Shes)
Forswear all Cabal, Lads!
Wakes, Unions and Rows;
Hot Drams and cold Sallads;
And don't pig in Styes that would suffocate Sows!
Quit Cobbet's, O'Connel's and Belzebub's banners,
And white-wash at once your Guts, Rooms, and Manners.

Here the advice is explicitly political. Echoing the popular belief that white-wash was an effective disinfectant of streets and dwellings, the speaker extends this recommendation to the diet and manners of the working class: "white-wash at once your Guts, Rooms, and Manners." Edmund Burke's "Swinish multitude"—already alluded to in previous references to hogs—is given its strongest echo in the implication that the poor live worse than pigs: "Don't pig in Styes that would suffocate Sows." Unusual here is the employment of "pig" as a verb, meaning "to huddle together in a disorderly, dirty, or irregular manner; to herd, lodge, or sleep together, like pigs" (*Oxford English Dictionary*). Few words capture so powerfully how the life of the poor in cholera districts was being described. The *Ecclesiologist,* for instance, speaks of "the six-and-thirty Irish families who pig in the adjoining alley" (*OED*). As if this were not enough, these are also the people most likely to want democratic reform. To cure cholera beforehand requires that the working class "Quit Cobbett's, O'Connel's, and Belzebub's Banners." Coleridge has his Cobbett-like doctor condemn himself in his own words.

Mention of the noted Irish statesman Daniel O'Connell, who founded the Catholic Association in 1823 and succeeded in getting the Catholic Emancipation Act passed in 1829, confirms that the poem is specifically directed toward the Irish poor, an immigrant population that was often blamed for the spread of epidemics, especially typhus and cholera.[13] A contemporary reader would hardly miss the inclusion of the potato in the list of foods to be avoided. Kay believed that the Irish had taught a "pernicious lesson" to the laboring classes of England, having shown them how to survive even the meanest of social conditions: "The system of cottier farming, the demoralization and barbarism of the people, and the general use of the potato as the chief article of food, have encouraged the population in Ireland more rapidly than the *available* means of subsistence have been increased" (21). Friedrich Engels adds to Kay's list, among other things, the idea that "the Irishman allows the pig to share his own sleeping quarters. This new, abnormal method of rearing livestock in the large towns is entirely of Irish origin. . . . The Irishman eats and sleeps with his pig, the children play with the pig, ride on its back and roll about in the filth with it" (106). The recommendation that these "dear Mud-larks" forswear "Wakes, Unions, and Rows" draws attention to the wave of rioting that occurred in primarily working-class Irish districts in March and April 1832 when Public Health authorities attempted to bury cholera victims before they had been given a proper funeral. Since the Irish poor frequently needed time to find the money for a funeral and were rarely able to bury their dead until the Sabbath, when they were free from work, British public health regulations, which insisted on burial in quicklime within twenty-four hours of death (normally reserved for criminals), produced violent ethnic conflicts, especially in London and Liverpool.[14] For people whose lives were often so miserable that their one hope was for a decent burial, the middle-class insis-tence on quick interment without a wake was a focal point of resistance.

Doctor Mudlark obviously claims to speak for the working class, for he refers to his ostensible audience as "my brethren." Grammar, spelling, and crude imagery mark the handbill as a parody of working-class language and culture. Words like "frisky" or "hallabaloo" are vernacular. "Never has see'd him" not only is ungrammatical but also powerfully captures Cobbett's view that the cholera scare is humbug. Probably most disturbing is the misspelling of "cholera morbus" as "Cholery morpus," which not only links the disease to coal miners through the pun on "colliery" but also suggests that the speaker has little medical training. Most obvious to a contemporary audience would have been the frequent appearance of Scottish and Irish dialect. The Irish or Scottish exclamation "Och!" is scattered throughout this poetic handbill. "Blethering" is a Scottish word meaning senseless talk, which ap-pears in Burns's *Tam O'Shanter:* "A bletherin, blusterin, drunken blellum" (2: 55). The use of "Honeys" as a term of endearment was almost exclusively an Irish and Scottish idiom.

As in Swift's satires of the Irish poor, Coleridge's adoption of the voice of a working-class democrat was not neutral or distanced. On a general level one might note that the satire is directed against both the ruling class and the working class, one for its failure to govern effectively, the other for its asser-tion of its right to a role in government, each side deriving its claims not from religion and tradition but from rationalistic economic and political theory ("the Bulls and Bears of the Stock Exchange"). The idea of linking politics with contagion came easily to hand, for Coleridge regularly drew this anal-

ogy, as in his argument in *The Statesman's Manual* that "the histories and
political economy of the present and preceding century partake in the general
contagion of its mechanic philosophy, and are the *product* of an unenlivened
generalizing Understanding" (*Lay Sermons* 28). Yet this abstract account of
the origins of the poem does not adequately address how its vitriolic energy,
at times almost out of control, largely derives from the disgust produced by
Coleridge's adoption of the language of reform, as used by those who would
employ the cholera epidemic for political purposes. The poem is essentially
an act of abjection. Coleridge consumes the language of those he dislikes in
order to spit it out; feeding on "offal" produces the disgust that cures. The
cholera handbill is thus a form of poetic inoculation, not so much against the
miserable conditions of the working class as against the unsuitability of allowing it to play a role in governing the nation. Thus, despite his own sympathy
for working-class people, Coleridge nevertheless sees them as being *abject*. By
adopting their voice in its most degraded form (in the representations and the
words of an Irish Doctor Mudlark), Coleridge seeks to produce a social cure.
The two voices in the poem—that of the pseudonymous doctor and that of
Coleridge—in their mutual antagonism and contradiction drive the poem
forward. "As much activated by indignation as by philanthropy," Coleridge
takes into himself the abject other from whom he seeks to separate himself.

Coleridge's health during the period leading up to the passage of the
Reform Bill further complicates the interpretation of the poem. Oddly, one
of the most popular remedies of the period—opium—is missing from his
handbill. Since one of the first signs of cholera was a "premonitory diarrhea,"
physicians often prescribed laudanum as an antidiarrheal to stop its progress.
The following notice posted by the Central Health Board of London in 1832
is typical:

Cholera Districts.—Looseness of bowels is the beginning of cholera; thousands of
lives may be saved by attending in time to this, a complaint which should on no
account be neglected by either old or young. In places where the disease prevails,
when cramps in the legs, arms, or belly are felt, with looseness or sickness at the
stomach, when medical assistance is not at hand, three tea-spoonsful of mustard-
powder, in half a pint of warm water, or the same quantity of warm water with as
much common salt as it would melt, should be taken as a vomit, and after the stomach
has been cleared out with more warm water, 25 drops of laudanum should be taken in
a small glass of any agreeable drink. (Cobbett 520–21)

There can be little doubt that Coleridge knew about the anticholeric aspects
of opium, for in the Crewe manuscript he indicates that "Kubla Khan" was

"composed, in a sort of Reverie brought on by two grains of Opium, taken to check a dysentary, at a Farm House between Porlock & Linton" (*Complete Poems* 525). Addicted to opium most of his life, the poet had had many lessons in its antidiarrheal powers.[15] On his return from Malta, he was so constipated that he resorted to asking the captain to use an instrument specifically designed to remove the obstruction in his bowels. On 18 November 1811 he writes that "Truly for 8 days together the Trunk of my poor Body was or seemed to be a Trunk which Nature had first locked, and then thrown away the Key" (*Collected Letters* 3: 347). On 14 May 1814 he remarks: "I used to think St. James's Text, 'He who offendeth in one point of the Law, offendeth in all,' very harsh; but my own sad experience has taught me it's aweful, dreadful Truth. . . . I have in this one dirty business of Laudanum an hundred times deceived, tricked, nay, actually & consciously LIED" (3: 490). In "Cholera Cured Before Hand," he appears to have been caught between two kinds of dirtiness—opium and cholera. Both were Eastern imports, both caused a loss of self-control, and both were understood as poisons that attacked the bowels, one causing constipation, the other extreme diarrhea. Thus, even as the poem participates in the public debates connected with Reform, which Coleridge not surprisingly refers to as a "huge tape-worm *Lie* of some 3 score & ten joints" (6: 902), it is also a culminating personal statement about more than thirty years of what the poet described as "intestine Conflict" (6: 589).

This conflict came to a crisis in the months just before passage of the Reform Bill. Over the previous decade, in addition to ongoing bronchial problems and erysipelas on the legs, Coleridge had suffered from an "all-absorbing Bowel-Complaint" (*Collected Letters* 6: 845). As if the East and the West were fighting it out for control of his body, whenever the bowel problem subsided, that of the bronchial tubes would reappear. "As my intestinal Canal has subsided into a Calm," Coleridge writes, "the Bronchia have set to work, all hands or glands rather, in the production and excretion of phlegm" (6: 870). In October 1831, just as the epidemic was gaining a foothold in England, Coleridge believed he had suffered a "retrocession of the morbid action to the intestinal Canal in a type resembling Cholera" (6: 874).[16] In February 1832, after eating two pork chops, he had an almost fatal bout of diarrhea: "From Noon till past six o'clock I never *once* sate down, but continued pacing to the tune of my own prayers & groans from the window of my own to that in the Room opposite" (6: 886). He probably did not actually contract epidemic cholera (though this possibility cannot be dismissed). Nevertheless, in a context in which the difference between modern cholera and the cholera morbus was not clear, his belief that the widely publicized epidemic was repeatedly victimizing him was not unreasonable.

Coleridge was also seeking at this time to be rid of his opium dependency even though his physician, James Gillman, warned against the effort, given his diarrheal state and the prevailing epidemic. In a letter to J. H. Green on 23 March 1832, Coleridge expresses his ambivalence in striking terms: "By the mercy of God I remain quiet; and so far from any craving for the poison that has been the curse of my existence, my shame and my *negro-slave* inward humiliation and debasement, I feel an aversion, a horror at the imagining: so that I doubt, whether I could swallow a dose without a resiliency, amounting almost to a convulsion" (*Collected Letters* 6: 892). Here the addiction to opium is described as a "curse," "shame," "humiliation," and "debasement." As someone who justifiably claimed that he had been "an ardent & almost life-long Denouncer of Slavery" (6: 940), Coleridge's suggestion that these feelings make him like a "negro-slave" derive from a deep sympathy for the oppressed. One month later, at a time when it appeared that he had indeed conquered his addiction, he speaks of the miracle of "a sudden emancipation from a 33 years' fearful Slavery" (6: 901). Nevertheless, it is also obvious that the "slave" represents a state of abjection that Coleridge was seeking to surmount. The situation where he found himself unable to let laudanum pass his lips, his feeling that he would vomit if he were to allow it to enter him, verges on the condition Kristeva calls the "abjection of self": that moment when the subject discovers that what it denies "constitutes its very *being, that it is* none other than abject" (5). Opium was a figure of his own abjection, his own unwilling participation in the dirtiness of life. In rejecting laudanum, therefore, Coleridge was seeking to reassert his own autonomy by separating his own abject, enslaved self from the others that embodied this abjection.

Yet as he rid himself of one Eastern poison (laudanum), the other Eastern poison (cholera) took its place. The abjection of one "new-imported Nabob" allowed the entrance of another. Less than a week after first announcing his decision to renounce opium, Coleridge writes that he continues to suffer from "a sad trial of intestinal pain and restlessness; but thro' God's Mercy, without any craving for the Poison, which for more than 30 years has been the guilt, debasement, and misery of my Existence" (6: 894). Despite this apparent improvement, however, a dramatic change appears simultaneously to have been taking place in his outward appearance, or at least in how he saw himself. Gillman assured him that he was healthier, but "when I look at myself in the Glass, I see almost the contrary." Harriet Macklin, a servant, confirmed his opinion, for when she saw him she exclaimed, "Sir! your face has not the same expression of Pain, Anxiety, and the being worn out by pain; [but] it is yellower, or brown and yellow, m[ore] than I have ever seen it" (6: 892). As Coleridge struggled to emancipate himself from the slavery of opium, his body seemed to be making him more like a "negro-slave."

On 17 May 1832 Coleridge suffered another bout of cholera. His health seemed improved, and he had enjoyed an afternoon in "high spirits" demolishing "a large number of incendiary 1 / 2d & penny flying sheets" supporting the Reform Bill and eulogizing Lord Grey, when, like the keelman William Sproat, he ate a mutton chop, which had an effect on his system equivalent to a "narcotic poison" (6: 907). Gillman prescribed morphine and mercury. Salivation occurred, but then Coleridge's head began to swell. "I will answer for it," Coleridge writes to J. H. Green, "that out of the foul Ward of a Hospital even you have never seen a Head so swoln, or a physiognomy so frightfully deformed as that of your poor friend at this moment. I have very nearly lost the voluntary power of ejecting the mucus from my Throat—& as to eating, it is impracticable. . . . I do not feel the slightest wish or craving for the Laudanum; nor do I believe, that it would even alleviate my sufferin[g]s. But yet I grieve for the too apparent failure of the experiment" (*Collected Letters* 6: 908). No longer able to eat or to expel phlegm, Coleridge seems to have gained mastery over opium at the cost of losing control over the upper part of his body and seeing his head become monstrous. The next day he provides a clearer picture of his physical appearance. His brother James came to visit him, but Coleridge refused him admittance. "I would not expose him to the fatigue of getting out of his Carriage, & climbing 5 flights of Stairs, in order to behold a Mask of Syphilis, as a Venus *sub* Medicis et Mercurio, when he had expected to see the Son of his Father" (6: 909). Coleridge's likeness to his family has disappeared, nor is it even clear any longer that he is male. Instead of seeing the "Son of his Father," James would have encountered the face of a syphilitic woman taking mercury. The poet's assertion in "Cholera Cured Before Hand," "my dear Honeys! / There is no Cure for you" would thus have had a deeply personal meaning for Coleridge, who only months before had seen himself as inhabiting the body of a syphilitic, cholera-ridden prostitute. By 10 June the poet's condition had improved. The "Virus Hermaphroditicum" was on the wane. His gums were no longer like "hillocks of sponge," the "bigness" and "aching" of his head had diminished, the salivation had stopped, and his breath was no longer fetid. He writes that now, when he looks in the mirror, "I no longer behold in my glass a Hottentot Venus sub medicis, with the characteristic Feature transplaced" (6: 913). Whether one sees Coleridge's illness as physical or psychological, it nevertheless suggests that he believed he had undergone the state of abjection that he associated with slavery and the working class. In "The Hottentot and the Prostitute," Sander Gilman suggests that nineteenth-century notions of female sexuality were read across the iconography of race, prostitution, and disease as European doctors, searching for physical signs of sexual deviancy in blacks and prostitutes, associated the "Hottentot Venus" Sarah Bartmann's characteristic feature, her protruding buttocks or steatopygia, with excessive sexuality. In an even stranger contribution to the psychopathology of disease, Coleridge outdoes Bartmann, seeing himself not only as a Hottentot Venus but as one whose buttocks have been transplanted to his face. In a situation in which the physicality of the lower stratum seems to have displaced his head and face, Coleridge has only to look in the mirror to see into the bottom of cholera—its link to dirt, slavery, blacks, and sexuality. "Cholera Cured Before Hand," written six weeks after Coleridge had recovered from this illness, is in many ways a highly personal document of his response to the shocking events taking place not only in the nation but in his personal life. In *Confessions of an English Opium Eater,* De Quincey magnified his own struggle with opium into an epic battle between East and West whose locus is the opium eater's imagination. In the 1856 revision of the *Confessions,* he even argues that opium has a "national value" inasmuch as it can delay the onset of "the great English scourge of pulmonary consumption" (209, 135). By assuming an Asian body, the opium eater is safeguarded from "our English hereditary complaint," but by so doing he loses the power of his mind to direct his body, falling under "the mortal languor of a relaxing disease" (102). In the phantasmic and unstable doublings of both his poem and his life, Coleridge fought a similar battle on multiple terrains: East/West, male/female, Irish/English, black/white, middle class/working class, lungs/bowels. As a poem that ultimately addresses the question of government, a subject that for more than thirty years had been a source of personal embarrassment for the poet, his pastiche of a working-class medical text constitutes a complex articulation of a special kind of middle-class hybridity, which struggles with feelings of dependency and vulnerability by abjecting them onto others. Having only just gained control over opium (thus allowing him to govern himself), and having recently inhabited a body that he would have excluded from universal suffrage, Coleridge must have wondered what else the conflict between his bowels and opium had in store for him.

"Tropical" England

> The great mass of the metropolitan community are as
> ignorant of the destitution and distress which prevail in
> large districts of London . . . as if the wretched creatures
> were living in the very centre of Africa.
> —James Grant, *Lights and Shadows of London Life*

The important role that Anglo-Indian physicians played in providing information on the characteristics and origins of cholera is well known.[17] Comparisons drawn between the conditions of the poor in India and those of the urban working class in England influenced how the British responded to cholera. Just as important, the British experience of cholera, in 1831–32, 1848–49, 1853–54, and 1866, also shaped how India came to be seen. There was a mutual refraction of colonial and metropolitan medical theory. The framing of "tropical disease" was thus not easily separated from the framing of the diseases of the urban poor, especially since that group was seen as the means by which the tropical or foreign diseases traveled into the very heart of the metropolitan city. The pathologizing of the urban working class occurred in tandem with the pathologizing of colonial peoples. Cholera has long been seen as the disease that brought the conditions of the working class to the attention of British public health authorities. Charles Greville, for instance, remarks that through the establishment of health boards "much of the filth and misery of the town will be brought to light, and the condition of the poorer and more wretched of the inhabitants can hardly fail to be ameliorated. The reports from Sunderland exhibit a state of human misery, and necessarily of moral degradation, such as I hardly ever heard of" (2: 20–21). At the same time as the British were discovering the dangers posed by colonial contact with the tropical world, they were also discovering the miserable conditions of the urban poor. As both populations simultaneously emerged as "health threats," the framing of each was refracted through the other. Rev. Newton Smart suggests the anxieties that were raised by the discovery of their similarities: "For several months it [cholera] had been creeping about the north, selecting for its prey the victims of intemperance and filth, of poverty and despair. And now it has appeared in the vast suburbs of London, inhabited, as they *partly* are, by perhaps the most destitute population on earth" (375). Smart contends that the "vast suburbs" of London, more impoverished than a Calcutta or a Bombay (both colonial cities built by the British), are likely to provide an ideal environment for the spread of the epidemic. In the literature of the 1830s, there is a mutual mirroring of the conditions of the urban working class and those of India: the "fever-nest" becomes a little piece of India in the heart of the colonial metropolis, while India increasingly appears as one vast "fever-nest," a subcontinent characterized by "filth . . . poverty, and despair."

Although Edwin Chadwick's *Report on the Sanitary Condition of the Labouring Population of Great Britain* (1842) is almost exclusively devoted to describing the pathogenic aspects of Britain, it too draws on the analogy between urban and colonial conditions. After describing the horrible state of the poor in the Mexican province of Guanaxuato, where the population is "half clothed, idle, stained all over with vices; in a word, hideous and known under the name of *leperos,* lepers," and pointing to the filthy conditions that make Alexandria "a seat of pestilence," Chadwick argues that people "are much mistaken who imagine that a similarly conditioned population is not to be found in this country; it is found in parts of the population of every large town; the description of the Mexican populace will recall features characteristic of the wretched population in the worst parts of Glasgow, Edinburgh, London, and Bath, and the lodging-houses throughout the country" (246–47). In fact Chadwick likens the city to a permanent barracks, except that by the 1840s the health conditions of the latter had improved significantly: "The towns whose population never change their encampment, have no such care, and whilst the houses, streets, courts, lanes, and streams, are polluted and rendered pestilential, the civic officers have generally contented themselves with the most barbarous expedients, or sit still amidst the pollution, with the resignation of Turkish fatalists, under the supposed destiny of the prevalent ignorance, sloth, and filth" (117). Rather than accepting disease, as they supposedly do in the East, he urges public health officers to follow the lead of colonial military physicians in actively improving city environments. The Sanitarian movement, one might argue, derived much of its authority from its transference of colonial medicine to the metropolis. In this context it is useful to recall the passage from Thomas Southwood Smith's *Treatise on Fever* that I cited in chapter 1, where he writes that "the room of a fever-patient, in a small and heated apartment in London, with no perflation of fresh air, is perfectly analogous to a stagnant pool in Ethiopia, full of the bodies of dead locusts. The poison generated in both cases is the same; the difference is merely in the degree of its potency." For Smith poverty mirrors the tropical environment: "Nature, with her burning sun, her stilled and pent-up wind, her stagnant and teeming marsh, manufactures plague on a large and fearful scale: poverty in her hut, covered with her rags, surrounded with her filth, striving with all her might, to keep out the pure air, and to increase the heat, imitates nature but too successfully; the process and the product are the same, the only difference is in the magnitude of the result. Penury and ignorance can thus at any time, and in any place, create a mortal plague" (364). The "fever-nest" is thus a social replication of tropical nature, a special kind of pathogenic microclimate that had emerged in manufacturing cities.

Alongside the "fever-nest," which is only the most extreme form of an increasing fear of the urban environment itself, one should also place the *factory* as a place increasingly associated with the tropics. In Coleridge's *Pamphlets on Children's Labour* the analogy is not fully developed, but it is implicit in his arguments about the long-term health impact of demanding that children stand "from thirteen to fifteen hours, in a foul air artificially heated" (*Shorter Works and Fragments* I: 716). At one point, to criticize the tendency of its supporters to speak only of the health of children at present working in a given factory, Coleridge draws a colonial analogy: "This is about as fair as it would be to decide on the healthiness of a Surinam Swamp by the number of slaves alive at any one moment, without distinguishing the new importations and without striking the balance between those who had perished and those who had stood the seasoning" (735). By the middle of the century, the analogy was commonplace. In Thomas Carlyle's *Latter-Day Pamphlets* (1850), British "industrial existence" is portrayed as "one huge hideous poison-swamp of reeking pestilence physical and moral." Carlyle sees the world produced by industrialism as another kind of colonialism, as pernicious as the systems in the West Indies and Ireland. "Between our Black West Indies and our White Ireland," he writes, "between these two extremes of lazy refusal to work, and of famishing inability to find any work, what a world have we made of it, with our fierce Mammon-worships, and our benevolent philanderings, and idle godless nonsenses of one kind and another!" (23–24).

Throughout the 1830s and 1840s, especially in the report of the Factories Enquiry Commission of 1833, the factory is frequently portrayed as an artificially produced tropical environment. Engels argues that by working in "the unwholesome atmosphere of the factories," which is "generally both damp and warm—usually warmer than is necessary," the "whole vitality of the worker is sapped, and this undermines his general physical condition as well as causing specific ailments" (174–75). A fear emerged that manufacturing operatives were physically and morally degenerating under these new conditions. It was believed that heat and the monotonous labor produced a host of bodily ailments, a general lassitude of the system, premature aging, stunted growth, and premature or excessive sexual activity. Speaking in the

House of Commons on 15 March 1844, Lord Ashley remarked that "if the present system of labour be persevered in, the county of Lancaster will speedily become a province of pigmies" (179n). Dickens's description of Coketown in *Hard Times* (1854) draws a similar tropical analogy. His first description of the town emphasizes its savage nature: "It was a town of red brick, or of brick that would have been red if the smoke and ashes had allowed it; but as matters stood it was a town of unnatural red and black like the painted face of a savage" (17). Later, colonial India provides the appropriate analogue for this new kind of urban space. "The atmosphere" of the mills, he writes, "was like the breath of the simoom: and their inhabitants, wasting with heat, toiled languidly in the desert." Dickens portrays the operatives as a desert people, who inhabit conditions no less poisonous than the hot air of the "simoom." Furthermore, the weather never changes. Describing the machinery of the mills, he declares that "no temperature made the melancholy mad elephants more mad or more sane. Their wearisome heads went up and down at the same rate, in hot weather and cold, wet weather and dry, fair weather and foul." Instead of the "summer hum of insects," the people of Coketown hear "all the year round . . . the whirr of shafts and wheels." When the sun does shine on Coketown, it produces the same fevered results as in the tropics. In such a pathogenic place, the sun is more dangerous than the frost; rarely does it look "intently into any of its [Coketown's] closer regions without engendering more death than life" (85).

There was also concern about what impact the factory might have on the sexuality of female operatives. In the early obstetrical manuals, it was generally believed that climate and morals had a significant effect on women's sexual development. Michael Ryan, for instance, summarizes conventional wisdom in his *Manual of Midwifery* (1841) when he remarks that "the eruption, or first appearance of the menstrual discharge or catemenia, generally occurs, in temperate climates, from the twelfth to the sixteenth year; in the meridional nations, from the eighth to the twelfth year; and in the polar regions, from the fifteenth to the twentieth year" (66). During the 1830s it was feared that the heat and immorality of the factory might have a similar effect on female operatives: "Heat has a considerable influence in bringing animals, as well as plants, to premature maturity. In the cotton mills of Manchester and Glasgow, and in many manufactories, which are kept at high temperatures, girls arrive early at a state of puberty" (60).[18]

In a chapter titled "Influence of Temperature and Manners upon Physical Development, &c., and upon Morals," Peter Gaskell suggests that the factory environment tropicalizes women's bodies: "The crowding together numbers

of the young of both sexes in factories, is a prolific source of moral delin-
quency. The stimulus of a heated atmosphere, the contact of opposite sexes,
the example of lasciviousness upon the animal passions—all have conspired to
produce a very early development of sexual appetancies. Indeed, in this respect, the female population engaged in manufactures, approximates very
closely to that found in tropical climates" (68–69). In 1844 Leon Faucher
cites Gaskell almost verbatim. By bringing "so many men, women, and
children together," he argues, "without any other object than Labour, there is
full scope for the birth and growth of passions which eventually refuse to
submit to constraint, and which end in unbridled license. The union of the
sexes, and the high temperature of the manufacturies, act upon the organisa-
tion like the tropical sun; and puberty is developed before age and education
have matured the moral sentiments" (46). The heat, crowding, and absence of
moral restraints in manufactories were producing tropical bodies and passions, and these were being assisted by the heavy use of opium among the
working class. Precocious sexual development was seen as a dangerous form
of sexual dysfunction, affecting women's capacity to reproduce. After also
noting that "the factory has the same effect as a tropical climate," Engels adds
that "in both cases nature revenges herself on precocious physical development by premature old age and debility" (183).

Reflecting the fears that were increasingly shaping colonial discussions of
the sexuality of British women in India and Africa, Engels then suggests that
the factory also produces the countereffect of "retarded physical development
among young women. . . . [T]he breasts mature late or not at all. Menstruation often does not begin until the seventeenth or eighteenth year, and occasionally is even postponed to the twentieth year. Often it does not occur at all.
Medical evidence is unanimous that girls in factories suffer from irregular
menstruation, coupled with great pain and various disorders, such as anaemia, which is particularly common" (183–84). In the context of a medical
geography that associated health with temperate states of the environment
and morals, the extremes of the factory—its physical and moral intemperance—manifested themselves in dysfunctional sexualities, in precocious sexual activity combined with premature aging, on one hand, or in reproductive
sterility on the other. Factories constituted a new and threatening urban
environment, a tropical microclimate situated within the temperate landscape
of England. Here British women were orientalized, becoming either a savage, sexualized hybrid race or its opposite, the anemic female whose reproductive capacity was fragile under the onslaught of tropical heat. Critics of
the factory system were in no doubt where, in Ann McClintock's phrasing,

the "porno-tropics" (21–24) were located; they were to be found in the English manufactories that were appearing everywhere in England.[19]

Looking at the recent rapid emergence of industrial centers in England, William Farr in his *Report on the Mortality of Cholera in England, 1848–49* (1852) drew an ominous comparison with the topography of the colonial world. Arguing that all plagues originate in the degenerative environments of colonial coastal lowlands, in cities built in the miasma-ridden atmospheres of the deltas, Farr concluded that the recent epidemic was a providential warning that by moving from the healthy rural and elevated environments (the equivalent of the hillside station?) that had fostered their strength as a people, the British were following the same path that had led to the degeneration and destruction of previous empires.

A large proportion of the population of England is now in the low seaports, manufacturing towns, and cities. . . . In addition to the inhabitants of the old towns, which have always been fatal, several millions of people are now in the seaports, in South Wales, in Staffordshire, in the mining districts of the north in the towns of the West Riding of Yorkshire, and in the dense districts of Lancashire; where the health of parents is depressed, and the circumstances are often so prejudicial to their offspring that of the coming generation five instead of two of every ten born are destroyed in the first five years of life, and the survivors, with a few happy exceptions, are left with shattered, feeble, febrile, and disorganized frames. The countenance of the children is painful in these districts; and in all the places where cholera has raged, presents the most striking contrast to the healthy, hardy aspect of the children in salubrious fields. (xciv–xcv)

Farr concludes that an urbanizing England is following the same path that led to the destruction of the great empires of the past—"the history of the nations on the Mediterranean, on the plains of the Euphrates and Tigris, the deltas of the Indus and the Ganges, and the rivers of China" (xciii). For Farr, the English were fast becoming a population of lowland coastal dwellers, crowded together in an atmosphere that weakened their constitutions and shortened their lives—and "no race of men, living in maremmas, marshes, deltas, low sea-coasts, low river-sides, could have acquired or wielded the Power of this Empire" (xcv).

The pathogenic framing of India provided the lens through which the British saw themselves. In this regard, it may be worthwhile to return to James Johnson's comments in the appendix to the British House of Commons *1828 Report of the Commissioners on the Supply of Water to the Metropolis.* Characteristically, he evaluates London's water supply by reference to India.

"We sneer at the delicacy of the Hindoo who slakes his thirst at the same tank where his neighbour is sacrificing to Cloacina; but what shall we say to the delicate citizens of Westminster, who fill their tanks and stomachs, with water from the Thames, at that very spot into which one hundred thousand cloacae, containing every species of filth, and all unutterable things, are daily disgorging their hideous and abominable contents?" Here the disgust produced by the lack of sanitation in India falls far short of the excretionary horror of London's water system. In the final analysis it is London, not India, that is the embodiment of a pathogenic environment. Johnson is astonished that "in these days of refinement, and in a metropolis whose inhabitants pride themselves on delicacy and cleanliness, a practice should obtain, at which posterity will shudder, if they can credit it. We do not believe that a parallel instance of bestial dirtiness can be cited from any part of the globe" (140).

Tropical Invalids

"There was yet a visit to the Doctor" (14). With these words, Marlow introduces the last requirement of his new employers before he can travel to Africa
in Joseph Conrad's *Heart of Darkness*. While waiting for the doctor to arrive,
he has a drink with a shabby company clerk. Over conversation that mainly
"glorified the Company's business," Marlow shows surprise "at him not
going out there." The clerk's blunt reply, "I am not such a fool as I look," says
much about the imperial ideal at the end of the nineteenth century. The
medical examination is no less discomfiting. First Marlow's pulse is checked.
"Good," the doctor says, but he follows it up with the ominous, "Good for
there." He then asks to measure Marlow's skull. "I always ask leave," he
declares, "in the interests of science, to measure the crania of those going out
there. . . . I have a little theory which you Messieurs who go out there must
help me to prove." By now, those who colonize have become as much the
object of scientific curiosity as the colonized. The focus of the doctor's study
is madness, specifically the "mental changes" that white colonists undergo in
the tropics. "Ever any madness in your family?" he asks. This kind of study
should be done "on the spot," but the doctor also knows the dangers. Naively,
Marlow asks whether he measures the employees' craniums "when they
come back too." "I never see them," he evasively replies, adding moreover
that "the changes take place inside, you know." Like Lamb joking about the
likelihood of Joseph Ritchie's ever returning from Africa, the doctor enjoys
his own brand of colonial humor, smiling "as if at some quiet joke." His
parting advice encapsulates the contemporary wisdom concerning the danger of tropical environments: "'Avoid irritation more than exposure to the
sun. Adieu. . . . In the tropics one must before everything keep calm.' . . . He
lifted a warning forefinger. . . . 'Du calme, du calme. Adieu'" (15).
   Although Marlow returned, others were not so lucky. James Martin recounts a typical case. "A gentleman of the civil service," he writes, "came

home after twenty years' residence in India, on private leave, not being considered sick. He arrived in October, and early in the following month he made a journey of four hours on a railway, with the window open. The lung next the window became that night completely engorged; and owing to the impoverished condition of the blood, and to the deficient powers of the system, the substance of the lung rapidly filled with serum. He died in a few days" (460). Colonial medical literature is replete with similar accounts of individuals who returned with their health ruined only to find that they no longer could survive the British climate. These were the "climate-struck," those whose colonial experience had made them "morbidly sensitive to all the changes of season" (461). Removed for too long from the tempering qualities of northern environments, their bodies had lost the capacity to adapt to change. For them a "change of air" no longer allowed a health-giving recovery of their original constitutions. Now it killed.

It is unnecessary to compound instances.[1] As Britain committed more people to the settlement, administration, and military control of tropical regions, more and more returned as invalids. Over the course of the nineteenth century, R. S. Mair observes in 1871, a predictable pattern had developed: "The young man proceeding to the East, was expected as a matter of course to return home, if he ever did return, a sallow, yellow coloured, emaciated invalid, with his liver sadly damaged, his mental energies and nervous system much enfeebled, and his constitution generally so shattered, as to render him unfit for any social intercourse or enjoyment" (213). Early in the century James Johnson coined the term "tropical invalid," being one himself. He also argued that special medical precautions were necessary if such people were to survive their native climate. He writes: "The powers of the constitution, however plastic, cannot immediately accommodate themselves to great and sudden changes of climate, even when the transition is from a bad to a good one; and the tropical invalid requires full as much caution and prudence in approaching the shores of England, as he did in landing at a former period, on the banks of the Ganges" (556). In the tropical invalid, nineteenth-century medical literature produced a unique condition, a new kind of colonial subjectivity, with specific medical problems and requirements. Such figures might seem to be part of the general literature of nineteenth-century invalidism. Diane Price Herndl and John Wiltshire have both noted that invalidism had become fashionable among the gentry. Wilde, in *The Importance of Being Earnest*, satirizes its popularity when Lady Bracknell, exasperated by the continuing ailments of the fictional Bunbury, complains: "Well, I must say, Algernon, that I think it is high time that Mr Bunbury made up his mind whether he was going to live or to die. This shilly-shallying with the question is absurd" (1.331–33). Whereas invalidism could be seen as a sign of refinement, especially when linked to consumption or nervous complaints, the literature on tropical invalids presents a much darker reflection on the epidemiological consequences of colonialism. In talking about these people, whose bodies registered in very personal terms the medical consequences of migration to tropical regions, European medicine addressed fundamental questions about the relation between biology and colonialism, seeing in these ruined bodies a dark allegory of imperial ambition and its limits.

Although the risks of an extended stay in tropical regions occasioned anxiety throughout the eighteenth century, it was generally believed that if Europeans could survive their first year they would become "seasoned" or acclimatized to the environment. Lind believed that "by length of time, the constitution of Europeans becomes seasoned to the East and West Indian climates, if it is not injured, by the repeated attacks of sickness, upon their first arrival." He therefore concluded that "Europeans, when thus habituated, are generally subject to as few diseases abroad, as those who reside at home" (*Essay on Diseases* 154–55). The 1813 publication of Johnson's *The Influence of Tropical Climates on European Constitutions,* however, increased doubts that Europeans could successfully adapt to new climates. Doctors began to speculate on a progressive deterioration of the European body in tropical regions. In 1821 Henry Marshall (who later served as chairman of the 1838 parliamentary inquiry on military deaths and invalidism) writes that in Ceylon most Europeans "undergo some change, both in their physical and mental functions. . . . Many of them soon sustain a deviation, more or less, from sound health, accompanied with a certain degree of emaciation. The skin loses the ruddy hue of robust health, and assumes a pale yellowish shade: moderate exercise becomes fatiguing, and the mind indisposed to much application" (*Notes on the Medical Topography* 74). By 1828 James Annesley is contending that a person who migrates to another region is like an "exotic" plant that has been "as it were, transplanted from the air and soil from which he has been, in a measure, formed, and in which he has longer vegetated." Here environmental medicine and early biogeography combine with an emergent racialism to suggest that "the European is constituted in a manner the best suited to the climate which he inhabits; and a similar conformation of the system of man to the circumstances of the country, may be traced in every part of the globe." Given the conformity between physical environments and human biology, Annesley concludes that when "man migrates from the climate which contributed to generate the peculiarities of his frame, to one which is remarkably different from that to which he is assimilated, then disorders of various kinds and grades may be expected" (6–7). Travel was thus intrinsically dangerous, no matter where one migrated to or from.

The negative effect of a long-term stay in a tropical region could be delayed through moral discipline, proper diet, frequent stays in the various hillside stations or sanitoriums, and periodic recuperative visits to temperate climates, but it could not be postponed indefinitely. As James Martin argued, there would inevitably be a decline under "the slow blight of the constitutional power" (434). He believed that the heat of tropical climates stimulated, and thus strained, the European body beyond its capacities. Under the continuing stress of a hot sun, both maturation and organic decline were "unnaturally and prematurely accelerated" (464). Employees of the East India Company, like British factory operatives, suffered from premature aging. Continuous sweating exhausted their bodies, producing atrophy first of the skin and then of the internal organs, notably the liver. Over time, the body lost its ability to respond to changes of weather, particularly cold, and this loss was increasingly seen as the cause of tropical diseases. The invalid succumbed to a "climate-struck" torpor that failed to respond to any medicine. The only resource was to return to England. By the 1870s, colonialism was guided by the assumption that lengthy stays in the tropics were to be avoided at all costs.[2] Military policy limited the time that officers and servicemen were stationed in tropical regions, and the preference was for establishing barracks in cooler elevated regions. White settlers, especially in India, were encouraged to make frequent visits home or to the hill stations. Mair in 1871 summarizes prevailing beliefs when he writes in *The European in India:* "Much has been said and written about acclimatizing the European in India; but the idea . . . for the reasons just given, is scarcely ever seriously entertained now-a-days by those who have carefully studied the influence of the climate generally. The number of those who do return to Europe with their constitutions unimpaired, after a long residence in India, is but small" (216).

Although during the seventeenth and eighteenth centuries women were generally assumed to be more suited to tropical climates than males, by the nineteenth century, despite statistical evidence to the contrary, there emerged a far more pessimistic view. As early as 1773 John Clark was arguing that in the intense heat of Madras women, like plants, lose their vigor: "The lively bloom and ruddy complexions they bring from Europe are soon converted into a languid paleness; they become supine and enervated, and suffer many circumstances of ill health peculiar to their sex, from mere heat of climate and relaxation of system" (41–42). By 1832 William Twining was arguing that "the influence of the climate of Bengal on the constitutions of European women, is a subject which requires the careful consideration of the practitioner. The effects of this climate on the constitution of the European female, will be observed in various morbid conditions of the function of menstruation, and in the state of the system at those periods when that secretion is going on" (27). In 1871 Mair is arguing the same point: "Females suffer perhaps even more than males. Their lives, especially those in affluent or easy circumstances, are generally torpid, and too little relieved by occupation. They have few necessities for exerting themselves; they take but little, often far too little, interest in domestic affairs; they become listless and apathetic and they succumb to the climate sooner than men" (216). Here stereotypes of Asiatic culture are applied wholesale to female colonists. In *Sketches of Brazil* (1852) Robert Dundas, who spent twenty-three years at the British Hospital in Bahia, Brazil, argues that "the European female, especially of the upper classes, feels the injurious influence of climate more sensibly, and at an earlier period, than the male" (99). Notwithstanding her "more regular and temperate habits" and "her exemption from many of the ordinary sources of tropical disease, as exposure to the sun, atmospheric vicissitudes, over-fatigue, &c., yet are these advantages more than counterbalanced by the inactivity and indolence almost necessarily connected with her position" (100). Given the widespread assumption that women were more prone to neurological disorders than men, colonial women were believed to be particularly predisposed to madness. Waltraud Ernst remarks that "the image of the grief-stricken widow in the prime of her life, left bereft of male connections and therefore going mad in a supposedly alien, dangerous and hostile, far-away place, emerged as a powerful organizing image of female insanity in the [British India] colony" ("European Madness" 362).

As in the controversies relating to female factory operatives, there was great concern about the impact that heat might have on sexual function. Edward J. Tilt concluded that women in India were "unusually prone to uterine diseases" (296) and that the longer they remained there "the more subject are they to deranged menstruation and to uterine affections" (293).[3] For bodies whose health depended on moral and physical temperateness, for bodies increasingly defined by their sexual function, tropical heat was seen as a danger. Indeed, Tilt proposes that in many cases the only cure for women "invalided by uterine disease" (309) is to move to a temperate climate. For female colonists, heat produced sexual dysfunction, not so much in the increase of sexual activity as in inflammations and sterility. Just as tropical heat was believed to intensify the virulence of most diseases, so too it magnified sexual pathologies. "*Sex* is a very important element in forming the statistics of sickness and mortality among Europeans in India," writes William Moore. "The functions of menstruation, parturition, and lactation exercise in all countries a powerful influence on female health, and this influence is most marked in the tropics. It must be recollected there are in the female system additional and important organs, specially subject to tropical influences, and, therefore, there are additional reasons why European women in the tropics should, as they so often do, break down sooner than men" (48–49). The division of West and East along the horizontal axis of upper and lower bodily disease, which I discussed in chapter 7, was also a gendered construction. Women's health, which had long been considered to be more subject to climatic and meterological influences than men's, was also believed to be more subject to the "tropical influences" because their biomedical identity was more profoundly linked to the lower sphere. The dangers of sexual dysfunction were thus heightened there. The organs differentiating female colonists from their male counterparts were believed to make them especially vulnerable. By the end of the nineteenth century, Rudolph Virchow was arguing that European acclimatization was not possible because of the negative effects of heat on female reproduction (744).

The dangers of a tropical environment were believed to be even more strongly manifest in children. Throughout most of the nineteenth century, the British regularly sent their children to England to be raised by relatives. "Children born of white or European parents in India," James Annesley remarks, "require to be sent to Europe in order to attain due maturity and strength. If allowed to remain in India, they seldom present the appearance of health, even when they arrive at puberty. A greater proportion of them also die before they reach this epoch of existence: and it seems probable that children, whose parents have both been the offspring of Europeans, but born and constantly resident in India, would be still weaker and less likely to arrive at maturity, or to reach the full physical development of the white variety of the species" (43–44n). Whereas adults could perhaps delay the inevitable decline into invalidism by producing an artificial "temperate" environment through frequent trips to Europe or the cooler hill stations, colonial children would have no "temperate" constitution to recover. Lady Emily Metcalfe speaks of the terrible toll on children in India:

During the period of British rule in India . . . hundreds of thousands of British children who were born in that country grew up barely knowing their parents. And year after year weeping mothers took their children down to the great trading ports of

Calcutta, Madras and Bombay, and handed them over to the care of friends or nurses to be taken "Home" and brought up by relatives, or in many cases (Rudyard Kipling and his sister Trix among them) by strangers. Such separations were one of the saddest aspects of the Raj; almost sadder than the terrible toll that heat and disease took yearly from the British who lived in India, and the fact that every mother expected to lose at least three children out of every five she bore. (49)

As in the 1830 debates over the employment of children in factories, fears were not simply for the physical health and proper growth of colonists' children, but also for their moral development. As Europeans separated themselves racially and culturally from the peoples they colonized, their anxiety about the impact these environments would have on their children increased. Andrew Davidson writes: "The child must be sent to England, or it will deteriorate physically and morally,—physically, because it will grow up slight, weedy, and delicate, over-precocious it may be, and with a general feebleness. . . . Morally, because he learns from his surroundings much that is undesirable, and has a tendency to become deceitful and vain, indisposed to study, and to a great extent unfitted to do so" (5). In 1832, in an ominous statement that would be repeated throughout the century, Twining reported that "all the inquiries which I have been able to make, afford no evidence that the third generation of pure European descent, exists in India" (29).

The medical literature on tropical invalidism was intrinsically a reflection on the feasibility of empire. The number of Europeans who were dying of tropical diseases had always raised questions about colonization of tropical environments. By the middle of the nineteenth century, there were serious doubts whether a global empire was possible, even if the idea seemed worth the sacrifice. After visiting the European botanical garden in Boorwa Saugor, Thomas Medwin thought it a fit emblem of the British Empire in India. "I could not help reflecting," he writes,

that we are exotics in the animal, as many of [the plants and shrubs in the garden] are in the vegetable kingdom, and sighed and exulted over the concluding paragraph from Gibbon, whilst speaking of the overthrow of the Mogul Empire. "Since the reign of Aurungzebe, their empire has been dissolved—their treasures of Delhi rifled by a Persian robber, and the richest of their kingdoms are now possessed by a company of Christian merchants, of a remote isle in the *Northern* ocean." The train of thought engendered by the recollection of this remarkable sentence, threw a gloom over my mind, that had till then been pretty tranquil. (*Angler in Wales* 2: 73)

Not only did tropical invalids raise doubts about Europeans' biological capacity to rule the globe, but their return posed a new set of problems for doctors practicing in England, because the changes their bodies had undergone did not appear to be easily reversible. In 1827, in the fourth edition of the *Influence of Tropical Climates on European Constitutions*, Johnson first included an essay titled "Observations on the Diseases and Regimen of Invalids on Their Return from Hot and Unhealthy Climates." He describes the pitiable state of these individuals. "It is really lamentable to see men returned from a tropical climate, walking about the streets of London, or going to places of amusement, in the cold raw evenings of winter, while the hacking cough, emaciated figure, and variegated countenance, proclaim a condition of the lungs which ill comports with this exposure to the vicissitudes of a northern climate" (576). Martin expanded this section in his edition of the book. "Strange as it may seem," he declares, such a person can no longer return to England without "serious risks to his health," because "he has undergone changes in his moral and physical nature but little considered or understood by his kinsmen and countrymen in general" (450). Returning home, "he now finds himself in middle, or more advanced life, differing in habits, associations, and pursuits, from those around him—his nearest relatives departed, and he an invalid and a stranger in the land of his birth" (450). Martin is here describing a new kind of cultural or biological hybridity. The tropical invalid is no longer a "native" either in his habits or in his "moral and physical nature." Having left the tropics because his body could no longer function in this new environment, he faces the prospect of being both an invalid and a stranger in England.

Robert Dundas in *Sketches of Brazil* declares that the "formidable maladies . . . to which Europeans are subject, apparently from change to the colder latitudes, on returning to their native land" were frequently brought to his attention "in a mode at once most momentous and alarming" (35). The subtitle of his book—*Including New Views on Tropical and European Fever, with Remarks on a Premature Decay of the System Incident to Europeans on Their Return from Hot Climates*—reflects its importance: "These individuals, in many instances, *break up*, as it is popularly termed, after a brief sojourn in their native land" (48). Much of the tragedy is that they appear to have lost the ability to live anywhere. As Dundas remarks, there comes a time when "a longer residence [in the tropics] cannot safely be permitted to the European" (107), a point in the life of every colonist "when the administration of medicinal agents proves either useless or hurtful" (111). Upon returning to England, however, the tropical invalid discovers he cannot live there either. This was hybridity with a vengeance: having lost the physiological capacity to adapt to a tropical region, yet having also departed from his native constitution, the "climate-struck" tropical invalid discovers that he inhabits a body fit for nowhere. In the end, imperial migration produces an epidemiological limbo, a permanent state of maladaptation and continued suffering in which the colonist, othered culturally and physically by migration elsewhere, can no longer adapt even to his native country.

As I have sought to demonstrate in discussing "The Brothers," the "Ancient Mariner," and Rousseau in *The Triumph of Life*, the tropical invalid constitutes a new kind of colonial subject, a hybridity not of the colonized, but of the colonizer. Bhabha has described the way the colonized, in mimicking the discourse of the European colonizer, produces a destabilizing uncertainty. As "a subject of a difference that is almost the same but not quite," mimicry is both "resemblance and menace" (86). Encounters with tropical invalids, people who had been othered by their colonial experience, produced a similar range of uncertainties and anxieties. This new kind of subjectivity—in which colonial hybridity, rather than producing two selves, two cultures, and two biologies, produced a subject in deadly contradiction with itself and its surroundings—challenged the authority of empire from within.

Jane Eyre *and Tropical Invalidism*

Although the tropical invalid emerges as a new kind of subject in the medical discourse of the Romantic period, the shadow cast on British culture by this figure grew as the nineteenth century progressed and as Britain committed more people to colonizing tropical regions. Charlotte Brontë's *Jane Eyre* (1847), a Victorian literary text, is useful in clarifying the trajectory of this discourse, one that will ultimately lead to *Heart of Darkness*. Recent criticism has demonstrated that *Jane Eyre* is a novel *of* and *about* empire.[4] That Brontë understood colonial spaces in terms of the language of medical geography can hardly be doubted. A striking example of such geographical mapping can be found in her description of Caroline Helstone's almost fatal fever in *Shirley*. Although Brontë admits that "mental excitement" and "habitual sadness" had predisposed Caroline to sickness, her fever comes from the East: "some sweet, poisoned breeze, redolent of honey-dew and miasma, had passed into her lungs and veins" (474). Entire Eastern weather fronts of plague, it seems, can sometimes settle over England: "The future sometimes seems to sob a low warning of the events it is bringing us, like some gathering though yet remote storm, which, in tones of the wind, in flushings of the firmament, in clouds strangely torn, announces a blast strong to strew the sea with wrecks; or commissioned to bring in fog the yellow taint of pestilence,

covering white Western isles with the poisoned exhalations of the East, dim-
ming the lattices of English homes with the breath of Indian plague" (473).
Brontë's depiction of plague in racial terms, as a "*yellow* taint of pestilence"
that covers "*white* Western isles" (emphasis added) is obvious here. More
interesting is her wholesale employment of meteorological language to establish a "geography of disease" that makes "fever" essentially a tropical import.
Politics, ideology, and weather are thus fused. Brontë blankets all of England
with the "breath of Indian plague," "the poisoned exhalations of the East."

That Brontë employs weather geopolitically is even clearer in the subsequent chapter, significantly titled "The West Wind Blows," which recounts
Caroline's recovery:

> It was the close of August: the weather was fine—that is to say, it was very dry and very
> dusty, for an arid wind had been blowing from the east this month past: very cloudless,
> too, though a pale haze, stationary in the atmosphere, seemed to rob of all depth of
> tone the blue of heaven, of all freshness the verdure of earth, and of all glow the light
> of day. . . . So long as the breath of Asiatic deserts parched Caroline's lips and fevered
> her veins, her physical convalescence could not keep pace with her returning mental
> tranquillity; but there came a day when the wind ceased to sob at the eastern gable of
> the Rectory, and at the oriel window of the church. A little cloud like a man's hand
> arose in the west; gusts from the same quarter drove it on and spread it wide; wet and
> tempest prevailed a while. When that was over the sun broke out genially, heaven
> regained its azure, and earth its green: the livid cholera-tint had vanished from the
> face of nature: the hills rose clear round the horizon, absolved from that pale malaria-
> haze. (499–500)

During the dog days of summer, England appears to have become another
Asia. Brontë imbues "the breath of Asiatic deserts" with a range of negative
meanings, portraying the eastern front as a "sob[bing]" breeze, "stationary,"
lacking "freshness" and "tone," devoid of "all glow." But a cloud, like a "man's
hand," rises in the west and with it a breeze that "ventilates" the English
atmosphere, ridding it of its "cholera-tint" and "malaria-haze" and allowing
the sun, the heaven, and the earth to recover. Like Keats in "To Autumn,"
Shelley in "Ode to the West Wind," or De Quincey is his account of the role
of winter in the "Science of Happiness," Brontë has succeeded in producing a
geopolitics of weather, one that draws an entire range of symbolic meanings
from English seasonal change.[5]

The appearance of the "man's hand" in the west points up that Brontë, like
Shelley, does not consider weather as strictly physical but sees it as expressing
social and moral relationships. "There is analogy," she writes, "between the
moral and physical atmosphere" (289). The same "hand" that could rid En-

gland of cholera and malaria might be employed elsewhere. On this level, in participating in a medical geography that implicitly favored European technologies and land use over those employed in tropical regions, Brontë shares much with nineteenth-century imperialists. Not surprisingly, her representation of West Africa as "the plague-cursed Guinea coast swamp" in *Jane Eyre* (397) is little different from Lind's. Yet this reading is a partial one, for the central tactic of *Jane Eyre* is to employ medical geography for anti-imperialist purposes: to question colonial optimism by demonstrating its immense cost in human lives and suffering.

The ambiguities in Brontë's use of European medical geography are explicit in the passage that deals with Rochester's decision to return to England. Brontë describes a night in Jamaica that might easily have been drawn from Lind's *Essay*. "It was a fiery West-Indian night," Rochester declares. "One of the description that frequently precede the hurricanes of those climates: being unable to sleep in bed, I got up and opened the window." Seeking fresh air, he finds no relief from the oppressive, tomblike atmosphere of the tropics. "The air was like sulphur-steams—I could find no refreshment anywhere. Mosquitoes came buzzing in and hummed sullenly round the room." In this state of despondency, "*physically influenced by the atmosphere*" (312, emphasis added) and by the screams of Bertha ("this the air—those the sounds of the bottomless pit!"), Rochester concludes that life in Jamaica is worse than hell. But just as he is about to commit suicide, suddenly "a wind fresh from Europe blew over the ocean and rushed through the open casement: the storm broke, streamed, thundered, blazed, and the air grew pure. . . . The sweet wind from Europe was still whispering in the refreshed leaves, and the Atlantic was thundering in glorious liberty: my heart, dried up and scorched for a long time, swelled to the tone, and filled with living blood. . . . I saw Hope revive— and felt Regeneration possible. . . . 'Go,' said Hope, 'and live again in Europe'" (312–13). In this enactment of atmospheric cleansing, as the muggy and mosquito-infested air of the tropics is radically dissipated by a European wind, Brontë produces one of the most powerful expressions in Victorian literature of an imperial ecological myth. Here liberty, purity, and health are expressed in a geographical symbolism of air and atmosphere. Even Rochester's body is given new life and new blood by this "change of air."

Rochester's quest for health might be said, then, to be a quest for fresh air. But he misunderstands the message conveyed by this wind, for he believes that hope is reinforcing the colonial myth that he can "travel yourself to what clime you will, and form what new tie you like" (313). What Rochester will learn—what Brontë believed the colonial experience should have taught the

British—is that he is *not* free to travel anywhere he desires. This is why the "sweet wind from Europe" passage anticipates and is structurally revised by the mythic communication between Rochester and Jane that will ultimately bring them together. Rochester describes it like this:

As I exclaimed "Jane! Jane! Jane!" a voice—I cannot tell whence the voice came, but I know whose voice it was—replied, "I am coming: wait for me!" and a moment after, went whispering on the wind, the words—"Where are you?"

I'll tell you, if I can, the idea, the picture these words opened to my mind: yet it is difficult to express what I want to express. Ferndean is buried, as you see, in a heavy wood, where sound falls dull, and dies unreverberating. "Where are you?" seemed spoken amongst mountains; for I heard a hill-sent echo repeat the words. Cooler and fresher at the moment the gale seemed to visit my brow: I could have deemed that in some wild, lone scene, I and Jane were meeting. In spirit, I believe, we must have met. (453)

Here Rochester seems not to have come any closer to finding a healthy environment than before, for the unventilated atmosphere of Ferndean is little better than that of Jamaica or, for that matter, tropical Guiana. And once again he is visited by a breeze that brings regeneration. Yet in this instance the wind comes not only from the hills but also from Jane. The heroine of the novel, then, is not just a person but the embodiment of an ecological myth, linking English places with English people: she is, indeed, Jane Air.[6]

Jane Eyre's curative power at the end of the novel should not surprise us, for she is named after the most important term in contemporary environmental medicine. Just as St. John Rivers is linked to water in the novel, Jane is associated with air, her surname at one point being written as "Aïre" (102). When Rochester, for instance, looks at Jane's painting of the evening star, itself both a landscape and a woman, what impresses him most is Jane's ability to represent the wind: "And who taught you to paint wind? There is a high gale in that sky, and on this hill-top" (127–28). This remark might constitute an allegorical statement about the novel itself, about its symbolization of an aspect of the physical environment as a woman. Similarly, when Jane attempts to determine why she should leave Rochester rather than live with him as his mistress, she understands her situation in enviromedical terms. She questions "whether is it better, I ask, to be a slave in a fool's paradise at Marseilles— *fevered* with delusive bliss one hour—*suffocating* with the bitterest tears of remorse and shame the next—or to be a village-schoolmistress, free and honest, in *a breezy mountain nook in the healthy heart of England*" (364, emphasis added). Here Jane articulates a powerful nativist myth, for even Marseilles, the traditional commercial gateway to the Levant, suffers from continuous "fevers" and "suffocating" airs. Rosamond Oliver is also described in terms of a nativist aesthetic as having "perfect beauty . . . as sweet features as ever the temperate clime of Albion moulded; as pure hues of rose and lily as ever her humid gales and vapoury skies generated and screened" (367). Yet it is equally obvious, even when Jane posits such ideals, that she does not feel they apply to her, for hers is a dark complexion, not unconnected with her association with Irishness, also explicit in the name "Eyre."

Jane Eyre can be read as a book on "tropical invalidism." Brontë's criticism of colonial missionary activity is quite clear in that St. John Rivers dies after only ten years in India. More good might have been done at home with the Olivers' "large fortune," Jane declares, than to lay "his genius out to wither, and his strength to waste, under a tropical sun" (377). Jane's view of this enterprise is clear. Perhaps with the recent history of Jewsbury or Roberts in mind, she adopts a gendered view of women's adaptability to a colonial climate, asserting that "if I go to India, I go to premature death" (409). Brontë does not provide any information about Rivers's last days, however, for like other writers discussed in this book, she is less interested in the impact of colonialism on other countries than in its effect on British social life. Her focus is primarily on figures of colonial return. One of the most notable of these is the Jamaican colonist Richard Mason. In portraying this "tropical invalid," Brontë recalled the guardian of a West Indian orphan, Melanie Hayne—"a sallow man doubtless suffering from the English cold" (Gérin 353). In him the reader sees the long-term impact of a tropical climate on a British body. Jane's description of Mason's first appearance intimates that he has passed through a process of othering, which makes him "a stranger" (191). Hybridity shapes her description. The first thing she notices is that his accent is "not precisely foreign, but still not altogether English." Mason appears attractive, but "on closer examination" Jane senses something that displeases, something lacking. His complexion is "sallow," betokening "tropical anaemia" and foreignness. Physiognomy is read as a symptom of moral integrity. The impact of the tropics is everywhere registered in his features: his face is "too relaxed," while his "eye wandered, and had no meaning in its wandering." A deathly figure, not without kinship to Wordsworth's Discharged Soldier or the Ancient Mariner, he embodies the region he comes from—"a tame, vacant life" (192). Hybridity is uncanny, for Jane continues to speak of Mason's attractiveness even as she is ultimately "repel[led]" by his disturbing and threatening otherness. An added problem is that he seems physiologically unable to keep warm. As he sits as close to the fire as possible, still wearing his overcoat, he "shiver[s] as some one chanced to open a door" and asks "for more coal to be put on the fire" (193). James Martin remarks that for the tropical invalid "the in-door temperature, carefully regulated during the winter and spring seasons, is that alone which is safe to him" (459).

Brontë's sophisticated employment in the novel of ideas drawn from tropical medicine is obvious in the episode when Rochester, having come upon Mason after he has been attacked by his sister Bertha, tries to administer a cordial to revive his spirits. In what seems an almost inexplicable gesture, Mason refuses the liquor, even though he is perilously close to death, fearing that it might produce a dangerous fever. "But will it hurt me?—is it inflammatory?" he asks (216). Such a statement, at such a time, demonstrates that Mason habitually observes the conventionally prescribed regimen for Europeans in the tropics. Since fevers were associated with a heightened blood temperature, physicians encouraged colonists to avoid anything that might "heat" the blood—all stimuli, such as liquor, venery, overeating, strong passions, or excessive exercise. Johnson writes: "The great secret, or fundamental rule, for preserving health in hot climates is, 'TO KEEP THE BODY COOL.' . . . On this principle, common sense alone would point out the propriety of avoiding heating and stimulating drink, for the same reasons that we endeavour to guard against the high temperature of the climate" (533). Set within the context of the various dietary and moral regimens imposed on the colonizing subject for survival in the tropics, this scene thus says a good deal about Richard Mason: he has done everything a European colonist was supposed to do and yet, as Brontë makes abundantly clear, is still physically ruined.

Mason has darker, more personal reasons for avoiding liquor, for we learn that he is the product, in Rochester's words, of "a mad family: idiots and maniacs through three generations." His mother was "both a mad woman and a drunkard" (294), and his sister, Bertha Mason Rochester, through a similar lack of concern for the dangers of moral laxity and liquor, has also gone mad. Recent criticism has tended to see Bertha's wildness, madness, and sexuality as signs of her being racially linked to blacks.[7] Her mother, they note, was a "creole." Although such a viewpoint allows readers to see Bertha as a voice of the colonized and conforms with present-day views on the fundamental social link between racial and sexual oppression, it is basically mistaken. Although the word "creole" was occasionally applied to blacks born in the West Indies, it was normally used to distinguish white Europeans born or naturalized there from those recently arrived. This interpretation also ignores the most obvious aspect of the Jamaican system of slavery, that in a society in which the fundamental distinction between master and slave was based on color, creole slaves did not marry their way to freedom, and manumission was rare. The idea of a black creole becoming a Jamaican plantation owner is a romantic fiction, even if it nicely mirrors the plot of *Jane Eyre* itself, the story of the dark outsider who comes into property. The major difficulty of this interpretive standpoint is that it stands in the way of our recognizing what is surely one of the most frightening examples of the "tropical invalid" in Victorian literature. By overemphasizing Bertha's "racial" otherness, contemporary criticism has ignored Brontë's real stress on the impact of the tropics on European female colonists.

Recognizing that Bertha is a European creole does not prevent us from also noting that Brontë's representation, like Coleridge's depiction of the Ancient Mariner, "blackens" Bertha, as it articulates anxieties about colonial disease by emphasizing her moral, intellectual, physical, and sexual link to popular stereotypes of black women. Bertha is tropicalized. Her body, like that of her brother, is hybrid (not by racial factors, but by colonial migration).[8] It is itself the site of colonial conflict in the text, and her madness expresses that conflict. In this connection, it is worth emphasizing that colonial physicians saw madness as a problem of colonists rather than of the colonized. Henry Marshall observes that though madness occurs in all parts of the world, "it is particularly prevalent among the *imported* inhabitants of low latitudes where the temperature of the atmosphere is high" ("Sketch" 348, emphasis added). Martin also stresses the increased prevalence of neurological disorders among tropical settlers: "Under exposure, excessive fatigue, mental depression, or neglect of temperance in diet, results ardent fever, with some serious local determination, and that very frequently to the cerebral organs" (38). Throughout the nineteenth century, as the anonymous doctor's comments to Marlow demonstrate, tropical madness was largely perceived as an occupational hazard for European colonists, linked to their maladaptation to a new environment. (The same arguments were applied to West Indian and southern slaves who had been uprooted from Africa.) From this perspective, Bertha's madness is itself a sign of her Europeanness. Feminist critics have noted that her madness reinforces Victorian notions of women's greater susceptibility to insanity.[9] As I have already noted, such ideas played a very significant role in a colonial context where this assumed "weakness of the sex" was believed to be exacerbated by tropical heat. Rochester maintains that under the influence of a tropical sun Bertha's disregard of a colonial regimen has had frightening consequences: "her character ripened and developed with frightful rapidity; her vices sprung up fast and rank . . . her excesses had prematurely developed the germs of insanity" (310–11). In a letter to

W. S. Williams, Brontë claimed that Bertha's illness was an example of "moral madness," caused by "a sinful life" (Wise 2: 173–74). In a colonial context, the madness of the colonist remained a lesson to Europeans of the crucial necessity of moral discipline.

In the family history of the Masons, Brontë provides a powerful illustration of the dangerous long-term impact of tropical climates on European bodies and minds and rejects the notion that European colonists can adapt to them. Rather than undermining imperialism by constructing a positive image of the colonial other to identify with, Brontë achieves a similar goal by othering the colonist, by producing a hybridity that is at war with itself. Adapted to neither English nor colonial environments, these people have lost the ability to live anywhere on earth.

Brontë also saw British imperialism in class terms, as an undertaking that was radically altering English social life. She consistently draws parallels between the English ruling class and the East, in references to Blanche Ingram's "oriental eye" (163), Rochester's Turkish despotism (271), and their charade in "oriental fashion" (185). Jill L. Matus argues that Brontë "uses Oriental images to probe questions of desire, sexuality, and representation" (140). These concerns are rarely removed from concerns about sexual and political enslavement. In response to Rochester's asking what she would do were he a pashaw bargaining for a harem—"so many tons of flesh and such an assortment of black eyes"—Jane responds that she would devote herself to liberating the "enslaved—your Harem inmates amongst the rest" (272). Brontë consistently associates tropical spaces with a loss of independence. Marseilles, as I noted earlier, is portrayed as a pathogenic environment, with "fevered" and "suffocating" air. Similarly, the attic at Thornfield, that "great plague-house" (143), not only replicates the suffocating heat of Jamaica but is just as strongly evocative of contemporary descriptions of the degenerative character of English factories. In this regard, there were even suggestions that the male factory owner wielded a despotic power over the persons of his female employees and could use it for immoral ends: "His factory is also his harem" (Engels 168). Rochester's illegitimate proposal to Jane in the "Eden-like" (250) orchard at Thornfield is undercut by an atmosphere redolent with the scents of a tropical New World, the smell of "honey-dew" and tobacco, so much so that it even seems to have fooled a species of moth that would normally be found in the tropics. "Look at his wings," says Rochester, "he reminds me rather of a West Indian insect; one does not often see so large and gay a nightrover in England" (251).

Although English imperial medicine might claim that English people breathe a "purer air," Brontë knew better. If "Jane Air" is as much a geograph-icomedical construct as a person, she is, throughout most of the novel, a homeless one. As the narrative charts her movement from the environs of Lowood, a place of endemic fever, through the illusory space of new begin-ning at "Marsh End" (a name that is itself a product of the extensive medical discourse on fevers), only to end in another pathogenic space, Ferndean, *Jane Eyre* constitutes a series of "medical topographies" set within the larger con-text of European colonial medical geography. The novel encourages us to read its representation of national health against the background of the exten-sive material written by proponents of the public health movement on the health of the working-class poor in the newly emerging industrial towns, for we learn that Jane's parents died from typhus, which her father contracted "while visiting among the poor of a large manufacturing town where his curacy was situated, and where that disease was then prevalent" (26). Jane Eyre's quest for health and home, then, had its beginning in a specifically urban, working-class context, and the novel might be said to draw its top-icality from its participation in what was essentially a discourse on the health of the working class.[10] In this regard, the ten-year controversy ushered in by Brontë's semiautobiographical description of the outbreak of fever at Lowood School (or Cowan Bridge, where she briefly attended school) was not simply a local dispute but reflected larger national debates initiated by the physicians connected with the Sanitarian movement. Brontë's resentment against au-thorities who were unwilling to take steps to improve the physical environ-ment at Cowan Bridge is similar to the indignation the Sanitarians felt at the needless suffering and the economic cost of disease among the urban working class. *Jane Eyre* deals with a twenty-five-year period that saw an epidemic rise of sickness among the poor, especially typhus, cholera, and tuberculosis. By 1838, as R. A. Lewis observes, "the steady annual stream of typhus cases swelled suddenly to flood proportions" (34). In Glasgow, during the typhus epidemic of 1846, the same year *Jane Eyre* was written, typhus alone caused a death rate of fourteen per thousand, close to the average annual death rate in England from all causes. (Glasgow's overall death rate that year was fifty-six per thousand, only slightly better than Jamaica's.)[11]

Susan Meyer has noted the centrality of "cleaning" in *Jane Eyre,* seeing it as Jane's symbolic attempt "at washing away oppression." Meyer, however, treats this issue as a limitation, as Brontë's attempt to create "a clean, healthy, middle-class environment as the . . . alternative to an involvement in oppres-sion" (264). We gain a different perspective if we understand Jane's insistence on cleanliness as part of the increasing demand, made not only by middle-class reformers but also by the working class, for healthier, more sanitary living conditions. Although Jane's effort to "clean down" Moor House (394) operates at a domestic level, her view of its importance is not far removed from the views of Edwin Chadwick, who claimed that "the various forms of epidemic, endemic, and other diseases caused, or aggravated, or propagated chiefly amongst the labouring classes by atmospheric impurities produced by decomposing animal and vegetable substances, by damp and filth, and close and overcrowded dwellings prevail amongst the population in every part of the kingdom, whether dwelling in separate houses, in rural villages, in small towns, in the larger towns—as they have been found to prevail in the lowest districts of the metropolis." By arguing that disease is not restricted to lower-class urban environments, Chadwick was not minimizing its severity there but was arguing, as Brontë also suggests, that public health was an issue of national importance. Chadwick goes on to claim that when "those circumstances are removed, by drainage, proper cleansing, better ventilation, and other means of diminishing atmospheric impurity . . . disease almost entirely disappears" (422). He thus sees sanitation and through it the production of clean "Eyre" as linked facets in the battle against disease.

Born into a family of Irish immigrants, a group frequently singled out as the purveyors of disease in England, Brontë would have had no difficulty recognizing that colonialism was not "over there, somewhere else" but was fundamental to the very being of Great Britain. *Jane Eyre* seems to suggest that England, in colonizing the world, had succeeded in transforming itself into a colonial environment, as much in need of curing as any other region of the world. The conclusion of the novel, in which Jane marries Rochester and settles at Ferndean, a place that "could find no tenant" because of its "ineligible and insalubrious site" (435), powerfully captures both the hope and the skepticism that shaped the public health movement in the years leading up to the Public Health Act. Brontë defines Jane Eyre's new beginning in terms of the language of "improvement," the curing of pathogenic places. She also shows an awareness that these changes will require a significant transformation in the attitudes of the ruling class. "It is time some one undertook to re-humanize you," Jane declares to Rochester (441).

In light of Brontë's personal experience, it would be difficult to see Jane's final settlement in the fog-ridden woods of Ferndean as more than the expression of a hope that England might be made more healthy for its people. One reason Brontë's comments on her experience at the Clergy Daughters' school at Cowan Bridge caused such controversy was that they challenged the popular national idea that, even if England's urban regions were sick, its rural heartland remained healthy. The Brontës' experience at Haworth belied such complacency. In her biography of Brontë, Gaskell employs the language of the Sanitarian movement to condemn the living conditions in this village. "Haworth is built with an utter disregard of all sanitary conditions," she writes. "The great old churchyard lies above all the houses, and it is terrible to think how the very water-springs of the pumps below must be poisoned" (92). Endemic sickness, poor health, and low fevers appear to have been the norm for people living at Haworth. Scattered throughout Gaskell's biography are continual references to sickness, as in the following passage: "Haworth was in an unhealthy state, *as usual;* and both Miss Brontë and Tabby suffered severely from the prevailing epidemics" (362, emphasis added). The small amount of statistical data available confirms Gaskell's impressions. As Lyndall Gordon observes in her recent biography of Brontë, "The Babbage Report on Haworth in 1850 notes that the annual mortality was 25.4 in a thousand, while that of a neighbouring village was only 17.6." Gordon points out that this average was little better than "some of the worst areas of London" (313, 347). Compared with Haworth, with its lack of sewerage and with a water supply that flowed through the graveyard, it is hard to imagine that the fictional Lowoods and Ferndeans were much worse. If one approaches English health from the perspective of the Brontë family, it is also difficult to believe that Charlotte Brontë shared a patriotic belief in the essential healthiness of England. All six children of Patrick and Maria Brontë died early, of diseases that probably took advantage of constitutions weakened by endemic fevers. Here the Brontës were probably not much different from their neighbors. In *Jane Eyre,* Charlotte Brontë drew on medical geography to ask whether "fever," the great killer of Europeans in tropical regions, was not just as much an ongoing part of the lives of the English at home, and she produced as her heroine a geomedical construct, a protagonist whose search for a healthy place to live comes to its conclusion and its new beginning in a place of endemic sickness. Thus Jane's options are quite circumscribed in the novel: it is not at all clear that marrying Rochester represents less of a threat to her health than going to India with St. John Rivers. Nor, it appears, was Jane's mother any more successful in her marriage choice, for she died of typhus brought on by her husband's missionary work among the poor of the manufacturing towns.

   Was Charlotte Brontë more successful? In her recent biography Lyndall Gordon has suggested that she died of a low-grade fever that had already killed her childhood nurse, Tabby, and that had been making its regular rounds through Haworth over the winter of 1853–54 (313).

NINE

"All the World Has the Plague": Mary Shelley's *The Last Man*

Midway through *The Last Man,* Mary Shelley's novel about the extinction of human beings by infectious disease at the end of the twenty-first century, Lionel Verney writes, "I spread the whole earth out as a map before me. On no one spot of its surface could I put my finger and say, here is safety" (188). Verney captures a critical moment in the history of epidemiology, which lies at the imaginative center of the novel: the recognition that modern diseases do not respect natural geographical boundaries. On an earth unified by the continual movement of people, goods, and pathogens, there are no safe places and nobody is exempt from possible contact. Paul Slack notes that epidemics "raise particularly broad issues in the history of ideas because they support, test, undermine or reshape religious, social and political as well as medical assumptions and attitudes. . . . Past epidemics continue to throw a peculiarly sharp light on the aideologies and mentalities of the societies they afflicted" (Ranger and Slack 3). Shelley's fictional epidemic serves a similar purpose by foregrounding the fundamental values and contradictions shaping English society. Yet the disease is also *pandemic,* and as such it illuminates imperial England's growing recognition that it was inescapably part of the world it helped bring into being, an anxious knowledge that was confirmed by the 1817 outbreak of cholera. By 1824, when Shelley began writing *The Last Man,* the disease had reached China, Southeast Asia, the Middle East, and Egypt. In another reference to maps, Verney describes the naïveté with which the British first responded to the pandemic.

We wept over the ruin of the boundless continents of the east, and the desolation of the western world; while we fancied that the little channel between our island and the rest of the earth was to preserve us alive among the dead. It were no mighty leap methinks from Calais to Dover. The eye easily discerns the sister land; they were united once; and the little path that runs between looks in a map but as a trodden footway through high grass. Yet this small interval was to save us: the sea was to rise a wall of adamant—without, disease and misery—within, a shelter from evil, a nook of the garden of paradise—a particle of celestial soil, which no evil could invade—truly we were wise in our generation, to imagine all these things!" (179–80)

Separated from the rest of the world by a "little channel," hardly more than "a trodden footway through high grass," the English believed they inhabited a "celestial soil," immune to the diseases ravaging other parts of the world. In *The Last Man* this illusion is finally shattered. Marlowe's Tamburlaine, embodying the expansionary vision of the sixteenth century, says, "Give me a map: then let me see how much / Is left for me to conquer all the world" (2.5.3.123–24). In the year 2094, in the face of a pandemic made possible by colonial expansion, Verney also calls for a map, this time looking for an escape. To his horror, he discovers there is none. "All the world has the plague!" (175).

Seen as both a development of and a critical departure from many of the ideas that shaped the Romantic understanding of disease, *The Last Man* provides an appropriate conclusion to this book. Shelley considered it a literary memorial to the Romantic period. In her journal she speaks of herself as "The last man! Yes I may well describe that solitary being's feelings, feeling myself as the last relic of a beloved race, my companions extinct before me" (*Journals* 2: 476–77). The novel looks backward to the writings of her husband Percy, Byron, and Godwin. It also looks anxiously toward the future. Verney writes his "history of the last man" in Rome, and by so doing pays homage to one of the novel's most important literary precursors, Gibbon's *Decline and Fall of the Roman Empire*, which Shelley read in 1815. "It was at Rome," Gibbon records, "on the 15th of October 1764, as I sat musing amidst the ruins of the Capitol . . . that the idea of writing the decline and fall of the city first started to my mind" (170). Like Gibbon's history, Shelley's is a critical elegy: both display admiration for an imperial city combined with a shrewd awareness of the limitations that have led to its collapse. Shelley's subject, however, is not Rome. Hers is the visionary task of writing the "decline and fall of the British Empire" proleptically, as a sibylline prophecy, a visionary postcolonialism. "Read your Fall!" writes Verney (339), as both the first and last great historian of the British Empire.

A distinctive aspect of Shelley's approach to this history, which differentiates it from similar meditations on the end of empire such as Anna Barbauld's *Eighteen Hundred and Eleven* (1812), is the importance she accords to disease.

The "plague" is more than a useful device for producing apocalyptic effects. In what is one of the first major works in the historical ecology of disease, a study that crystallizes colonial disease experience, Shelley reflects on the important role empire has played in the global spread of diseases. She recognizes that England is not removed from the epidemiological forces that are radically reshaping the globe. Being an advanced industrial nation provides no guarantee of immunity from epidemics. The novel also dismantles the idea of a world in which diseases are limited to discrete biomedical environments or "climates." Neither does nature guarantee the well-being of certain peoples over others or even the well-being of humans in general.

The Plague and Empire

The plague appears at a significant moment in the novel, just as Lord Raymond is about to enter the deserted city of Constantinople (Stamboul). The historical significance of this event is made clear by Raymond, who sees it as the culminating moment in "the mighty struggle ... between civilization and barbarism" (110). Through his actions "antique barbarism" will be expelled from Europe, "a power which, while every other nation advanced in civilization, stood still" (127). Raymond's conquest is inextricably bound up with egocentrism. Perdita, for instance, who is unwilling "to oppose any of his desires," suggests that "love of the Greek people, appetite for glory, and hatred of the barbarian government ... stimulated him." She is also the first to voice the fear that contact with the East might pose an epidemiological risk: "One word, in truth, had alarmed her more than battles or sieges, during which she trusted Raymond's high command would exempt him from danger. That word, as yet it was not more to her, was PLAGUE. This enemy to the human race had begun early in June to raise its serpent-head on the shores of the Nile; parts of Asia, not usually subject to this evil, were infected" (127). To the Europeans plague is only a word, a foreign disease of little relevance to them. Raymond responds that it has always been endemic to the East, so the current outbreak is not out of the ordinary. What he does not recognize is that his own actions are transforming the ecology of the disease, as the fall of Stamboul erases its traditional boundaries. Just as the British influence in India unleashed cholera, Raymond's conquering the city produces a catastrophe for Europe. It brings into being a new disease—or perhaps an old one with increased virulence—that takes advantage of the disappearance of the boundary between East and West to spread first into Thrace and Macedonia, then into Thessaly and Athens, and from there to the rest of the globe.[1]

Shelley's understanding of the epidemic as a product of both colonial contact with the East and the breakdown of boundaries is paralleled in Raymond's affair with Evadne Zaimi. Several critics, attending only to those instances in the novel where the plague is gendered as a female, as "Queen of the World" (252), have further suggested that Evadne personifies its ambiguities. It is her witchlike curse that initiates the plague: "Fire, and war, and plague, unite for thy destruction—O my Raymond, there is no safety for thee!" (131).[2] As Mary Poovey and others have proposed, Evadne is the displaced voice of Shelley's anger about her lack of power as a female writer (*Proper Lady and the Woman Writer* 114–42). But she also stands in opposition to the concept of female propriety that Shelley, like other British women during the period, was constructing for herself. The antithesis and rival of Perdita, Evadne is a "foreigner" (23) who destabilizes boundaries in her cross-dressing, her murky political past, and her fluid national and class affiliations. Even her architectural designs for the National Gallery orientalize the West, since they are drawn from "her remembrance of the edifices which she had seen in the east" (83). Thus, even though Shelley identifies with Evadne, whose genealogy can be traced back through Safie of *Frankenstein* to Mary Wollstonecraft, she also associates her with a dangerous moral contagion that is undermining British society. Through contact with her, Raymond loses the ability to recognize boundaries: "His spirit was as a pure fire, which fades and shrinks from every contagion of foul atmosphere: but now the contagion had become incorporated with its essence, and the change was the more painful. Truth and falsehood, love and hate lost their eternal boundaries" (91). In *The Last Man,* Evadne's uncertain nationality, superimposed on her uncertain morality, is looked on with suspicion, and her explicit sexuality is viewed as a threat. The contrast between Evadne's Hellenic ideals and her living conditions in England is striking. When Raymond meets her she is living in "one of the most penurious streets in the metropolis. . . . Poverty, dirt, and squalid misery characterized its appearance" (77–78). Evadne's life in London draws attention to the "drear and heart sickening poverty" (78) of the urban working class. Crossing the boundary between the East and the pathogenic world of the urban laboring classes, she thus emblematizes their epidemiological link. As Raymond enters her apartment he notices not only poverty, but within the threshold "a pair of small Turkish slippers" (78).

Shelley draws on other plague narratives, such as Defoe's *Journal of the Plague Year* (1722), Boccaccio's *Decameron* (1348–53), and Charles Brockden Brown's *Arthur Mervyn* (1799). Yet these narratives consider disease in local terms, as part of their respective urban contexts, rather than as a world-historical phenomenon. A more important influence was provided by the nineteenth-century imperial context, most notably the link between cholera and Hastings's Grand Army in India and the role that disease played in the failure of Napoleon's imperial ambitions. By his own admission, Raymond's conquest of Stamboul is a reprise of Napoleon's expedition to the East. "My first act when I become King of England," he declares, "will be to unite with the Greeks, take Constantinople, and subdue all Asia. I intend to be a warrior, a conqueror; Napoleon's name shall vail to mine" (40). Like Bonaparte in *Napoleon Visiting the Pesthouse at Jaffa*, Raymond sees the plague as ideopathological, a "base superstition" (140). He also seeks to rally his troops by the grand gesture of entering the disease-ridden city alone. For Raymond, the East and disease are fused into a single image, the primary obstacle to a perfect social order. Here he follows the more radical strands of Enlightenment social philosophy represented by Adrian and by Percy Bysshe Shelley. "Oh, that death and sickness were banished from our earthly home! that hatred, tyranny, and fear could no longer make their lair in the human heart!" declares Adrian. "The choice is with us; let us will it, and our habitation becomes a paradise. For the will of man is omnipotent, blunting the arrows of death, soothing the bed of disease, and wiping away the tears of agony" (54). As lord protector of England, Raymond sought to bring into being this new social order, based on science and reason:

Raymond was occupied in a thousand beneficial schemes. Canals, aqueducts, bridges, stately buildings, and various edifices for public utility, were entered upon; he was continually surrounded by projectors and projects, which were to render England one scene of fertility and magnificence; the state of poverty was to be abolished. . . . The physical state of man would soon not yield to the beatitude of angels; disease was to be banished; labour lightened of its heaviest burden. Nor did this seem extravagant. The arts of life, and the discoveries of science had augmented in a ratio which left all calculation behind; food sprung up, so to say, spontaneously—machines existed to supply with facility every want of the population. An evil direction still survived; and men were not happy, not because they could not, but because they would not rouse themselves to vanquish self-raised obstacles. Raymond was to inspire them with his beneficial will, and the mechanism of society, once systematised according to faultless rules, would never again swerve into disorder. (76)

Both Adrian and Raymond see disease as a form of disorder, an expression of the failure of science and society to perfect the means by which life can be rid of "self-raised obstacles." Like poverty, it is a social condition and, as such, has a social cure.

When Raymond discovers that renovating British society is beyond his ca-

pacity, he renews his devotion to the theme of Greek independence, a concern not unconnected with the "extensive commercial relations [of] every
European nation" (115) with Greece. The idea of imperial conquest thus has
its origin in the failure of English domestic politics and, even more decisively,
in Raymond's inability to govern his own passions: "one who seemed to govern the whole earth in his grasping imagination, and who only quailed when
he attempted to rule himself" (40). Here *The Last Man* displays its debt to
Percy's analysis of the psychopathology of empire in *The Triumph of Life*. "I
was overcome / By my own heart alone," says Rousseau, "which neither
age / Nor tears nor infamy nor now the tomb / Could temper to its object"
(240–43). In his final days, even Raymond recognizes that the grand gesture is
hollow. Having seen in 1814 the devastation produced in France by the Napoleonic Wars, Shelley had no difficulty recognizing that war and plague were
associated more than metaphorically. She writes: "Nothing could be more
entire than the ruin which these barbarians had spread as they advanced; perhaps they remembered Moscow and the destruction of the Russian villages;
but we were now in France, and the distress of the inhabitants, whose houses
had been burned, their cattle killed, and all their wealth destroyed, has given a
sting to my detestation of war, which none can feel who have not travelled
through a country pillaged and wasted by *this plague,* which, in his pride, man
inflicts upon his fellow" (*History of a Six Weeks' Tour* 19, emphasis added). In
drawing a picture of the destruction produced by the plague, Shelley must
have had these war-torn landscapes in mind. When Verney surveys the battle-
field near Kishan, he sees a world that anticipates the one produced by the
plague: "From the top of the mound, I looked far round—all was silent and
deserted" (130). War and plague are united not only in their effects, but also
ecologically, for the plague is spread, as cholera was, by the movement of
armies, those large pools of bodies that make possible the transmission of
infectious diseases over long distances. Shortly after Raymond's death, Verney
has a dream in which his friend reappears as "a gigantic phantom, bearing on
its brow the sign of pestilence" (146). Read in terms of the history of plague
and the major epidemiological consequences of Britain's massive military
presence in India, Shelley's identification of Raymond with the pandemic
displays a profound social understanding of the dynamics of colonial disease.
As a narrative in the psychopathology of empire, *The Last Man* articulates
Britain's darkest fears, that colonialism has unleashed forces that dwarf European medical, technological, and social know-how. What is an anxiety in this
novel has become an important critical perspective at the end of the twentieth
century. As David Arnold suggests, "European colonialism, once praised for

having freed much of Africa, Asia, and the Pacific from the scourge of disease, is now widely regarded as having been (as Donald Denoon puts it) a 'health hazard,' unleashing a crisis of mortality that it was medically powerless, until relatively recently, to efface" ("Medicine and Colonialism" 1404).

Deconstructing the Boundaries of Disease

Volume 3 of *The Last Man* opens with a valedictory apostrophe to an England that no longer exists, as the small remnants of its population prepare to leave the island in search of a climate that will support them. Shelley envisions that extraordinary moment in the history of England when it is no longer an adequate human habitat. Like other Romantics, she understands the story of England as that of the social control of nature, the historical transformation of a cold island in the midst of the Atlantic into a socially constituted temperate environment. The production of England was expensive, "the labour of hundreds of thousands alone could make this inclement nook fit habitation for one man" (235), but the social organization of labor achieved results. Shortly after Adrian's recovery from madness and fever, he and Verney tour England on the way to Windsor Castle. Writes Verney: "We passed through busy towns and cultivated plains. The husbandmen were getting in their plenteous harvests, and the women and children, occupied by light rustic toils, formed groupes of happy, healthful persons, the very sight of whom carried cheerfulness to the heart" (53). Adrian climbs a hill and seeing the landscape below offers a hymn to the "benignant spirit" that has "built up the majestic fabric we inhabit, and framed the laws by which it endures" (53). The spirit that Adrian evokes is not God, but the social order embodied in a republican England. For Shelley, England was an extraordinary social product—"the triumph of man!" (235). It began as a "ragged canvas naturally," offering only "clouds, and cold, and scarcity," and was "painted by man with alien colours" (235). England comes to embody the idea of "civilization" because its status as a habitable environment is totally dependent on the maintenance of the social order.

The education of Lionel Verney at the beginning of the novel indicates that the same social forces that transformed the English landscape have also transformed its people. He is initially portrayed as wild, "rough as the elements, and unlearned as the animals I tended" (9), the moral equivalent of the harsh landscape he inhabits. Strikingly, Shelley employs colonial language to describe Verney's change from his "savage habits" (12). "My life was like that of an animal, and my mind was in danger of degenerating into that which informs brute nature," he writes (12). In contrast to this brute physicality, Adrian is portrayed as both a civilizing and a climatic force: "He came up the while; and his appearance blew aside, with gentle western breath, my cloudy wrath: a tall, slim, fair boy, with a physiognomy expressive of the excess of sensibility and refinement stood before me; the morning sunbeams tinged with gold his silken hair, and spread light and glory over his beaming countenance" (17). Under Adrian's benevolent influence, Verney undergoes a radical bodily and intellectual transformation. "He had touched my rocky heart with his magic power," writes Verney. "I . . . felt myself as much changed as if I had transmigrated into another form, whose fresh sensorium and mechanism of nerves had altered the reflection of the apparent universe in the mirror of mind" (19, 21). Verney undergoes an education that colonizes him, yet strikingly he sees his "trans*migration*" as equivalent to coming out of the "jungle" to recover his own native ground: "The trim and paled demesne of civilization, which I had before regarded from my wild jungle as inaccessible, had its wicket opened by him; I stepped within, and felt, as I entered, that I trod my native soil" (18). Shelley reinforces the association between Verney's education and colonialism elsewhere by drawing a parallel between his heart and the uncultivated landscape of America: "Friendship, hand in hand with admiration, tenderness and respect, built a bower of delight in my heart, late rough as an untrod wild in America, as the homeless wind or herbless sea" (24). Most strikingly, Verney likens his education to Columbus's discovery of the New World: "I felt as the sailor, who from the topmast first discovered the shore of America; and like him I hastened to tell my companions of my discoveries in unknown regions. . . . I had lived in what is generally called the world of reality, and it was awakening to a new country" (21). Shelley thus applies a colonial model to England itself, seeing it as a colonial prototype, a region whose landscape and people have submitted to a civilizing process that has transformed them.

Like Percy, Shelley insists that one must understand disease in global terms. But she is far more pessimistic about the ability of Western civilization and technology to control nature and the epidemiological consequences of colonial contact. As the epidemic approaches England, she demolishes every argument brought forward to support the idea of British insularity. The metaphor of England as a "vast and well-manned ship, which mastered the winds and rode proudly over the waves" (5) establishes at the beginning of the novel that it is not an "island nation" isolated from the rest of the world but an empire based on maritime trade. The cost of maintaining Britain as a social environment prevents it from isolating itself from the rest of the world. Despite the news that the epidemic was producing "havoc and death . . . on a scale of fearful magnitude," British merchants "connected with these countries" (162) continue to trade with them. Typical of advanced nations, however, the British assume that their scientific and commercial sophistication will provide immunity from this worldwide epidemic. "Can it be true, each asked the other with wonder and dismay, that whole countries are laid waste, whole nations annihilated, by these disorders in nature? The vast cities of America, the fertile plains of Hindostan, the crowded abodes of the Chinese, are menaced with utter ruin. . . . As yet western Europe was uninfected; would it always be so?" Surprisingly, there is general agreement: "O, yes, it would—Countrymen, fear not!" (169). Colonial geography supports the idea that ecological catastrophes are a "natural" occurrence elsewhere: "In the still uncultivated wilds of America, what wonder that among its other giant destroyers, Plague should be numbered! It is of old a native of the East, sister of the tornado, the earthquake, and the simoom, Child of the sun, and nursling of the tropics, it would expire in these climes" (169). The British believe that agricultural and technological development, climate, and Western social organization are prophylactics against disease. During the early stages of the plague, they assume that England's "salubrious" air will prevent the disease from establishing itself. When this hope fails, they look to the "temperateness" of their seasons, placing their faith in the coming winter: "Winter was hailed, a general and never-failing physician. . . . The effects of purifying cold were immediately felt; and the lists of mortality abroad were curtailed each week. . . . We breathed again" (172). Ideas of race reinforce a sense of security: the plague "drinks the dark blood of the inhabitant of the south, but it never feasts on the pale-faced Celt. If perchance some stricken Asiatic come among us, plague dies with him, uncommunicated and innoxious" (169). Fused with ideas of race are concepts of national character, of the greater moral discipline of the British. Verney declares, "Remember that cleanliness, sobriety, and even good-humour and benevolence, are our best medicines" (178).[3] Safely ensconced in a colonialist framework that sees epidemics as intrinsically foreign to Britain's "celestial soil," the British can look on the total devastation of the globe with apparent equanimity. Trade continues while whole countries—entire continents—are being devastated.

   The Last Man examines a question that was central during the colonial period and that is becoming of paramount importance today as one looks at political states struggling to survive in the face of an epidemic rise in diseases. Does society constitute a defense against epidemics? How well can a state respond to a massive rise of disease when its resources are limited? Adrian rightly recognizes that society provides human beings with the best means of responding to epidemics: "It was only through the benevolent and social virtues that any safety was to be hoped for the remnant of mankind" (222). Yet epidemics by their nature test and undermine these resources. Verney's history details the progressive breakdown of British social institutions under the onslaught of the plague. As in previous plagues, many political leaders flee, among them the Lord Protector Ryland. New political arrangements emerge, sometimes for the better. Manufacturing and trade decline, resulting in unemployment, food shortages, and a scarcity of medical aid. Agriculture also fails, as rural laborers find it "impossible to enter on the task of sowing seed, and other autumnal labours" (222). Most important, the plague destroys Britain's primary resource—its people. Without people to reproduce and maintain it, English social space disappears. Verney describes the deterioration of the roads, the decline of the cities, and the changes in the rural landscape. Eventually British society collapses through depopulation. Writes Verney: "Man existed by twos and threes; man, the individual who might sleep, and wake, and perform the animal functions; but man, in himself weak, yet more powerful in congregated numbers than wind or ocean; man the queller of the elements, the lord of created nature, the peer of demi-gods, existed no longer" (233). With the disappearance of social organization, the physical environment created by human labor can no longer be maintained, and the remnants of British society decide to emigrate. England is dead, and Verney writes its eulogy:

It was not for the rose of Persia thou wert famous, nor the banana of the east; not for the spicy gales of India, nor the sugar groves of America; not for thy vines nor thy double harvests, nor for thy vernal airs, nor solstitial sun—but for thy children, their unwearied industry and lofty aspiration. They are gone, and thou goest with them the oft trodden path that leads to oblivion,—

Farewell, sad Isle, farewell, thy fatal glory
Is summed, cast up, and cancelled in this story. (235–36)

The disappearance of England might seem to pale in comparison with the subsequent extinction of the human race, but it remains an extraordinary moment in the literature of empire.

Although the portrayal of the end of the human race is a remarkable theme, which Shelley shared with other writers, one should not miss how the novel also narrates the collapse of an entire society in the face of disease. Here Shelley was not engaging in visionary speculation. Such things were happening all around her, as native societies crumbled under the combined attack of epidemics and European settlement. This is one of the first lessons learned by the monster in *Frankenstein* as he hears "of the discovery of the American hemisphere, and wept with Safie over the hapless fate of its original inhabitants" (115). Southey's contemporaneous *Tale of Paraguay* (1825) tells a similar story of the total destruction of the Guarani people through smallpox. What makes *The Last Man* unique is that Shelley redirects this knowledge of the precariousness of societies in the face of colonial disease back on England itself, suggesting that it too is susceptible to total social collapse. She undercuts the fallacy that it is "natural" for colonial societies to undergo continual epidemiological crises whereas advanced societies find ways to withstand epidemics. The novel examines a scenario that was being acted out elsewhere and applies it to England. The plague reverses the progress of empire. Initially, as the plague subdues other nations, "crowds of emigrants inundated the west of Europe" and England became "the refuge of thousands" (168). Anxiety about "foreigners" and "immigrants" runs as a leitmotiv through the novel.

England is also forced to deal with colonial return on a massive scale: "The English, whether travellers or residents, came pouring in one great revulsive stream, back on their own country; and with them crowds of Italians and Spaniards" (171). The plague is undoubtedly a democratizing force, which levels "all distinction of rank" (212). But it is also a force of devolution. Verney's metaphor of a "revulsive stream" suggests his ambivalence as he looks on the reflux of the colonial world back on its origins. Not only does the British Empire contract into itself, but it suffers a form of *reverse colonialism*. Weakened by disease, it is at one point even invaded by "strangers" (213). Several hundred people from North America, augmented by the Irish, "poured with one consent into England. . . . They swept the country like a conquering army, burning—laying waste—murdering" (214–15). In England they are joined by "the lower and vagabond English" (215). "Calling to mind the long detail of injuries which had for many years been forgotten," they are intent on "taking London, conquering England" (215). Adrian defuses conflict by accepting these strangers and sharing the land, a policy analogous to that of many native populations who were also in no condition to repulse outsiders. In this case, however, since both populations are in a state of decline, the consequences of this policy, in its insistence on the higher importance of human allegiances over national ones, are diminished. As the plague further depopulates England, those remaining conclude that they must leave England and establish a colony elsewhere. Without the labor that made this "alien" environment habitable, England returns to its original state: "Thy soil will be birth-place of weeds, thy sky will canopy barrenness" (235). *The Last*

Man is indeed both the first and last history of the British Empire. Because aboriginal societies were collapsing everywhere under the onslaught of disease and the opportunistic incursions of European colonists, the novel, like other works I have discussed, is a strangely doubled text, one that allows its readers to grasp the meaning of the disappearance through social collapse of an entire people and their way of life. H. G. Wells was right to allude to *The Last Man* in his *War of the Worlds,* for the novel records imaginatively a collective experience that frequently left no records, as it reads England's future through the lens of contemporary colonial history. And like Wells, Shelley too sees colonial disease doubling back on those who colonize. What one might call visionary prophecy, in other words, is actually colonial history writ large, the colonial metropole read from the perspective of the periphery.

A New Disease

The Romantic period saw the emergence of a deepening concern about the epidemiological consequences of colonialism. Initial concern was with the epidemic rise of disease in the places of colonial contact, its impact not only on native populations but also, increasingly, on Europeans. Ambivalence about colonialism was especially manifest when the colonists returned home as invalids. The worldwide outbreak of cholera in the 1820s crystallized apprehension about the impact of colonialism on those who stayed at home, especially as physicians found it harder and harder to establish "natural" or "climatic" boundaries between an ostensibly healthy England and the pathogenic colonial world. As the similarities between the diseases suffered by the urban working class and those of other regions of the world became more apparent; as epidemics became associated with poverty and ignorance rather than climate or geography; as Britain seemed to be invaded by "foreigners" and "immigrants," the British middle class felt less sure that they were safe from epidemics. By the 1820s, more writers began to look at the rapid travel of diseases across the globe with alarm, since the boundaries of colonial contact no longer were clear.

Shelley is among a vanguard of writers focusing on disease as a primary problem of the modern world. Strikingly, she presents the plague that destroys humankind as a *new* disease, whose origins and mode of transmission are never discovered. Nothing that public authorities do to reduce losses has any effect. The pandemic breaks out mysteriously in the East, and just as mysteriously disappears seven years later in the vale of Chamonix. After the 1817 outbreak of cholera, the idea that a new disease might appear and rapidly spread along the commercial arteries of empire was hardly visionary. For many physicians, who believed that diseases responded in different ways to changing circumstances, the appearance of cholera raised the prospect that an entire range of new diseases were on the horizon. Colonial physicians were particularly aware of the dynamic nature of diseases and their ecologies because they lived in regions that were undergoing rapid environmental change with consequent observable changes in the behavior and impact of diseases. Benjamin Moseley, for instance, in his *Treatise on Sugar* (1799), remarks that in commercial societies "it is impossible that the type of their diseases should remain stationary, or that some will not appear and others disappear. . . . The science of medicine therefore has not improved,—it has changed: because diseases change" (161–62). "It is certain," he remarked twelve years earlier, "that diseases undergo changes and revolutions. Some continue for a succession of years, and vanish when they have exhausted the temporary, but secret, cause which produced them. Others have appeared and disappeared suddenly; and others have their periodical returns" (*Treatise on Tropical Diseases* 43). James Kennedy, one of the most important contemporary authorities on cholera, concluded that the 1817 outbreak of cholera was not the first instance of a new disease coming into being. A year earlier, he remarks, Bengal was visited by the "'Malignant Sore Throat' [probably diphtheria], a contagious disease previously unknown, unless by name, in this portion of the globe" (15–16). Colonialism opened new channels for the spread of diseases into new regions. He notes that "the majority of the severe contagious diseases which have from time to time afflicted Europe were imported from the East" (13). Smallpox, he believed, came into being under circumstances quite similar to those of cholera, through a combination of "the crowded population of China, and the coincidence of famine [and] a distempered atmosphere" (13). Instead of blaming China for these diseases, however, he concludes that "every age may be expected to modify the registered maladies, as it modifies the habits and genius of the inhabitants; and new diseases may be expected to arise, and old diseases to decline, as the natural consequence of a change in the physical and moral condition of the people" (13–14). Although a contemporary epidemiologist would also include changes in the physical environment as a factor, Kennedy shows a very modern understanding of the dynamics of disease etiology. Colonial physicians showed a good deal of uncertainty about the identity and causes of many diseases, yet some of it reflected their impressive understanding of the dynamic and changing aspects of the new disease environments they were encountering.

In *Sir Thomas More* (1831), Robert Southey declared that every passing year increased the likelihood of England's suffering a devastating epidemic. "The importation" of the plague, asserts More in his colloquy with Montesinos, "is as possible now as it was in former times: and were it once imported, do you suppose it would rage with less violence among the crowded population of your metropolis, than it did before the Fire, or that it would not reach parts of the country which were never infected in any former visitation?" The urban working class remains a source of tremendous health anxieties. But not all epidemics are imported. More asks, "What if the sweating-sickness, emphatically called the English disease, were to show itself again?" The sweating sickness, or sudor anglicus, remains an enigma for historical epidemiology because its symptoms correspond to no modern disease. Five successive epidemics took place between 1485 and 1551, then it mysteriously disappeared. More, who brought the disease to the attention of Cardinal Wolsey in 1508, quite rightly asks if "any cause can be assigned why it is not as likely to break out in the nineteenth century as in the fifteenth?" Microbes are unpredictable. Diseases suddenly appear and just as easily disappear only to return when human beings think they finally have gained control over them. The sweating sickness was also enigmatic because its victims were almost exclusively English, both at home and abroad. In Britain the Irish, Welsh, and Scots were spared. More also wonders whether the British factory system might not "generate for you new physical plagues, as they have already produced a moral pestilence unknown to all preceding ages." After noting that inoculation may not guarantee "certain security" if smallpox should assume "a new and more formidable character," More draws attention to the naturalization of yellow fever in America and its apparent spread to Spain in 1800. Despite their ostensibly greater medical knowledge, the British in Gibraltar "found themselves as unable to stop its progress, or mitigate its symptoms, as the most ignorant empirics in the peninsula." In an ominous declaration, More states that "you have hitherto escaped it, speaking with reference to secondary causes, merely because it has not yet been imported. But any season may bring it to your own shores; or at any hour it may appear among you home-bred" (1: 50–53). Southey's anxieties, which were shared by others during the 1820s and 1830s, are deeply expressive of one strand of modernity. New diseases or new varieties of old diseases, home-grown or imported, are always looming just over the horizon.

At the end of the twentieth century, as each year seems to usher in a new health threat and one can hardly be confident in the power of medicine and social institutions to meet these challenges, especially in regions where the social and intellectual resources of states are weak, *The Last Man* seems amazingly prescient. Over the past half century a panoply of new diseases have gained public attention: Lyme disease, Legionnaires' disease, toxic shock syndrome, mad cow disease, flesh-eating infections, the Hong Kong chicken influenza; a long list of hemorrhagic fevers (Korean, Argentine, Bolivian, Venezuelan; Marburg, Lassa, and Ebola; Chikungunya); various forms of viral encephalitis; AIDS. Simultaneously, diseases that once seemed under control are reviving and becoming more widespread: malaria, dengue, tuberculosis, hepatitis, cholera, diphtheria, pneumonic plague, measles, chlamydia, genital herpes, and syphilis. For many Romantic writers, the ever-present chance of infectious disease produced conservative responses. "I saw the danger in its whole extent," writes Southey (1: 56). For him, and for De Quincey, Coleridge, and Wordsworth, these fears fostered an insistence on the need to maintain traditional moral and political values in the face of the enormous changes taking place both in England and abroad. Wordsworth's visit to London in book 7 of *The Prelude* powerfully expresses the fear that the colonial "contact zone" no longer exists on the periphery but occupies the commercial heart of England. The metropole is the embodiment of colonial uncertainties, where "all specimens of man / Through all the colours which the sun bestows" (1805 *Prelude* 7.236–37) produce a confusion of nations and peoples promiscuously mixing, the antithesis of an organic, native community:

> The Swede, the Russian; from the genial south,
> The Frenchman and the Spaniard; from remote
> America, the hunter Indian; Moors,
> Malays, Lascars, the Tartar and Chinese,
> And Negro ladies in white muslin gowns.
>
> (239–43)

De Quincey thought that England might be swallowed up or drowned by the East. He even imagined that the pastoral landscapes of England owed their being to a time when all of continental Europe was India! "Even within our domestic limits,—even where little England, in her south-eastern quarter, now devolves so quietly to the sea her sweet pastoral rivulets,—once came roaring down, in pomp of waters, a regal Ganges, that drained some hyperbolical continent, some Quinbus Flestrin of Asiatic proportions, long since gone to the dogs" (*Collected Writings* 8: 10–11). Recalling the scene in Lilliput when Gulliver, the "man-mountain" (Quinbus Flestrin), relieves himself in a mighty torrent, De Quincey imagines England as having come into being as the polluting Ganges poured its waters into the Atlantic, before Asia had "gone to the dogs." In Asia, De Quincey saw an image of both the origin and end of mankind. In these writers fear of the world produced by colonialism gives rise to a fear of contact with outsiders, foreigners, and immigrants, a fear of the traveling populations increasingly associated with disease and poverty. Disease also heightened class anxieties, as the working class came to be perceived as the equivalent of a colonial population within England. The diseases of poverty looked the same, so it was difficult to see much difference between the fevers of Calcutta and those of Manchester. Just as the different morbidity rates of colonizers and colonized exacerbated social conflict in the colonial world, a similar gap was registered between the well-off and the poor in England. The notion of the "sanitary district" did not apply, therefore, solely to the urban geographies of colonial regions. It shaped nineteenth-century ideas of urban social space.

In this context, Percy and Mary Shelley stand out as writers who insist that Western societies cannot isolate themselves from the world they have helped create. As Arno Karlen observes, "In our time, because of mobility and high-speed travel and trade, no disease is irrelevant to the rest of the world" (229). Percy Shelley felt it crucial to retain a faith in humans' capacity to gain control over disease through science and social progress. He was unwilling to separate humankind's struggle against disease from the struggle against social inequality. There can be little doubt that he looked on the global rise of diseases with apprehension, as his fears about elephantiasis demonstrate. Yet his was a fear not of other peoples or other races, but of the power of kings, priests, and commerce to desolate the globe. It was a fear of the politics and ecological degradation of the colonial world, not of its peoples. Nowadays, when human beings are destroying species and ecologies at an almost inconceivable rate, his belief in the necessity to work toward producing a healthy world remains an enduring legacy:

> man has lost
> His terrible prerogative, and stands
> An equal amidst equals: happiness
> And science dawn though late upon the earth;
> Peace cheers the mind, health renovates the frame;
> Disease and pleasure cease to mingle here.
> (*Queen Mab* 8.225–30)

Percy Shelley would have had no difficulty recognizing that health is a global problem that cannot be addressed without social change on a worldwide level. He would have looked with horror on our present world, which has seen the gap widen between those regions where people expect a relatively healthy life and those where epidemic diseases are producing misery on a terrible scale. Vast regions of the globe are currently undergoing epidemiological crises beyond imagining, as developed nations seem satisfied with treating health as a business rather than a social responsibility and show very little concern about instituting policies and programs that might alleviate problems elsewhere. Shelley would have had no difficulty diagnosing why large portions of the globe are being decimated by socially preventable diseases. The fallacy of "colonial geography," which assumes that disease is "natural" or "the norm" elsewhere, continues to shape the contemporary world and the West's dealings with the less fortunate regions of the globe. In such a context, it should not surprise us if contemporary health anxieties mirror those of the 1820s and 1830s: the similarities are greater than the differences.

Mary Shelley modifies his social theory of disease with a more pessimistic view of the chances that human beings will ever gain control over diseases. Indeed, it is Victor Frankenstein's attempt to "banish disease from the human frame, and render man invulnerable to any but a violent death" (34) that ushers in the horrors of *Frankenstein*. For Mary Shelley disease is not something that will someday recede from human life. She has less faith either in the power of modern science to gain complete control over diseases or in the prospect of addressing health on a global scale. Her experience of disease was largely one of its inevitable unpredictability. Having gone to Italy for her husband's health, she lost her daughter Clara there to dysentery in 1818 and her son William to an enteric fever (probably typhoid) in 1819. "We came to Italy thinking to do Shelley's health good—but the Climate is not any means warm enough to be of benefit to him & yet it is that that has destroyed my two children (*Letters* 1: 101). More than any other text of the Romantic period, *The Last Man* examines the limits of the social control of disease. When the epidemic takes root on the island, the British discover to their dismay that their social institutions do not constitute a safeguard. The image of Adrian struggling to maintain his society in the face of this epidemic is an extraordinary one. Other colonial societies must have had their own Adrians (or their Saynadays), who continued to recognize that society constitutes the best hope against epidemic destruction, yet many of them also lost their battle against disease. Mary Shelley argued against human complacency, the assumption that technology and science guarantee the continuance of Western social life.

For her disease is permanent, obscure, and dark, and human beings must learn to live in its shadow. It is in this sense that the novel constitutes a literary memorial to the Romantic period and perhaps also a memorial to the confidence that shapes twentieth-century medicine. She questions the confidence that underlay Romantic conceptions of nature and of human life, the notion that nature has selected human beings for preferential treatment and that ultimately the earth was made to serve human needs. What might seem a sad irony in the novel, that nature itself from the beginning of the novel to its end remains healthy, opens up a new perspective on nature, one not centered on humans. Everything in nature continues as it should—yet human beings are destroyed by a disease that affects only them. Disease, in other words, might ultimately be natural and an expression of order. How you see it depends on whether you are a human or a microbe.

What follows from this recognition? Human beings have always lived with disease, even in those periods when they thought it was about to be eliminated from the earth. As Garrett notes, microbes, "humanity's ancient enemies . . . didn't go away just because science invented drugs, antibiotics, and vaccines (with the notable exception of smallpox)" (10). Certainly, more than ever we should be cognizant that we live in a world that over time could see human beings disappear just as they have eliminated and are eliminating other species. Nature remains a horizon governing human life even as humans typically refuse to accept any limits to their destruction of the natural world. Recognizing disease as something that will continue to shape human destiny may also produce greater humility among the technologically advanced nations and perhaps lead to greater efforts to assist the many societies that are currently undergoing enormous epidemiological crises. In *The Last Man,* Verney is infected by his encounter with a black man: "I lowered my lamp, and saw a negro half clad, writhing under the agony of disease, while he held me with a convulsive grasp. With mixed horror and impatience I strove to disengage myself, and fell on the sufferer; he wound his naked festering arms round me, his face was close to mine, and his breath, death-laden, entered my vitals" (245). This episode powerfully embodies the fear of contagion that shaped European encounters with others over so much of the colonial period. Encounter brings with it disease, and Verney struggles to "disengage" himself from the embrace of this impoverished other. Yet Verney survives! Perhaps Shelley wanted this embrace, which functions as inoculation rather than contagion, to serve as an allegory of the fearful embrace of colonial encounters.[4] In a world where everyone is now in the same biopathological soup, where there is no place diseases cannot reach, there is perhaps another implicit lesson. Our diversity, the different biological immunities that populations have developed over time in different disease ecologies, may ultimately hold the key to our survival. The biological diversity—the "foreignness"—that caused so much pain and suffering in the colonial world might also hold within it something that will preserve at least some of us somewhere from the coming plague that Shelley prophesies.

NOTES

Introduction: Colonialism and Disease

1. For discussions of this myth, see Crosby, *Ecological Imperialism;* Stannard, "Disease."

2. Darwin is citing Rev. John Williams's *Narrative of Missionary Enterprises in the South Sea Islands* (1837).

3. My thanks to Julia M. Wright for bringing this passage to my attention. For the politics of yellow fever, see Pernick.

4. See esp. Fanon 102–58; MacLeod and Lewis; Arnold, *Imperial Medicine* and his excellent essay "Medicine and Colonialism." For good studies of colonial medicine and disease in the West Indies, see McClellan; Sheridan; Pluchon; and Dunn 263–334. For America, see Shryock. For India, see Arnold, "Cholera" and *Colonizing the Body;* M. Harrison; Ernst, "European Madness" and *Mad Tales;* and Ramasubban. For Africa, see Curtin, *Death by Migration, Image of Africa, Disease and Empire,* and "White Man's Grave"; Scott 1: 64–80; D. Kennedy, *Islands of White;* J. Davies; Ransford; Farley; and Vaughan.

5. See the important work of Curtin: *Atlantic Slave Trade, Death by Migration,* "Epidemiology," *Image of Africa,* and "White Man's Grave." Equally influential has been the work of Crosby, most notably *Ecological Imperialism* and *Columbian Exchange.* For more general discussions of the role of disease in history, see Sigerist; Cartwright; McNeill, *Plagues and Peoples;* Kiple, "Ecology of Disease"; and Karlen.

6. Gilman's work is important in this regard; see, *Difference and Pathology* and *Health and Illness.*

7. See Ramenofsky; Dobyns, *Their Number Become Thinned;* Crosby, *Columbian Exchange* and *Ecological Imperialism;* Curtin, *Image of Africa* and *Death by Migration;* Stannard, *American Holocaust* and "Disease and Infertility"; V. King; Kiple and Beck; and McNeill, *Plagues and Peoples.* Hulme provides a valuable study of colonial discourse on the native Caribbean.

8. Originally published by James Johnson in 1813, it went through a series of editions until 1841, when James Martin became first a cowriter and then, after Johnson's death in 1845, its author. Martin served twenty-two years in military service in Bengal and as physician to the Council of India. He was the author of *Notes on the Medical Topography of Calcutta* (Calcutta: Huttman, 1837) and was also a major author of the *Report of the Commissioners Appointed to Enquire into the Sanitary State of the Army in India, Parliamentary Papers,* vols. 1 and 2 (1863).

9. The term "biomedical" came into use during the 1950s; I use it anachronistically throughout the book to refer to the interaction of biology, environment, and medicine during the period discussed.

10. See Curtin, "End of the 'White Man's Grave'?" Mark Harrison reaches a similar conclusion about the continuing anxieties relating to morbidity: "Morbidity rates . . . were a major cause of anxiety well into the twentieth century. It was not mortality from diseases such as cholera, but the persistent incapacitating effects of malaria, typhoid, and venereal disease which most concerned colonial authorities" (2–3).

11. In 1825 Henry Nelson Coleridge, Samuel's nephew, visited the Caribbean and later published *Six Months in the Caribbean* (1841).

12. Austen's mother's brother, James Leigh Perrot, married into a Barbados estate, which was passed on to his son. Her father's sister, Philadelphia, went to India, where in 1753 she married a surgeon of the East India Company, Tysoe Saul Hancock. Her only daughter, Eliza, a valued member of the Austen circle, was perhaps also the child of a liaison with Warren Hastings.

13. Landon died in mysterious circumstances less than two months after arriving on the Gold Coast of Africa.

14. Though I would emphasize more the conflicts that shaped the formation of an idea of the British nation, I agree with Linda Colley that Britain was an "invented" nation, as the British "came to define themselves as a single people not because of any political or cultural consensus at home, but rather in reaction to the Other beyond their shores" (6). Whereas Colley focuses on the role of military conflict and religion in this process, my goal is to suggest the ways a continuing experience with colonial disease fostered a biological and cultural conception of Britishness and the anxieties underlying its formation.

15. Timothy Brennan makes a powerful case for the importance of the voice of the "colonized" rather than the "colonies" in imperial literature after the Second World War.

16. See Sontag, *AIDS and Its Metaphors*, esp. 60–71.

17. Medicine during this period was international in range, so a complete understanding of colonial medicine would need to encompass the important work of European physicians and their colonial counterparts.

18. For the role of medicine in Romantic literature, see de Almeida; Goellnicht; and Logan. For a study of the role of health in Austen's novels, see Wiltshire. See Haley and Vrettos for examinations of health in Victorian literature.

19. See also Makdisi and the essays collected in Richardson and Hofkosh, Arac and Ritvo, and Fulford and Kitson.

20. For work on colonialism and gender, see L. Brown; Nussbaum; Young; Sharpe; and de Groot. Hyam provides a wide ranging and flexible examination of sex and imperialism.

Chapter 1. Romantic Medical Geography: *Empire, Disease, and the Construction of Pathogenic Environments*

1. For current theoretical work on the politics of landscape, see Cosgrove and Daniels; W. Mitchell; Barrell; Bermingham; and Daniels. For feminist studies of

landscape, see Kolodny and Merchant. For a discussion of landscape and colonialism, see Bohls, *Women Travel Writers*.

2. See esp. Levine's valuable chapter "The Landscape of Reality" 204–26.

3. For discussions of Finke's work in the context of eighteenth-century medical geography, see Rosen; Barrett, "Medical Geographical Anniversary"; Jordanova, esp. 28–30; and Sargent. For further discussion of medical geography, see Grmek and Hannaway.

4. Barrett discusses relevant passages, such as Finke's claim that the essay is "the first medical geography ever written" ("Medical Geographical Anniversary" 705).

5. For an overview of the range of positions available to contagionists and anti-contagionists, see Pelling; Pickstone; Hamlin; Eyler 97–122; and Rosenberg, *Explaining Epidemics*, esp. 293–302. Rosenberg employs "contamination" in an unusual manner, as a term that has affinities with "contagion" theories. For the eighteenth century, see Riley.

6. The first "spot map" was prepared by Valentine Seaman in "An Enquiry into the Cause of the Prevalence of the Yellow Fever in New York," *Medical Repository, New York* 1 (February 1798): 315–72. For Brockden Brown's response to yellow fever outbreaks in America during this period, see Krieg 41–69. By the 1830s disease maps were being used to understand outbreaks of cholera in England, as in Shapter, *History of Cholera,* and Snow. For discussions of early disease mapping, see Howe, "Disease Mapping"; E. Gilbert; and Meade, Florin, and Gesler 19.

7. Recent studies of tropical medicine generally focus on its emergence as a recognized field of medical study during the 1890s, during the apex of British imperialism. This emphasis obscures the fact that for far more than two centuries, in writing and practice, colonial physicians had recognized that tropical climates were unique medical environments requiring specific medical knowledge. Thomas Trapham's *A Discourse of the State of Health in the Island of Jamaica* (1679) is the first book written by an English physician dealing with tropical medicine. For useful material on early tropical medicine in addition to Scott, see Balfour; Cook; and Sheridan. For discussions of tropical medicine and imperialism, see Worboys; Farley; MacLeod and Lewis; and Arnold, *Colonizing the Body* and *Imperial Medicine*.

8. For discussions of Lind's medical geography, see Barrett, "'Scurvy' Lind's Medical Geography"; Curtin, *Image of Africa* 72–79; and Sargent, who refers to him as a "pioneer in tropical medicine" (197). This James Lind is the naval physician who played a key role in the development of antiscorbutic medicines; another James Lind, who served in India, was physician to George III and was a major influence on P. B. Shelley.

9. For Lind's understanding of the relation between medicine and colonialism, see Lawrence.

10. In *Ecology, Climate, and Empire,* esp. 5–36, and *Green Imperialism* 168–308, Grove discusses the early emergence of ideas about the link between deforestation and climate change, particularly rainfall reduction.

11. William Ferguson believed it was not excess of moisture in colonial soils that produced miasmas, but instead the process of drying in areas once covered by water. However, he too agreed that the only true remedy "must be found in the powers of cultivation, ever opening the surface for the escape of pestilential gases, and exhausting the morbific principle by a constant succession of crops." This model produces a hierarchy of colonial topographies: "Wherever malaria prevails, the uncultivated savannah, even though used for pasture, becomes infinitely more pestiferous than the plantation, and the depopulated country falls completely under its dominion" (294).

12. Curtin notes that since the major vector of malaria, the *Anopheles gambiae* mosquito, breeds in small natural collections of water exposed to sunlight, "Clearing and cultivation were precisely the measures most likely to increase its numbers" (*Image of Africa* 81). See also McNeill, *Plagues and Peoples* 47.

13. For studies of disease, dirt, and colonialism, see Pickstone; Chakrabarty; and Anderson, "Excremental Colonialism."

14. De Almeida notes that in their course outlines for the practice of medicine, Babington and Curry "devoted over fifty-six pages to the various natures of fever," and the 1810 *Encyclopaedia Britannica* "allocated fifty-two pages in its entry 'Medicine' to febrile disease" (208).

15. Noting that there was relatively little typhus fever in mainland England during the first two decades of the nineteenth century, Pickstone indicates that "the journal articles on fever were chiefly about exotic and military experience" (141).

16. Jerome J. McGann argues: "To read Wordsworth's re-telling of this pitiful story is to be led further and further from a clear sense of the historical origins and circumstantial causes of Margaret's tragedy. The place of such thoughts and such concerns is usurped, overgrown. Armytage, poet, and reader all fix their attention on a gathering mass of sensory, and chiefly vegetable, details. Hypnotized at this sensational surface, the light of sense goes out and 'the secret spirit of humanity' emerges" (*Romantic Ideology* 83). Alan Liu is also critical, noting that "it is precisely 'close reading' that has most loved the humanity of imagery" (312). Liu sees Wordsworth's vegetation as camouflage that must be penetrated to get at the history concealed behind it. "What is the cash value of spear-grass?" he asks, as he claims that the Romantic lyric makes money through this substitution.

17. In "Ruth," Wordsworth drew extensively on Bartram in his description of the flowers of the magnolia, "that with one scarlet gleam / Cover a hundred leagues and seem / To set the hills on fire" (*Lyrical Ballads* 58–60).

18. For the historical impact of disease on the regional identity of the American South, see Savitt and Young.

19. Schoenfield notes this possibility (152).

20. In discussing the impact of scurvy on aesthetics during the colonial period, in "'The Rime of the Ancient Mariner,' a Ballad of the Scurvy" (unpublished), Jonathan Lamb discusses Trotter's view that calenture was a symptom of scurvy: "scorbutic Nostalgia" was "the first symptom" of "the disease in all its stages" (*Observations* 44).

21. Pillar Mountain is suggestive of the Pillars of Hercules, the headlands of Gibraltar and Jebel Musa, which were seen by the ancient world as the gateway to the unknown.

22. Wordsworth cites *The Hurricane* in a note to a passage in book 3, lines 930–40, of *The Excursion*.

23. For an examination of Gilbert's influence on Romanticism, see Kaufman.

24. See her discussion of "When first I journey'd hither" (pp. 130–33). Her not yet published work on siblings is extremely valuable and adds substantially to our understanding of the economics of "corporate families."

Chapter 2. *"Voices of Dead Complaint": Colonial Military Disease Narratives*

1. For contemporary war poetry, see B. Bennett. For an argument that the representation of domestic women allowed Romantic writers to articulate conflicting attitudes toward the public and private aspects of war and soldier's bodies, see Favret.

2. See Nash 3–25; Linebaugh, *London Hanged* 123–42 and "Atlantic Mountains"; Rediker; Linebaugh and Rediker. Linebaugh notes estimates that "by the end of the eighteenth century fully a quarter of the complement of the Royal Navy consisted of men of African origin. . . . The ship, if not the breeding ground of rebels, became a meeting place where various traditions were jammed together, an extraordinary forcing house of internationalism. African, Briton, quashhee, American (not to mention Portuguese, lazar, and Spanish) would have cooperated, for their lives depended on it, in the rigging and on the decks, in the fo'c'sle and the mess" ("Atlantic Mountains" 112). Gilroy draws on this work in developing the idea of the "Black Atlantic" as a space that dissolved "the structures of the nation state and the constraints of ethnicity and national particularity" (19); this concept is weakened by its reintroduction of the racial categories that he claims to be avoiding.

3. For an even more celebratory poem, see "Brave News from Admiral Vernon" (1740) (Masefield 133–36).

4. Gradish notes that "according to one set of statistics compiled midway through the war, 7,377 seamen died and another 4,031 were discharged on account of disease during the years 1755–1757. At the same time, however, only 413 died from wounds received in combat or in accidents" (120).

5. Guerra provides a good summary of this period. For a more detailed discussion of the occupation of St. Domingue, see Geggus.

6. C. L. R. James downplays the importance of disease in the success of the revolution, arguing instead that the success of the blacks is attributable to "the decree of abolition, the bravery of the blacks, and the ability of their leaders" (214).

7. The cholera epidemic that reached England in 1831 is estimated to have killed 23,000 people in England and Wales. This number not only is relatively small compared with those who died of common fevers and childhood diseases but also is less than half of those who died in the British effort to gain control of St. Domingue in the

1790s. Nevertheless it was an epidemic that was the focus of extensive public attention and anxiety. See Underwood 168.

8. For a brief discussion of disease among sailors, see Lloyd 258–66.

9. See Knollenberg.

10. In "Answer to a Craftsman," Swift contemplates satirically the benefits of French and Spanish recruitment of Irishmen to serve in their armies. If they were to recruit six thousand men, he remarks, "Here will be Thirty Thousand Pounds *per annum* saved clear to the Nation, for they can find no other Employment at Home, beside begging, robbing, or stealing." If more were recruited, and France and Spain happened to be at war with each other, additional advantages would be accrued: "How soon would those Recruits be destroyed, then what a Number of Friends would the Pretender lose, and what a Number of Popish Enemies all true Protestants get rid of" (*Prose Works* 12: 174).

11. See Linebaugh, *London Hanged* 94–97.

12. Gradish notes that "there were many eighteenth-century Englishmen who regarded the armed forces as a means of ridding towns and parishes of the unwanted inhabitants" (83).

13. See also Western.

14. Roderick's decision to stay in the West Indies is not as foolhardy as it might seem: his previous exposure to yellow fever obviously has increased his chances of survival there.

15. See also Brooks, "Goldsmith's 'Private Centinel.'"

16. See Erdman 213–23 and editor's introduction to *Narrative*.

17. In 1792, of Great Britain's eighty-one battalions of foot soldiers, nineteen were stationed in the West Indies; nine were in India, and twenty-five were in Gibraltar, Nova Scotia, and Ireland, leaving only twenty-eight for service in Great Britain (McGuffie 16).

18. For English Romantic interest in the West Indies, see Richardson. M. Ferguson provides a detailed discussion of English feminist responses to events in St. Domingue (209–48).

19. Although discussions of the important impact of colonialism on the "Rime" can be traced back to Lowes, the most developed and strongest political readings are those of Empson, "Ancient Mariner," and Ebbatson. See also B. Smith; Keane; McKusick; and Baum 1–56.

20. See also H. Brown.

21. Coleridge wrote a review of this book when it appeared.

22. See also Klein 197; Rediker 43; and K. Davies.

23. In the verse of the 1790s, the slave and the soldier are regularly associated with each other, as in Robert Merry's "The Wounded Soldier," which speaks of the "savage hearts" of those who send "the *slave* to fight against the *free*" in colonial regions (B. Bennett 242–45).

24. John Stedman displays a similar fear in seeing a group of newly landed slaves in

Suriname: they "were such a set of living atomatons, such a resurrection of Skin and bones, as justly put me in mind of the last trumpet; seeming that moment to be rose from the grave, or deserted from the Surgeons Hall at the old Bailey—and of which no better discription can be given than by comparing them to walking Skeletons covered over with a piece of tand leather" (166).

25. In both the lecture and essay on the slave trade, Coleridge claims that the disease atmosphere produced in a slave ship by overcrowding actually rots its timber frame as it destroys its human cargo: "We may form some idea of the hot & pestilent vapours arising from their [the slaves'] confinement between the decks by the fact that the very timbers of the vessel are rotted by them, so that a slave ship is considered as lasting only half the time of another—so dreadful is this confinement between the decks, that slaves who have been thrust down at night in health have been brought up dead in the morning" ("Lecture on the Slave-Trade," *Lectures* 241–42).

26. For a valuable discussion of yellow fever in the poem, especially its dissolution of the boundaries of race, slavery, and empire, see Lee, "Yellow Fever."

27. Crook and Guiton suggest that the poet may have been drawing on the belief put forward by Giolamo Fracastor and by the orientalist William Jones that leprosy was a tropical form of syphilis, caused by heat and sun (120–21).

28. Jonathan Lamb, in "'The Rime of the Ancient Mariner,' a Ballad of the Scurvy" (unpublished), provides persuasive evidence that Coleridge drew on medical representations of scurvy in his representation of "Life-in-Death."

29. In discussing the *Journal* of Janet Schaw, Bohls notes that an extreme whiteness of skin was valued by West Indian plantation women. Island ladies, notes Schaw, "want only color to be termed beautiful. . . . Yet this I am convinced is owing to the way they live, excluded from proper air and exercise. From childhood they never suffer the sun to have a peep at them, and to prevent him are covered with masks and bonnets, that absolutely make them look as if they were stewed" ("Aesthetics of Colonialism" 386).

30. I am drawing this term from Barrell: see also Leask's broader employment of the term.

31. For parallels between the "Rime" and *Salisbury Plain,* see Magnuson 76–78; Eilenberg 47–49; and Modiano. Collings argues that *Salisbury Plain* is a defining text in a "poetics of cultural dismemberment" (1–34).

32. Wordsworth declared that "all that relates to her [the Female Vagrant's] sufferings as a soldier's wife in America, & her condition of mind during her voyage home, were faithfully taken from the report made to me of her own case by a friend" (*Salisbury Plain Poems* 221). In the light of what we currently know of the experience of Europeans in military service in the West Indies, there seems little need to question this assertion.

33. In "Andrew Jones," another poem of 1798, Wordsworth dramatizes the antithetical viewpoint of a speaker who looks forward to the day when the army or press-gang will rid the village of this man:

> I hate that Andrew Jones: he'll breed
> His children up to waste and pillage.
> I wish the press-gang or the drum
> With its tantara sound would come,
> And sweep him from the village!
>   (*Lyrical Ballads* 1–5)

The cause of this anger is that Jones stole money from a vagrant! An additional interpretive twist comes from the fact that the poem probably alludes to John Scott's widely known and reprinted antiwar poem "The Drum," which begins: "I Hate that drum's discordant sound, / Parading round, and round, and round" (*Cambridge Intelligencer* 3 August 1793). The poem was originally ode 13 of John Scott's *Poetical Works* (1782), 201; see B. Bennett 80.

34. Gilbert Blane notes: "During the war, which broke out with France in 1778, and with Spain in 1779, the West Indies was the principal seat of naval operations, and much greater fleets were then employed in that quarter of the world than in any former period" ("Observations" 139).

35. On 1 March 1796 Coleridge recounts the story of the Eighty-eighth Regiment, which after serving on the Continent for two years, was reduced from 1,100 men to 250. They embarked for the West Indies with Christian's convoy but suffered from a fever that carried "off about five a day," so they were forced to return home. When they arrived, now reduced to 100 men, they "marched under the command of an officer of the 80th, for Portsmouth, where they will probably be drafted into some other corps" (*Watchman* 43–44).

36. For recent work on Wordsworth's representation of vagrants, see G. Harrison; Simpson 160–84; and Langan.

37. Anthony Jackson, a late mariner of HMS *Warwick,* might have been among the beggars Wordsworth saw when he visited Bartholomew Fair. In 1783 Jackson published his own broadside titled "Large Sieves and Plain Truths." Opening with "Attend you Seamen all unto the Lines I have here penn'd; the Truth doth speak," he goes on to deplore the impoverished condition of discharged sailors: "I'll tell you how we are rewarded for all our pains, to go in the streets and beg, thieve, or starve and be Hanged for what they care what become of us." He concludes this short tract with an appeal for charity: "The above Seaman is stabb'd in his left Breast with a Bayonet, shot in this right arm, and wounded in his head, having a wife and one child, humbly hopes for generosity" (qtd. in Morley 358–59). Is it possible that the Blind Beggar, whom Wordsworth saw in London, having in nautical terms "far travelled . . . beyond the reach of common indications" (1805 *Prelude* 7. 608–09), carried a story like that of Jackson pinned to his chest? Perhaps the "might of waters" (617) is not simply a biblical allusion.

38. For evidence that the soldier is named Robert Walford, see Gill in Wordsworth, *Salisbury Plain Poems* 11–12; for the story of John and Jenny Walford, see Bewell, *Wordsworth and the Enlightenment* 51–54.

39. Arnold Schmidt argues that the hanging of the soldier draws on contemporary interest in the naval mutinies of 1797 led by Richard Parker.

40. Edwards employs language similar to Glover's when he interprets colonial death as a scandal: "What numbers have perished—not in the field of honour—but on the bed of sickness!—not amidst the shouts of victory—but the groans of despair!—condemned to linger in the horrors of pestilence; to fall without a conflict, and to die without renown!" (3: 181).

41. See Jacobus's suggestive discussion of Wordsworth's silent response to the slave trade (74).

42. The revision of the poem is discussed by Butler (Wordsworth, *"Ruined Cottage"* 3–35) and by J. Wordsworth.

43. See, for instance, Charles Lamb's comment to Wordsworth on 9 August 1814, that he had "known the story of Margaret . . . even as long back as I saw you first at Stowey" (3: 95).

44. See also Southey's "Hannah," "The Soldier's Wife," and especially the account of the abandoned woman in *Joan of Arc*, 7. 320ff. Contemporary navy songs dealing with this topic are legion.

45. For material on the Seamen's Hospital Society, see Manson-Bahr and also Cook.

46. The initial impetus for these efforts came from the influx of destitute sailors into many cities at the end of the Napoleonic Wars. For Leigh Hunt's effort to direct attention to this problem, see the series of articles titled "Distressed Seamen."

Chapter 3. Colonial Dietary Anxieties

1. In the final version of the plate, the only symbols of adversity are the pawn-broker's shop (which is no longer needed) and the sign painter, in the upper left-hand corner, who is significantly painting a "gin bottle," which hangs from the signpost.

2. See, for instance, Leask's discussion of this episode, 209–15.

Chapter 4. Keats and the Geography of Consumption

1. Keats's medical knowledge has been the subject of three excellent studies: Goellnicht; de Almeida; and Roe 160–201. For a discussion of "consumption" as a metaphor in Keats's letters, see Michael.

2. The first edition was titled *The Influence of Climate in the Prevention and Cure of Chronic Diseases, More Particularly of the Chest and Digestive Organs: Comprising an Account of the Principal Places Resorted to by Invalids in England and the South of Europe; a Comparative Estimate of Their Respective Merits in Particular Diseases; and General Directions for Invalids While Travelling and Residing Abroad* (London: Underwood, 1829). In 1835 Clark published *A Treatise on Pulmonary Consumption*.

3. Sir Hugh Beevoir observed that for the incidence of tuberculosis "the Strand

and St Giles triple the [death] rate for Lewisham and Hampstead. London stands almost alone in its tremendous contrasts" (i).

4. Keats's comments can usefully be compared with Austen's humorous send-up of this medical discourse in her unfinished novel of 1817, *Sanditon*. There Mr. Parker speaks of the absolute necessity of a six-week seaside stay for the maintenance of health: "The Sea air & Sea Bathing together were nearly infallible, one or the other of them being a match for every Disorder, of the Stomach, the Lungs or the Blood; They were anti-spasmodic, anti-pulmonary, anti-sceptic, anti-bilious, & anti-rheumatic. Nobody could catch cold by the Sea, Nobody wanted Appetite by the sea, Nobody wanted Spirits, Nobody wanted Strength.—They were healing, softing, relaxing—fortifying & bracing—seemingly just as was wanted—sometimes one, sometimes the other.—If the Sea breeze failed, the Sea-Bath was the certain corrective; & where Bathing disagreed, the Sea Breeze alone was evidently designed by Nature for the cure" (qtd. in Wiltshire 207).

5. Almost two centuries earlier Thomas Gage had made the same complaint about the "little substance and virtue" of food in Mexico, which left people's stomachs "gaping and crying, Feed, feed" (200).

6. See Elaine Scarry's arguments about the impossibility of expressing one's own pain or that of another.

7. Fry and Gurney write: "Where large numbers of poor persons are obliged to inhabit a single, wretched, building, half-fed, half-clothed, and in the midst of filth it cannot be a matter of surprise that low fever should be generated, nor that, when generated, it should spread to every class in society" (52). For a discussion of the "fever nest," see Hardy, esp. 193–203.

8. For the ambiguities in the mythic representation of Apollo, see de Almeida 17–21.

9. As Welch argues, for instance, late in the century, "It is the vulnerability of tissue that is inherited, not the actual disease" (229).

10. See also Barnes 33–37.

11. Severn writes, "His mental exertions and application have I think been the sources of his complaints—If I can put his mind at ease I think he'll do well" (Rollins 1: 186).

12. For an extensive discussion of the period's confusion of poisons with contagion and its importance in Keats's writings, see de Almeida 182–202.

13. See Goellnicht 203–7; and Dubos and Dubos 44–66.

14. Edward Said's argument in *Orientalism* that Europe constructed the East as a female object of desire has been extremely influential. See, for instance, Chaudhuri and Strobel; McClintock; Nussbaum; and de Groot.

15. See Aske for an insightful discussion of the role of envy in this criticism.

16. See also E. Jones, "Keats in the Suburbs."

17. In his *Autobiography*, Hunt is quite proud of his West Indian and Philadelphian

origins. His father, a "true exotic" from Barbados, "ought not to have been transplanted" to America, he writes (10–11). In explaining both his family's and his own financial difficulties, he argues that the fault lay in "the West Indian blood of which we all partake, and which has disposed all of us, more or less, to a certain aversion from business" (17).

18. See, for instance, W. Bate 581. For a valuable discussion of the importance of weather in the poem, see J. Bate.

19. Temperate climates, however, were defined not by homogeneity, but by variability. Benjamin Rush, for instance, remarks: "Perhaps there is but one steady trait in the character of our climate, and that is, it is uniformly variable" ("Account of the Climate of Pennsylvania" 90). Philadelphia is "a compound of most of the climates of the world. Here we have the moisture of Britain in the spring, the heat of Africa in summer, the temperature of Italy in June, the sky of Egypt in the autumn, the cold and snows of Norway and the ice of Holland in the winter, the tempests (in a certain degree) of the West-Indies in every season, and the variable winds and weather of Great-Britain in every month of the year" (97).

20. For a suggestive discussion of the political valences of "conspiring" in the context of the recent events at Manchester, see Roe 253–57.

21. See also Keach, "Cockney Couplets."

22. McGann's "Keats and the Historical Method" has established the dominant view that politics is repressed or evaded in "To Autumn." For other relevant work, see Cox; A. Bennett; and Newey, "Alternate Uproar."

23. Annesley, for instance, argues that "the low grounds at the mouths of rivers, or along their course, are rendered thus particularly insalubrious by the deep, rich, and moist soil which form them; by the quantity of rich mud and slime deposited upon them, particularly after inundations, and by the luxuriant vegetation, part of which must necessarily in a warm climate be always undergoing decay, with which they abound" (13).

24. As it turned out, he did not live long enough to recover his investment.

25. Babington and Curry note that yellow fever produces a "yellow suffusion of the skin, varying in degree from a sallow hue to a deep orange tint" (55). In his *Examination of the Prejudices Commonly Entertained against Mercury*, Curry also notes that "there are few inter-tropical complaints, in which the liver is not either primarily or secondarily a considerable partaker" (26). He had also planned to write a larger treatise on the liver titled *Treatise on the Nature of the Hepatic Function; the Purposes It Serves in the Animal Oeconomy; and the Powerful Influence Which a Disordered State of It Exerts, in Exciting, Aggravating, and Modifying Various Forms of Disease, both General and Local*. Also, James Johnson dedicated the *Influence of Tropical Climates* to Curry, who was his physician when he returned from India as an invalid.

26. See, for instance, Browne's reference to tuberculosis as a "soft Death" (4: 39).

27. Keats was considering moving to Teignmouth in May 1819 (*Letters* 2: 112–

13); for Keats's comments on the "femminine [*sic*] Climate" of Devonshire ("I fancy the very Air of a deteriorating quality") and his preference for the "Sinews" of a "long brown plain," see *Letters* 2: 241–42.

28. Less than a month later, Keats became a vegetarian, explaining that "I have left off animal food that my brains may never henceforth be in a greater mist than is theirs by nature" (*Letters* 2: 225).

29. For a good assessment of this aspect of the poem, see also Newey, "Keats, History, and the Poets" 185–90.

30. The subheading above is from the epitaph on Keats's tomb.

31. One should also mention, especially within the context of Keats and the reviews, Henry Kirke White, who, it was believed, also died of consumption brought on by bad reviews.

32. For information on death rates and their decline during the nineteenth century, see Frederick Hoffmann and F. Smith.

33. During the early years of the AIDS epidemic, it was seen in similar terms as a disease of the young.

34. See also Barnes 29; Hutcheon and Hutcheon 40–48. Sontag typically overstates her case in arguing that "the Romantic invented invalidism as a pretext for leisure, and for dismissing bourgeois obligations in order to live only for one's art" (*Illness as Metaphor* 33–34).

35. In the 1835 *Table Talk* (325n), Coleridge changed "loose" to "slack" and thus occasioned Leigh Hunt's denial of that "appearance of 'laxity,' that has been strangely attributed to him in a late publication."

36. See Wolfson, *Questioning Presence* 296–300; Swann 81–92.

37. Joseph Severn indicates that during the final stages of his illness Keats "found many causes of his illness" in Fanny Brawne's "exciting and thwarting of his passions" (Rollins 2: 92). "I should have had her when I was in health, and I should have remained well," he wrote to Brown in 1820 (*Letters* 2: 351). In a July 1820 letter to Fanny Brawne, he inverts the traditional language of disease transmission, its being caused from the exhalations of fevered bodies, to suggest the more important role that desire plays in causing fever. He declares, "You are to me an object intensely desireable—the air I breathe in a room empty of you is unhealthy" (2: 304). The "feverish unrest" (244) of love is a central concern of *Isabella,* a poem in which Lorenzo's desire heats his blood, which "fever'd his high conceit of such a bride" (46).

38. For more on the relation between consumption and the ambiguities of Romantic desire, see de Almeida 203–15; see also Graves's discussion of consumption as the white goddess (425–29); Goellnicht 223; and Brink 144–95. For its biographical sources in a cruel trick played on Tom Keats, which the poet thought brought on Tom's consumption, see Gittings's discussion of "Amena Bellefila," esp. 355–56.

39. For a valuable discussion of the complexity of form in these poems, see Wolfson, *Formal Charges* 164–92.

40. See also Wolfson's discussion of "the cultural processing of 'the death of John

Keats' " ("Keats Enters History" 19) and her excellent earlier study, "Feminizing Keats." See also Roe's discussion of the critical emphasis on Keats's childishness (202–29) and James Heffernan's argument that Shelley largely "invented the strange story of Keats's death" (295). For the political ambivalence shaping Shelley's representation of Keats, see Cox.

41. See Sweetser 41–43; for the French experience, see Barnes 9–10, 37–41.

42. See Wasserman 463–466.

43. Compare this description, for instance, with an analogous one used by Mrs. Ellis in her 1838 obituary notice for Maria Jane Jewsbury: "The author of 'The Enthusiast' has, in that story, bequeathed to the world a striking and most melancholy picture of the ceaseless conflict, the insatiable thirst for what is unattainable, and the final wretchedness necessarily attendant upon the ungoverned ambition of superior intellect, when associated with the weakness, natural dependence and susceptibility of women" (qtd. in Clarke 59).

44. The colonial discourse on *sati* has been the focus of recent postcolonial criticism. See, for instance, Spivak, "Can the Subaltern Speak?" Mani, "Contentious Traditions" and "Cultural Theory, Colonial Texts"; Sunder Rajan 15–63; and Sharpe 49–52, 103–10.

Chapter 5. Joseph Ritchie and "The Diseased Heart of Africa"

1. For relevant studies, see my introduction, note 4.

2. For discussions of epidemiology in colonial Africa, see, esp. Hartwig and Patterson; Curtin, *Death by Migration, Image of Africa,* and "White Man's Grave"; Scott 1: 64–80; Gelfand; J. Davies; Ransford; Farley; D. Kennedy, *Islands of White;* and Vaughan.

3. For an excellent discussion of cartography during the Romantic period, see Lee, "Mapping the Interior."

4. Kingsley died of enteric fever in South Africa in 1900 while serving as a nurse to Boer prisoners.

5. See Peterson 25–26; Curtin, *Image of Africa* 483.

6. The Sierra Leone Company drew the same conclusions in its account of the epidemic. Noting that only four of the twenty-six upper servants died, the company suggested that the high mortality rates among lower servants (twenty-nine out of fifty-nine) derived from their being intemperate, poorly lodged, and without adequate medical attention. Thirteen out of eighteen settlers died, the writers claimed, from the consumption of liquor. The explanation for the high mortality rate of the soldiers of 69 percent (eleven out of sixteen), that they were "almost universally intemperate" (48), reflects middle-class assumptions about this group. See Sierra Leone Company 47–49.

7. The *Dictionary of National Biography* notes that Ritchie "wrote many elegant pieces of verse besides his 'Farewell to England,' which is entitled by power of expression and depth of feeling to a permanent place in literature."

8. For further accounts of Ritchie's expedition, see Bovill; Bohen 48–52; and the *Dictionary of National Biography* entry for Ritchie.

9. See Pratt; Jardine, Secord and Spary; and Brockway.

10. Lee, in "Poetic Voodoo," suggests that *Lamia* shows Keats's interest in Africa, perhaps stimulated by his having heard an account of Edward Bowdich's soon-to-be-published *A Mission from Cape Coast Castle to Ashantee* (1819). Bowdich (1791–1824) was instrumental in negotiating peace with the kingdom of Ashanti for the African Company of Merchants. He later donated his African collections to the British Museum. After studying natural science and mathematics in Paris with Humboldt and Cuvier, he published geographic studies of Africa, among these *An Essay on the Geography of North-Western Africa* (1821), *An Essay on the Superstitions, Customs and Arts, Common to the Ancient Egyptians, Abyssinians, and Ashantees* (1821), and *An Account of the Discoveries of the Portuguese in . . . Angola and Mozambique* (1824). Shortly after arriving at Bathurst, at the mouth of the Gambia River, intending to explore the interior of Africa via Sierra Leone, he died of malaria at age thirty-three.

11. Lyon notes: "The allowance of £2000, which was made to Mr. Ritchie, had already been expended, in buying Merchandize, Instruments, Arms, &c. and otherwise making provision for the welfare of the Mission; but the merchandize was selected in England, and unfortunately was such as could be of little utility in the interior, of which circumstance we were not aware until too late" (57).

Chapter 6. Percy Bysshe Shelley and Revolutionary Climatology

1. See also Farley 13–30.

2. "When last [I] saw you I was about to enter into the profession of physic," he wrote to Elizabeth Hitchener on 8 October 1811 (*Letters* 1: 144).

3. See Condorcet's celebration of a medical utopia in the "Tenth Epoch" of his *Esquisse d'un tableau historique des progrès de l'esprit humain* (1793); for an excellent discussion of the work of Cabanis, see Staum.

4. For Shelley's interest in agriculture, see Morton, *Shelley and the Revolution in Taste* 232–34.

5. For more on colonialism and ecology, see R. Grove's work.

6. Morton uses the word "technotopianism" in "Shelley's Green Desert" 417. For an argument that Shelley is a "confirmed orientalist and liberal imperialist," see Leask 70.

7. The "Ode to the West Wind" has not been recognized as a poem shaped by the politics of environment, yet when read in the context of passages like these, it is clear that the wind itself is more than simply a meteorological effect. It is an enviromedical concept, as it drives the "pestilence-stricken multitudes" before it, making possible not only rebirth but the cure of the earth's primary population groups: "yellow, and black, and pale, and hectic red" (4–5).

8. Current climatological studies suggest that the Romantics were correct in

recognizing that a major climatic change had occurred in the region. Between A.D. 300 and 800, two major drought periods saw the collapse of several of the cities along the Great Silk Road to the East. "In Arabia," H. H. Lamb notes, "places where agriculture had been carried on with the aid of elaborate irrigation works, which had survived earlier periods of desiccation, were abandoned around AD 600" (168).

9. Since population increase is a sign of good government, Shelley cannot conceive of a social revolution that does not lead to an increase in pleasure and erotic fulfillment—in Scrivener's words, "a renovated erotic nature" (69). In the ideal world that concludes *Queen Mab*, "impotence" is in the catalog of evils (the others being crime, languor, disease, and ignorance) that are exiled from earth (see 9.9–10).

10. The idea that a total global climatic change might make health universally available to all human beings continued to fascinate Shelley throughout his career. In *Prometheus Unbound*, the union of Promethean science with the love of Asia makes possible the recovery of a temperate world:

> a soft influence mild;
> Shall clothe the forests and the fields—aye, even
> The crag-built desarts of the barren deep—
> With ever-living leaves and fruits and flowers.
> (3.3.120–24)

11. See Morton's discussion of "greening the desert" (*Shelley and the Revolution in Taste* 219–27); see also his "Shelley's Green Desert."

12. Neil Fraistat has identified the source as Sir George Stuart Mackenzie's *Travels in the Island of Iceland during the Summer of the Year MDCCCX* (Edinburgh: Archibald Constable, 1811); see his notes to *Queen Mab* in volume 2 of the *Complete Shelley* (Baltimore: Johns Hopkins UP, forthcoming).

13. Shelley reinforces the symbolic association of the landscape of Mont Blanc with that of the East when he speaks of "snowy pyramids" (152) and "horrible desarts" (166). The waterfall near Maglans is described as falling "from the overhanging brow of a black precipice on an enormous rock, precisely resembling some colossal Egyptian statue of a female deity" (*History of a Six Weeks' Tour* 145).

14. In the *History of a Six Weeks' Tour*, Mary Shelley also adopts the language of an ideopathologist as she emphasizes that the Swiss children "appeared in an extraordinary way deformed and diseased. Most of them were crooked, and with enlarged throats" (110). Those living in Evian, then under the control of the King of Sardinia, are even "more wretched, diseased and poor, than I ever recollect to have seen." Mary concludes that the difference between the Swiss and the Chamoniards is "a powerful illustration of the blighting mischiefs of despotism, within the space of a few miles" (116–17). In her *Journal* entry for 26 March 1818, she returns to this theme, remarking that "under the dominion of this tyranny the inhabitants of the fertile vallies bounded by these mountains are in a state of the most frightful poverty & diseases" (1: 200).

15. For the argument that the poem is about the uncertainty of conceiving origins, see Tetrault 63–85.

16. For relevant material on the "Little Ice Age," see Le Roy Ladurie, *Times of Feast;* J. Grove; and H. H. Lamb 211–40.

17. See J. Grove 187; and Pfister.

18. For material on the Tambora volcano, see Harington. For a discussion of the impact of this event on Byron and Keats, see J. Bate.

19. Through an analysis of the extensive use of rhyme in the poem, Keach suggests that the poem produces "an order of language that accepts the arbitrary and submits it to the deliberations of art" (*Shelley's Style* 200).

20. James Johnson draws a similar analogy: "There is no unmixed good in this world, the inundations of the Nile and the Ganges, while they scatter fertility over the valley of Egypt, and the pains of Bengal, sow with a liberal hand, at the same time, the seeds of dreadful diseases!" (47).

21. See also Kennedy, *Islands of White* 109–27.

22. See his discussion of Medwin (Leask 68–71, 154–71). Shortly after ordering a copy of James Mill's *History of British India,* Shelley inquired into the possibility of gaining employment at the court of a native prince, not with the East India Company. For material on Shelley's Indian circle, see Mazzeo.

Chapter 7. Cholera, Sanitation, and the Colonial Representation of India

1. See Curtis 85–89.

2. Though most present-day historians agree that the comma-shaped bacterium *Vibrio cholerae,* which causes epidemic cholera, was probably endemic to India, they also agree that 1817 was a turning point in its history. As Richard Evans has observed, cholera has "a good claim to be regarded as the classic epidemic disease of the nineteenth century," a "creation of the industrial age" ("Epidemics and Revolution" 151–52, 150).

3. See also Headrick 145–70.

4. See, for instance, Morris; Evans, *Death in Hamburg* and "Epidemics and Revolution"; Durey; Briggs; Pelling; and Charles E. Rosenberg, *Cholera Years.*

5. See Pelling: "As the cause of death and debility in mid-nineteenth-century England, cholera was surpassed among epidemic diseases by 'common continued fever' (chiefly typhoid, relapsing fever, and some typhus), scarlet fever, smallpox, and measles, and accounted for only a very small proportion of the area of highest mortality, which occurred among infants and young children" (4).

6. Three versions of the poem exist in separate letters, one to Coleridge's physician friend J. H. Green, 26 July 1832, Coleridge, *Collected Letters* 6: 916–18; the second, to Henry Nelson Coleridge, 28 August 1832, 6: 922–25; and another, dated 5 September 1832, to the surgeon J. H. B. Williams (not published in *Collected Letters* but available in Stephens). Unless otherwise noted, I will be referring to the version sent to H. N. Coleridge. The poem appeared in Coleridge's *Poetical Works* in a group titled "Jeux d'Esprit."

7. The September version is signed "Philodemus Coprophilus, Physician extraordinary to their sovereign Majesties, the People."

8. J. Jackson notes that the NCSTC CD-ROM produces 305 titles including the word "cholera" between 1820 and 1832.

9. For Coleridge's knowledge of contemporary medicine, see Harris; Levere 36–57, 201–21; H. Jackson, "Coleridge on the King's Evil" and "Coleridge's Collaborator"; and Vickers.

10. In a marginal comment added sometime around 1815 to the flyleaf of John Walker's *A Dictionary of the English Language, Answering at Once the Purposes of Rhyming, Spelling, and Pronouncing . . .* (London: 1775), Coleridge writes: "Contagious Typhus—originates, at least is always aggravated by impure air—especially human Effluvia—General treatment, applicable to all cases = Cleanliness, Ventilation, plentiful dilution—partial fomentation, friction" (see *Marginalia*, vol. 6 [forthcoming]). Anthony Harding has drawn my attention to a passage from *Notebook* 49 (British Museum Add. MS 47544) in which Coleridge, referring to James Welsh's *Military Reminiscences, from a Journal of Nearly Forty Years' Active Service in the East Indies* (1830), reflects on the puzzling selectivity of cholera in its victims and its apparent disregard for environmental barriers: "When we read so often (& who that reads military history can do otherwise of the Fevers, Cholera Morbus, &c &c evidently occasioned by particular states of the Atmosphere, sometimes in connection with the Soil—marsh or swamp-land—but often, where no such accessory influences can be traced—as where the Disease tacks & veers its mysterious Course from India to Russia, over soils & lands of the most various & opposite conditions & characters—how forcibly does not the sense of the dependence of our Lives on a directing Providence present itself to the Mind!"

11. *Wesleyan Methodist Magazine* 3rd ser. 11 (1832): 204–5.

12. For a discussion of this legislation in the context of colonial India, see P. Levine.

13. In a letter to Henry Coleridge, Coleridge describes "O'Connel, & the gang of Agitators" as but symptoms of the popular unrest of the "agitated Mass." O'Connell fares better than does Joseph Hume, leader of the radical party, who is described as being "more mischievous," as "a *fermenting* Virus" (885). For the association of the Irish with the spread of disease, see Kraut 31–49; Stallybrass and White; and Poovey, *Making a Social Body* 55–72.

14. Lord Greville notes that "furious contests have taken place about the burials, it having been recommended that bodies should be burned directly after death, and the most violent prejudice opposing itself to this recommendation" (2: 79). See Morris 104–14; Durey 163–70.

15. Heather Jackson has brought it to my attention that Coleridge also experimented with Indian bhang, a form of hashish, which he smoked and ate in 1803. See the *Marginalia*, under Robert Percival's *An Account of the Island of Ceylon* (1803) (vol. 5).

16. Thomas Poole notes that Coleridge suffered "two very severe attacks of the prevailing cholera, & suffered dreadfully under them" (*Collected Letters* 6: 874n).

17. In addition to the writings of James Johnson, James Kennedy, and James Annesley, whose *Sketches of the Most Prevalent Diseases of India* (London, 1825) was influential, the following list represents only a small part of the works published by physicians who had had some experience in India: A. T. Chirstie, M.D. (of Madras), *Observations on the Nature and Treatment of Cholera* (Edinburgh, 1828); Charles Searle (of Madras), *Cholera, Its Nature, Cause and Treatment* (London, 1830); George Hamilton Bell, *Treatise on Cholera Asphyxia or Epidemic Cholera as It Appeared in Asia and More Recently in Europe* (Edinburgh, 1831); Reginald Orton, *An Essay on the Epidemic Cholera of India* (1st ed. Madras, 1820; 2nd ed. London: Burgess and Hill, 1831); and T. Mollison, *Remarks on the Epidemic Cholera of India* (London, 1830).

18. For a discussion of the role of these ideas in the Victorian construction of motherhood, see Matus 56–70.

19. Throughout the 1830s John Roberton, the surgeon at the Manchester Lying-in Hospital, wrote several articles in the *Edinburgh Medical and Surgical Review* that sought to provide "a physiological inquiry concerning the period of female puberty in different climates" (15). These essays were collected in his *Essays and Notes on the Physiology and Diseases of Women* (1851). By 1842 Roberton had concluded in "On the Period of Puberty in Negro Women" that "there was no truth in the alleged forcing effect of heated cotton factories on the female constitution" (31).

Chapter 8. Tropical Invalids

1. For an evaluation of the available statistical data, see Curtin, *Death by Migration*.

2. For discussions of colonial acclimatization, see Curtin, *Death by Migration;* D. Arnold, *Colonizing the Body;* D. Kennedy, *Islands of White* and "Perils of the Midday Sun"; M. Harrison 36–59; Sargent; and Anderson, "Race, Disease, and Tropical Medicine."

3. Chapter 13, titled "Influence of India and Hot Climates on the Health of Women," was also published separately in 1875 as *Health in India for British Women*.

4. See Spivak, "Three Women's Texts"; Meyer; Azim; and Brantlinger 12.

5. It is possible that Brontë was thinking of Thomas Winterbottom's description of the tornadoes of Sierra Leone; the account begins thus: "A dark cloud, not larger than 'a man's hand,' is first observed on the verge of the eastern horizon" (1: 25).

6. Compare this scene, for instance, with Rochester's association of Bertha's cries and breath with Jamaican air: "Something of her breath (faugh!) mixed with the air I breathed" (311).

7. See Spivak, "Three Women's Texts" 247–48; Azim 183; and Meyer 252–53. See also Gilman's discussion of racial stereotypes in *Difference and Pathology,* esp. 76–149.

8. Over the nineteenth century, "creolization" also took on a biological meaning, as in Lafcadio Hearn's reference to "those extraordinary influences of climate and environment which produce the phenomena of creolization" (416).

9. See Matus; Showalter; and Gilbert and Gubar. For an examination of the way middle-class British women displaced their anxieties about their perceived powerlessness in their representations of slaves, see M. Ferguson, *Subject to Others.*

10. The publications of Thomas Southwood Smith, James Kay, Neil Arnot, and Edwin Chadwick, notably the Poor Law Commission reports of 1838 and the Royal Commission document of 1845, *Health of Towns and Populous Places,* are relevant here. During the nineteenth century, it should be stressed, typhus was a class-specific disease, "not inaptly . . . termed," as Richard Millar observed in his *Clinical Lectures,* "the *poor man's disease*" (11).

11. See M. W. Flinn's "Introduction" to Edwin Chadwick's *Report on the Sanitary Condition of the Labouring Population of Great Britain* 10.

Chapter 9. "All the World Has the Plague": Mary Shelley's The Last Man

1. For an insightful discussion of the relation between imperialism and disease in the novel, see Cantor 193–96.

2. See Fisch 273–77; Mellor, in M. Shelley, *Last Man* xxiv; Aaron 17; and S. Goldsmith 149. Shelley's gendering of the plague is actually much more fluid, since she frequently portrays the disease in gender neutral or masculine terms: "the brother of death" (192), "earth's desolator . . . enthroned himself" (177), "the enemy had tortured, before he murdered" (203–4). The plague stands apart from the categories that humans apply to it, even those of gender.

3. The British response to epidemic finds a parallel in the optimism of Americans toward cholera. Charles Rosenberg notes the confidence that initially shaped American health policies in the period leading up to the outbreak of the disease: "Filth, misery, vice, and poverty conspired to produce its unfortunate victims. Few such could be found in a land enjoying those unique blessings granted the United States. The healthy farmers and sturdy mechanics of the United States could, Americans believed, never provide such hecatombs of victims as cholera had claimed from among the pagans, Moslems, and papists of Europe and the East. America had no class to compare with the miserable slumdwellers of Paris and London or with the brutalized serfs of Nicholas' Russia. Even New England mill hands were as well fed and clothed as any class in the world, their habits perfectly regular and temperate. 'With clean persons and clean consciences,' Americans were prepared to meet the disease without trembling" (*Cholera Years* 15–16).

4. Ann Mellor makes a similar point, though from an essentially moralistic standpoint: "If one were forced to embrace the Other rather than permitted to define it exclusively as 'foreign' and 'diseased,' one might escape this socially constructed plague" (M. Shelley, *Last Man* xxiv).

WORKS CITED

Aaron, Jane. "The Return of the Repressed: Reading Mary Shelley's *The Last Man.*" *Feminist Criticism: Theory and Practice.* Ed. Susan Sellers. Toronto: U of Toronto P, 1991. 9–21.

Abrams, M. H. "The Correspondent Breeze: A Romantic Metaphor." *English Romantic Poets: Modern Essays in Criticism.* Ed. M. H. Abrams. New York: Oxford UP, 1960. 37–54.

Adair, James. *Medical Cautions Chiefly for the Consideration of Invalids.* 2nd ed. Bath: Cuttwell, 1787.

Addison, Joseph. *Works.* Ed. Richard Hurd. 5 vols. London: Bohn, 1854.

Rev. of *Adonais,* by P. B. Shelley. *Literary Gazette and Journal of Belles Lettres* 255 (8 Dec. 1821): 772–73.

Adorno, Theodor. "Commitment." *New Left Review* 87–88 (1974): 75–91.

Alloula, Malek. *The Colonial Harem.* Trans. Myrna Godzich and Wlad Godzich. Minneapolis: U of Minneapolis P, 1986.

Anderson, Warwick. "Disease, Race, and Empire." *Bulletin of the History of Medicine* 70 (1996): 62–67.

———. "Excremental Colonialism: Public Health and the Poetics of Pollution." *Critical Inquiry* 21 (1995): 640–69.

———. "Race, Disease, and Tropical Medicine." *Bulletin of the History of Medicine* 70 (1996): 94–118.

Annesley, James. *Researches into the Causes, Nature, and Treatment of the More Prevalent Diseases of India, and of Warm Climates Generally.* 2nd ed. London: Longman, Brown, Green, and Longmans, 1841.

Arac, Jonathan, and Harriet Ritvo, eds. *Macropolitics of Nineteenth-Century Literature: Nationalism, Exoticism, Imperialism.* Philadelphia: U of Pennsylvania P, 1991.

Arnold, David. "Cholera and Colonialism in British India." *Past and Present* 113 (1986): 118–51.

———. *Colonizing the Body: State Medicine and Epidemic Disease in Nineteenth-Century India.* Berkeley: U of California P, 1993.

———. "Medicine and Colonialism." *Companion Encyclopedia of the History of Medicine.* Ed. W. F. Bynum and Roy Porter. London: Routledge, 1993. 2: 1393–1416.

———, ed. *Imperial Medicine and Indigenous Societies.* Manchester: Manchester UP, 1988.

Aske, Martin. "Keats, the Critics, and the Politics of Envy." *Keats and History.* Ed. Nicholas Roe. New York: Cambridge UP, 1995. 46–64.

Austen, Jane. *Emma.* Harmondsworth, Eng.: Penguin, 1966.

———. *Sanditon, an Unfinished Novel by Jane Austen, Reproduced in Facsimile from the*

Manuscript in the Possession of King's College, Cambridge. Ed. B. C. Southam. Oxford: Clarendon, 1975.

Azim, Firdous. *The Colonial Rise of the Novel.* London: Routledge, 1993.

Babington, William, and James Curry. *Outlines of a Course of Lectures on the Practice of Medicine, as Delivered in the Medical School of Guy's Hospital.* London: Bensley, 1802–6.

Balfour, Andrew. "Some British and American Pioneers in Tropical Medicine and Hygiene." *Transactions of the Royal Society of Tropical Medicine and Hygiene* 19 (1925): 189–231.

Barnes, David S. *The Making of a Social Disease: Tuberculosis in Nineteenth-Century France.* Berkeley: U of California P, 1995.

Baron-Wilson, Cornwall (Mrs.). *The Life and Correspondence of M. G. Lewis.* 2 vols. London: Henry Colburn, 1839.

Barrell, John. *The Infection of Thomas De Quincey: A Psychopathology of Imperialism.* New Haven: Yale UP, 1991.

Barrett, Frank A. "A Medical Geographical Anniversary." *Social Science and Medicine* 37 (1993): 701–10.

——. " 'Scurvy' Lind's Medical Geography." *Social Science and Medicine* 33 (1991): 347–53.

Bate, Jonathan. "Living with the Weather." *Studies in Romanticism* 35 (1996): 431–47.

Bate, Walter Jackson. *John Keats.* Cambridge: Harvard UP, 1963.

Baum, Joan. *Mind-Forg'd Manacles: Slavery and the English Romantic Poets.* North Haven, CT: Archon Books, 1994.

Beevoir, Hugh. "The Declension of Phthisis." *Lancet* 2 (1899): 1005–20.

Beier, A. L. *Masterless Men: The Vagrancy Problem in England, 1560–1640.* London: Methuen, 1985.

Bennett, Andrew. *Keats, Narrative and Audience: The Posthumous Life of Writing.* Cambridge: Cambridge UP, 1994.

Bennett, Betty T. *British War Poetry in the Age of Romanticism: 1793–1815.* New York: Garland, 1976.

Bermingham, Ann. *Landscape and Ideology: The English Rustic Tradition, 1740–1860.* Berkeley: U of California P, 1986.

Bewell, Alan. "*Jane Eyre* and Victorian Medical Geography." *Journal of English Literary History* 63 (1996): 773–808.

——. "The Political Implications of Keats's Classicist Aesthetics." *Studies in Romanticism* 25 (1986): 220–29.

——. *Wordsworth Nature, Man, and Society in the Experimental Poetry.* New Haven: Yale UP, 1989.

Bhabha, Homi K. *The Location of Culture.* London: Routledge, 1994.

Bigland, Eileen. *Lord Byron.* London: Cassell, 1956.

Blake, William. *The Poetry and Prose of William Blake.* Ed. David V. Erdman. Garden City, NY: Doubleday, 1965.

Blane, Gilbert. "Observations on the Diseases of Seamen." *The Health of Seamen: Selections from the Works of Dr. James Lind, Sir Gilbert Blane, and Dr. Thomas Trotter.* Ed. Christopher Lloyd. London: Navy Records Society, 1965.

——. "On the Comparative Health of the British Navy, from the Year 1779 to the Year 1814, with Proposals for its Farther Improvement." *The Health of Seamen: Selections from the Works of Dr. James Lind, Sir Gilbert Blane, and Dr. Thomas Trotter.* Ed. Christopher Lloyd. London: Navy Records Society, 1965.

——. *A Short Account of the Most Effectual Means of Preserving the Health of Seamen.* N.p.: n.p., 1780.

Bloom, Harold. "The Internalization of Quest-Romance." *Romanticism and Consciousness: Essays in Criticism.* New York: Norton, 1970.

Bohen, A. Adu. *Britain, the Sahara, and the Western Sudan, 1788–1861.* Oxford: Clarendon, 1964.

Bohls, Elizabeth A. "The Aesthetics of Colonialism: Janet Schaw in the West Indies, 1774–1775." *Eighteenth-Century Studies* 27 (1994): 363–90.

——. "Mimicry, Hybridity, and Violence in Stedman's *Narrative of a Five Years' Expedition against the Revolting Negroes of Surinam.*" 1995 ASECS Conference.

——. *Women Travel Writers and the Language of Aesthetics, 1716–1818.* New York: Cambridge UP, 1995.

Boswell, James. *Boswell's Life of Johnson.* Ed. George Birkbeck Hill. 2nd ed. 6 vols. Oxford: Clarendon, 1964.

Boucé, Paul-Gabriel. *The Novels of Tobias Smollett.* New York: Longman, 1976.

Bovill, E. W. *The Niger Explored.* London: Oxford, 1968.

Bradford, William. *Bradford's History of Plymouth Plantation, 1606–1646.* Ed. J. Franklin Jameson. *Original Narratives of Early American History.* New York: Scribner, 1908.

Bradley, A. C. "Notes on Shelley's 'Triumph of Life.'" *Modern Language Review* 9 (1914): 441–56.

Brantlinger, Patrick. *Rule of Darkness: British Literature and Imperialism, 1830–1914.* Ithaca: Cornell UP, 1988.

Brennan, Timothy. "The National Longing for Form." *Nation and Narration.* Ed. Homi K. Bhabha. London: Routledge, 1990. 44–70.

Briggs, Asa. "Cholera and Society in the Nineteenth Century." *Past and Present* 19 (1961): 76–96.

Brink, Andrew. *Loss and Symbolic Repair: A Psychological Study of Some English Poets.* Hamilton, ON: Cromlech, 1977.

British House of Commons Parliamentary Papers. *1828 Report of the Commissioners on the Supply of Water in the Metropolis* (21 April 1828), 9: 1–155.

Brockway, Lucille H. *Science and Colonial Expansion: The Role of the British Royal Botanic Gardens.* New York: Academic, 1979.

Brontë, Charlotte. *Jane Eyre.* Ed. Margaret Smith. Oxford: Oxford UP, 1975.

——. *Shirley.* Ed. Herbert Rosengarten and Margaret Smith. Oxford: Clarendon, 1979.

Brooks, Christopher. "Goldsmith's 'Private Centinel' and the Rejection of Imperialism." *University of Dayton Review* 20 (1989): 21–32.

——. "'Guilty of Being Poor': Goldsmith's 'No-Account' Centinel." 1996 American Society for Eighteenth-Century Studies Conference.

Brown, Huntington. "The Gloss to *The Rime of the Ancient Mariner.*" *Modern Language Quarterly* 6 (1945): 319–24.

Brown, Laura. *The Ends of Empire: Women and Ideology in Early Eighteenth-Century English Literature.* Ithaca: Cornell UP, 1993.

Browne, Thomas. "A Letter to a Friend." *The Works of Sir Thomas Browne.* Ed. Simon Wilkin. 4 vols. London: Bohn, 1846.

Burg, C. L. van der. "L'alimentation des Européens et des travailleurs indigènes aux pays chauds." *Janus* 10 (1905): 88–94.

Burke, Edmund. *The Writings and Speeches of Edmund Burke.* Ed. Paul Langford. Oxford: Clarendon, 1991.

Burns, Robert. *The Poems and Songs of Robert Burns.* Ed. James Kinsley. 3 vols. Oxford: Clarendon, 1968.

Burt, Adam. *A Tract on the Biliary Complaints of Europeans in Hot Climates; Founded on Observations in Bengal; and Consequently Designed to Be Particularly Useful to Those in That Country.* Calcutta: Hay, 1785.

Bury, M. R. "Social Constructionism and the Development of Medical Sociology." *Sociology of Health and Illness* 8 (1986): 137–79.

Busey, Samuel S. *Immigration: Its Evils and Consequences.* 1870. New York: Arno, 1969.

Butler, James A. "Tourist or Native Son: Wordsworth's Homecomings of 1799–1800." *Nineteenth-Century Literature* 51 (1996): 1–15.

Bynum, W. F., and Roy Porter, eds. *The Companion Encyclopedia of the History of Medicine.* 2 vols. London: Routledge, 1993.

Byron. Ed. Jerome J. McGann. Oxford: Oxford UP, 1986.

Byron's Letters and Journals. Ed. Leslie A. Marchand. 12 vols. London: Murray, 1978.

Caldwell, Charles. *An Oration on the Causes of the Difference, in Point of Frequency and Force, between Two Endemic Diseases of the United States of America, and Those of the Countries of Europe.* Philadelphia: Bradford, 1802.

Cantor, Paul A. "The Apocalypse of Empire: Mary Shelley's *The Last Man.*" *Iconoclastic Departures: Mary Shelley after "Frankenstein."* Ed. Syndy M. Conger, Frederick S. Frank, and Gregory O'Dea. Cranbury, NJ: Associated UP, 1997. 193–211.

Carlyle, Thomas. *Latter-Day Pamphlets.* 1850. London: Chapman and Hall, 1872.

Cartwright, Frederick F. *Disease and History.* New York: Thomas Y. Crowell, 1972.

Chadwick, Edwin. *Report on the Sanitary Condition of the Labouring Population of Great Britain.* 1842. Ed. M. W. Flinn. Edinburgh: Edinburgh UP, 1965.

Chakrabarty, Dipesh. "Open Space/Public Space: Garbage, Modernity and India." *South Asia* ns 14 (June 1991): 15–31.

Chalmers, Albert J. "Two Early Eighteenth Century Treatises on Tropical Medicine." *Proceedings of the Royal Society of Medicine (sec. Hist. Med.)* 7 (1914): 98–106.

Chaudhuri, Nupur, and Margaret Strobel, eds. *Western Women and Imperialism: Complicity and Resistance.* Bloomington: Indiana UP, 1992.

Cheyne, George. *Essay of Health and Long Life.* London: Strahan, 1724.

Chisholm, Colin. *An Essay on the Malignant Pestilential Fever Introduced in the West Indian Islands from Boullam, on the Coast of Guinea, as It Appeared in 1793–1794.* Philadelphia: Thomas Dobson, 1799.

"The Cholera in the Gazette." *New Monthly Magazine* 31 (1831): 490.

Clairmont, Claire. *The Journals of Claire Clairmont.* Ed. Marion Kingston Stocking. Cambridge: Harvard UP, 1968.

Clark, James. *The Sanative Influence of Climate: With an Account of the Best Places of Resort for Invalids in England, the South of Europe, etc.* 3rd ed. London: Murray, 1841.

——. *A Treatise on Pulmonary Consumption Comprehending an Inquiry into the Causes Nature Prevention and Treatment of Tuberculous and Scrofulous Diseases in General.* London: Sherwood Gilbert and Piper, 1835.

Clark, John. *Observations on the Diseases in Long Voyages to Hot Countries, and Particularly on Those Which Prevail in the East Indies.* London: Wilson and Nicol, 1773.

Clarke, Norma. *Ambitious Heights: Writing, Friendship, Love: The Jewsbury Sisters, Felicia Hemans, and Jane Welsh Carlyle.* New York: Routledge, 1990.

Clarkson, Thomas. *An Essay on the Impolicy of the African Slave Trade.* 2nd ed. London: Phillips, 1788.

——. *The History of the Rise, Progress, and Accomplishment of the Abolition of the African Slave-Trade by the British Parliament.* 2 vols. 1808. London: Cass, 1968.

Clemesha, William Wesley. *Sewage Disposal in the Tropics.* London: Thacker, 1910.

Clifford, Brendan, ed. *"Billy Bluff and the Squire" (a Satire on Irish Aristocracy) and Other Writings by Rev. James Porter.* Belfast: Athol, 1991.

Cobbett, William. "Cholera Morbus." *Cobbett's Weekly Political Register* 75.9 (25 Feb. 1832): 513–23.

Coleman, William. *Yellow Fever in the North: The Methods of Early Epidemiology.* Madison: U of Wisconsin P, 1987.

Coleridge, Samuel Taylor. *Collected Letters of Samuel Taylor Coleridge.* Ed. Earl Leslie Griggs. 6 vols. Oxford: Clarendon, 1956–71.

——. *The Complete Poems.* Ed. William Keach. London: Penguin, 1997.

——. *Lay Sermons.* Ed. R. J. White. *The Collected Works of Samuel Taylor Coleridge.* Princeton: Princeton UP, 1972.

——. *Lectures 1795 on Politics and Religion.* Ed. Lewis Patton and Peter Mann. *The Collected Works of Samuel Taylor Coleridge.* Princeton: Princeton UP, 1971.

——. *Marginalia.* Ed. Heather Jackson and George Whalley. 6 vols. *The Collected Works of Samuel Taylor Coleridge.* Princeton: Princeton UP, 1980–.

——. *Notebooks of Samuel Taylor Coleridge.* Ed. Kathleen Coburn. Princeton: Princeton UP, 1957–.

——. *Samuel Taylor Coleridge.* The Oxford Authors. Ed. H. J. Jackson. Oxford: Oxford UP, 1985.

———. *Shorter Works and Fragments*. Ed. H. J. Jackson and J. R. de J. Jackson. 2 vols. *The Collected Works of Samuel Taylor Coleridge*. Princeton: Princeton UP, 1995.

———. *Table Talk*. Ed. Carl Woodring. 2 vols. *The Collected Works of Samuel Taylor Coleridge*. Princeton: Princeton UP, 1990.

———. *The Watchman*. Ed. Lewis Patton. *The Collected Works of Samuel Taylor Coleridge*. Princeton: Princeton UP, 1970.

Colley, Linda. *Britons: Forging the Nation, 1707–1837*. New Haven: Yale UP, 1992.

Collings, David. *Wordsworthian Errancies: The Poetics of Cultural Dismemberment*. Baltimore: Johns Hopkins UP, 1994.

Comaroff, Jean. "The Diseased Heart of Africa: Medicine, Colonialism and the Black Body." *Knowledge, Power, and Practice: The Anthropology of Medicine and Everyday Life*. Ed. Shirley Lindenbaum and Margaret Lock. Berkeley: U of California P, 1993. 305–29.

———. "Medicine: Symbol and Ideology." *The Problem of Medical Knowledge: Examining the Social Construction of Medicine*. Ed. P. Wright and A. Treacher. Edinburgh: Edinburgh UP, 1982. 49–69.

Conder, Josiah. Rev. of *Lamia, Isabella, the Eve of St Agnes, and Other Poems*, by John Keats. *Eclectic Review* ns 14 (Sept. 1820): 158–71.

Conrad, Joseph. *Heart of Darkness*. Ed. Robert Kimbrough. 3rd ed. New York: Norton, 1988.

Constable, Thomas. *Archibald Constable and His Literary Correspondents*. Edinburgh: Edmonton and Douglas, 1873.

Cook, G. C. *From the Greenwich Hulks to Old St Pancras: A History of Tropical Disease in London*. London: Athlone, 1992.

Cooter, Roger. "Anticontagionism and History's Medical Record." *The Problem of Medical Knowledge; Examining the Social Construction of Medicine*. Ed. P. Wright and A. Treacher. Edinburgh: Edinburgh UP, 1982. 87–108.

Corbin, Alain. *The Foul and the Fragrant*. Cambridge: Harvard UP, 1986.

Cornwall, Barry. "Recollections of Books and Their Authors.—No. 6. John Keats, the Poet." *Olio, or Museum of Entertainment* 1 (1828): 391–94.

Cosgrove, Denis, and Stephen Daniels, eds. *Iconography of Landscape: Essays on the Symbolic Representations, Design and Use of Past Environments*. Cambridge: Cambridge UP, 1988.

Cotton, Richard Payne. *The Nature, Symptoms and Treatment of Consumption*. London: Churchill, 1852.

Cowper, William. *The Poems of William Cowper*. Ed. John D. Baird and Charles Ryskamp. 3 vols. Oxford: Clarendon, 1980–95.

Cox, Jeffrey N. "Keats, Shelley, and the Wealth of the Imagination." *Studies in Romanticism* 34 (1995): 365–400.

Creighton, Charles. *A History of Epidemics in Britain*. 2 vols. 1891. New York: Barnes and Noble, 1965.

Crook, Nora, and Derek Guiton. *Shelley's Venomed Malady*. Cambridge: Cambridge UP, 1986.

Crooks, J. J. *Historical Records of the Royal African Corps*. Dublin: Browne and Nolan, 1925.

Crosby, Alfred W. *The Columbian Exchange: The Biological Consequences of 1492*. Westport, CT: Greenwood, 1972.

——. *Ecological Imperialism: The Biological Expansion of Europe, 900–1900*. Cambridge: Cambridge UP, 1986.

Currie, James. *Medical Reports on the Effects of Water, Cold and Warm, as a Remedy in Fever and Other Diseases*. 2nd ed. Liverpool: M'Creery, 1798.

Curry, James. *Examination of the Prejudices Commonly Entertained against Mercury, as Beneficially Applicable to the Greater Number of Liver Complaints and to Various Other Forms of Disease, as Well as to Syphilis*. London: M'Creery, 1810.

Curtin, Philip D. *The Atlantic Slave Trade: A Census*. Madison: U of Wisconsin P, 1969.

——. *Death by Migration: Europe's Encounter with the Tropical World in the Nineteenth Century*. Cambridge: Cambridge UP, 1989.

——. *Disease and Empire: The Health of European Troops in the Conquest of Africa*. Cambridge: Cambridge UP, 1998.

——. "The End of the 'White Man's Grave'?: Nineteenth-Century Mortality in West Africa." *Journal of Interdisciplinary History* 21 (1990): 63–88.

——. "Epidemiology and the Slave Trade." *Political Science Quarterly* 83 (1968): 191–216.

——. *The Image of Africa: British Ideas and Action, 1780–1850*. Madison: U of Wisconsin P, 1964.

——. "The White Man's Grave: Image and Reality, 1780–1850." *Journal of British Studies* 1 (1961): 94–110.

Curtis, Charles. *An Account of the Diseases in India, as They Appeared in the English Fleet, and in the Naval Hospital at Madras, in 1782 and 1783; with Observations on Ulcers, and the Hospital Sores of That Country*. Edinburgh: Laing, 1807.

Daniels, Stephen. *Fields of Vision: Landscape Imagery and National Identity in England and the United States*. Cambridge: Polity, 1993.

Darwin, Charles. *The Voyage of the "Beagle."* New York: Signet, 1988.

Darwin, Erasmus. *Zoönomia*. 2 vols. London: Johnson, 1794–96.

Davidson, Andrew. *Hygiene and Diseases of Warm Climates*. Edinburgh: Pentland, 1893.

Davies, J. N. P. *Pestilence and Disease in the History of Africa*. Johannesburg: Witwatersrand UP, 1979.

Davies, K. G. "The Living and the Dead: White Mortality in West Africa, 1684–1732." *Race and Slavery in the Western Hemisphere: Quantitative Studies*. Ed. Stanley L. Engerman and Eugene D. Genovese. Princeton: Princeton UP, 1975. 83–98.

Davy, Humphry. *The Collected Works of Sir Humphry Davy.* Ed. John Davy. 9 vols. London: Smith, Elder and Cornhill, 1839.

Dawson, P. M. S. *The Unacknowledged Legislator: Shelley and Politics.* Oxford: Clarendon, 1980.

de Almeida, Hermione. *Romantic Medicine and John Keats.* New York: Oxford UP, 1991.

Defoe, Daniel. *Robinson Crusoe.* New York: Norton, 1975.

de Groot, Joanna. " 'Sex' and 'Race': The Construction of Language and Image in the Nineteenth Century." *Sexuality and Subordination: Interdisciplinary Studies of Gender in the Nineteenth Century.* Ed. Susan Mendus and Jane Rendall. London: Routledge, 1989. 89–128.

Delaporte, François. *Disease and Civilization: The Cholera in Paris, 1832.* Trans. Arthur Goldhammer. Cambridge: MIT P, 1986.

De Quincey, Thomas. *The Collected Writings of Thomas De Quincey.* Ed. David Masson. 14 vols. London: Black, 1896–97.

——. *Confessions of an English Opium Eater.* Ed. Alethea Hayter. Harmondsworth, Eng.: Penguin, 1971.

——. *De Quincey as Critic.* Ed. John E. Jordan. London: Routledge and Kegan Paul, 1973.

——. *Selected Writings of Thomas De Quincey.* Ed. Philip van Doren Stern. New York: Random, 1937.

Dickens, Charles. *Hard Times.* New York: Norton, 1966.

——. *The Life and Adventures of Nicholas Nickleby.* Ed. Dame Sybil Thorndike. London: Oxford UP, 1950.

[Dickson, Samuel]. *Memorable Events in the Life of a London Physician.* London: Virtue, 1863.

Dobyns, Henry F. "An Outline of Andean Epidemic History to 1720." *Bulletin of the History of Medicine* 37 (1963): 493–515.

——. *Their Number Become Thinned.* Knoxville: U of Tennessee P, 1983.

Douglas, Mary. *Purity and Danger: an Analysis of Concepts of Pollution and Taboo.* London: Routledge, 1966.

Dubos, René, and Jean Dubos. *The White Plague: Tuberculosis, Man, and Society.* 1952. New Brunswick: Rutgers UP, 1987.

Dundas, Robert. *Sketches of Brazil: Including New Views on Tropical and European Fever, with Remarks on a Premature Decay of the System Incident to Europeans on Their Return from Hot Climates.* London: Churchill, 1852.

Dunn, Richard S. *Sugar and Slaves: The Rise of the Planter Class in the English West Indies, 1624–1713.* Chapel Hill: U of North Carolina P, 1972.

Durey, Michael. *The Return of the Plague: British Society and the Cholera, 1831–2.* Dublin: Gill and Macmillan, 1979.

Ebbatson, J. B. "Coleridge's Mariner and the Rights of Man." *Studies in Romanticism* 11 (1972): 171–206.

Edwards, Bryan. *The History, Civil and Commercial, of the British West Indies.* 5 vols. London: Miller, 1819.

Eilenberg, Susan. *Strange Power of Speech: Wordsworth, Coleridge and Literary Possession.* New York: Oxford UP, 1992.

Empson, William. "The Ancient Mariner." *Critical Quarterly* 6 (1964): 289–319.

——. Introduction. *Coleridge's Verse: A Selection.* Ed. William Empson and David Pirie. London: Faber, 1972.

Rev. of *Endymion,* by John Keats. *Baldwin's London Magazine,* Apr. 1820, 380–89.

Engels, Friedrich. *The Condition of the Working Class in England.* Trans. and ed. W. O. Henderson and W. H. Chaloner. Oxford: Blackwell, 1958.

Equiano, Olaudah. *The Life of Olaudah Equiano or Gustavus Vassa the African.* Ed. Paul Edwards. London: Dawsons, 1969.

Erdman, David V. *Blake: Prophet against Empire: A Poet's Interpretation of His Own Times.* Rev. ed. Princeton: Princeton UP, 1969.

Erikson, Kai. "Notes on Trauma and Community." *Trauma: Explorations in Memory.* Ed. Cathy Caruth. Baltimore: Johns Hopkins UP, 1995. 183–99.

Ernst, Waltraud. "European Madness and Gender in Nineteenth-Century British India." *Social History of Medicine* 9 (1996): 357–82.

——. *Mad Tales from the Raj: The European Insane in British India, 1800–1858.* London: Routledge, 1991.

"Europeans in the Tropics." *British Medical Journal* (9 Jan. 1897): 93–94.

Evans, Richard J. *Death in Hamburg: Society and Politics in the Cholera Years, 1830–1910.* Oxford: Clarendon, 1987.

——. "Epidemics and Revolution: Cholera in Nineteenth-Century Europe." *Epidemics and Ideas: Essays on the Historical Perception of Pestilence.* Ed. Terence Ranger and Paul Slack. Cambridge: Cambridge UP, 1992. 149–73.

Everest, Kelvin. " 'Ozymandias': The Text in Time." *Percy Bysshe Shelley: Bicentenary Essays.* Ed. Kelvin Everest. Cambridge: Brewer, 1992. 24–42.

Eyler, John M. *Victorian Social Medicine: The Ideas and Methods of William Farr.* Baltimore: Johns Hopkins UP, 1979.

Falconbridge, Maria. *Narrative of Two Voyages to the River Sierra Leone during the Years 1791–1793.* 1794. London: Cass, 1967.

Fanon, Frantz. *A Dying Colonialism.* Trans. Haakon Chevalier. Harmondsworth, Eng.: Penguin, 1970.

Farley, John. *Bilharzia: A History of Imperial Tropical Medicine.* Cambridge: Cambridge UP, 1991.

Farr, William. *British House of Commons Parliamentary Papers. Ninth Annual Report of the Registrar General* (1847–48).

——. *Report on the Mortality of Cholera in England, 1848–49.* London: Clowes, 1852.

Faucher, Leon. *Manchester in 1844: Its Present Condition and Future Prospects.* Trans. by a member of the Manchester Athenaeum. 1844. London: Cass, 1969.

Favret, Mary A. "Coming Home: The Public Spaces of Romantic War." *Studies in Romanticism* 33 (1994): 539–48.

Fayrer, Joseph. *On the Climate and Fevers of India.* London: Churchill, 1882.

Ferguson, Moira. *Subject to Others: British Women Writers and Colonial Slavery, 1670–1834.* New York: Routledge, 1992.

Ferguson, William. "On the Nature and History of Marsh Poison." *Transactions of the Royal Society of Edinburgh* 9 (1823): 273–96.

Fielding, John. *A Brief Description of the Cities of London and Westminster.* London: Wilkie, 1776.

Finke, Leonhard Ludwig. *Versuch einer allgemeinen medicinish-praktischen Geographie: Worin der historische Thiel der einheimschen Völker- und Staaten-Arzneykunde vorgetragen wird.* 3 vols. Leipzig: Weidmann, 1792–95.

Fisch, Audrey A. "Plaguing Politics: AIDS, Deconstruction, and *The Last Man.*" *The Other Mary Shelley: Beyond "Frankenstein."* Ed. Audrey Fisch, Anne Mellor, and Esther Schor. New York: Oxford UP, 1993. 267–86.

Fletcher, Charles. *A Maritime State Considered, as to the Health of Seamen; with Effective Means for Rendering the Situation of British Seamen More Comfortable.* 2nd ed. London: Vinct, 1791.

Ford, George H. *Keats and the Victorians: A Study of His Influence and Rise to Fame, 1821–1895.* New Haven: Yale UP, 1944.

Fortescue, J. W. *A History of the British Army.* 13 vols. London: Macmillan, 1899.

Foucault, Michel. "The Politics of Health in the Eighteenth Century." *Power / Knowledge: Selected Interviews and Other Writings.* Trans. Leo Marshall. Ed. Colin Gordon. New York: Pantheon, 1980.

Frank, Johann Peter. *A System of Complete Medical Police: Selections from Johann Peter Frank.* Ed. Erna Lesky. Baltimore: Johns Hopkins UP, 1976.

Friedlaender, Walter. "Napoleon as 'Rois Thaumaturge.'" *Journal of the Warburg and Courtauld Institutes* 4 (1940–41): 139–41.

Fry, Elizabeth, and John Gurney. *Report Addressed to the Marquess Wellesley.* London: Arch, 1827.

Fry, Paul. "History, Existence, and 'To Autumn.'" *Studies in Romanticism* 25 (1986): 211–19.

Frye, Northrop. *The Great Code: The Bible and Literature.* Toronto: Academic, 1982.

Fulford, Tim, and Peter Kitson, eds. *Romanticism and Colonialism: Writing and Empire, 1780–1830.* Cambridge: Cambridge UP, 1998.

Gage, Thomas. *The English-American, His Travail by Sea and Land, or A New Survey of the West-Indie's. . . .* London: Cotes, 1648.

Garnett, David. "Books in General." *New Statesman and Nation* 10 June 1933: 763.

Garrett, Laurie. *The Coming Plague: Newly Emerging Diseases in a World out of Balance.* New York: Farrar, 1994.

Gascoigne, John. *Joseph Banks and the English Enlightenment: Useful Knowledge and Polite Culture.* Cambridge: Cambridge UP, 1994.

Gaskell, Elizabeth. *The Life of Charlotte Brontë.* Ed. Margaret Lane. London: Lehmann, 1947.

Gaskell, Peter. *The Manufacturing Population of England, Its Moral, Social, and Physical Conditions, and the Changes Which Have Arisen from the Use of Steam Machinery.* London: Baldwin and Cradock, 1833.

Gaulter, Henry. *The Origins and Progress of the Malignant Cholera in Manchester.* London: Longman, 1833.

Geggus, David Patrick. *Slavery, War, and Revolution: The British Occupation of Saint Dominique, 1793–1798.* Oxford: Clarendon, 1982.

Gelfand, Michael. *Rivers of Death in Africa.* London: Oxford UP, 1964.

Gérin, Winifred. *Charlotte Brontë: The Evolution of Genius.* Oxford: Clarendon, 1967.

Gibbon, Edward. *Memoirs of My Life and Writings.* Ed. A. O. J. Cockshut and Stephen Constantine. Hartnolls, Bodmin: Keele UP, 1994.

Gilbert, E. W. "Pioneer Maps of Health and Disease in England." *Geographical Journal* 124 (1958): 172–83.

Gilbert, Sandra M., and Susan Gubar. *The Madwoman in the Attic: The Woman Writer and the Nineteenth-Literary Imagination.* New Haven: Yale UP, 1979.

Gilbert, William. *The Hurricane: A Theosophical and Western Eclogue to Which Is Subjoined a Solitary Effusion in a Summer's Evening.* London: Edwards, 1796.

Gilfillan, George. *Gallery of Literary Portraits.* 2 vols. Edinburgh: Hogg, 1856.

Gill, Stephen. *William Wordsworth: A Life.* Oxford: Clarendon, 1989.

Gillespie, Leonard. *Observations on the Diseases Which Prevailed on Board a Part of His Majesty's Squadron on the Leeward Island Station, between Nov. 1794 and April 1796.* London: Cuthell, 1800.

Gillett, Eric. *Maria Jane Jewsbury: Occasional Papers, Selected with a Memoir.* London: Oxford UP, 1932.

Gilman, Sander L. *Difference and Pathology: Stereotypes of Sexuality, Race, and Madness.* Ithaca: Cornell UP, 1985.

——. *Disease and Representation: Images of Illness from Madness to AIDS.* Ithaca: Cornell UP, 1988.

——. *Health and Illness: Images of Difference.* London: Reaktion, 1995.

——. "The Hottentot and the Prostitute: Toward an Iconography of Female Sexuality." *Difference and Pathology: Stereotypes of Sexuality, Race, and Madness.* By Sander L. Gilman. Ithaca: Cornell UP, 1988. 76–108.

Gilroy, Paul. *The Black Atlantic: Modernity and Double Consciousness.* Cambridge: Harvard UP, 1993.

Gittings, Robert. *John Keats.* Harmondsworth, Eng.: Penguin, 1968.

Godwin, William. *Enquiry concerning Political Justice and Its Influence on Modern Morals and Happiness.* London: Robinson, 1793. Harmondsworth, Eng.: Penguin, 1985.

——. *Of Population.* 1820. New York: Kelley, 1964.

Goellnicht, Donald C. *The Poet-Physician: Keats and Medical Science.* Pittsburgh: U of Pittsburgh P, 1984.

Goldsmith, Oliver. *The Collected Works of Oliver Goldsmith.* Ed. Arthur Friedman. Oxford: Clarendon, 1966.

Goldsmith, Steven. "Of Gender, Plague, and Apocalypse: Mary Shelley's *Last Man.*" *Yale Journal of Criticism* 4.1 (1990): 129–73.

Goode, S. W. *Municipal Calcutta: Its Institutions in Their Origin and Growth.* Calcutta: Constable, 1916.

Gordon, Lyndall. *Charlotte Brontë: A Passionate Life.* London: Chatto and Windus, 1994.

Gradish, Stephen F. *The Manning of the British Navy during the Seven Years' War.* London: Royal Historical Society, 1980.

Grainger, James. *An Essay on the More Common West Indian Diseases, and the Remedies Which That Country Itself Produces. To Which Are Added Some Hints on the Management of the Negroes.* London: Becket and De Hondt, 1864.

Grant, James. *Lights and Shadows of London Life.* 2 vols. London: Otley, 1842.

Graves, Robert. *The White Goddess: A Historical Grammar of Poetic Myth.* 3rd ed. London: Faber, 1952.

Green, Martin. *Dreams of Adventure, Deeds of Empire.* New York: Basic, 1979.

Greville, Charles. *The Greville Memoirs.* Ed. Henry Reeve. 2 vols. New York: Appleton, 1875.

Grmek, Mirko. "Géographie médical et histoire des civilisations." *Annales: Economies, Sociétés, Civilisations* 18 (1963): 1071–87.

Grove, Jean M. *The Little Ice Age.* London: Methuen, 1988.

Grove, Richard H. *Ecology, Climate, and Empire: Colonialism and Global Environmental History, 1400–1940.* Cambridge, Eng.: White Horse, 1997.

———. *Green Imperialism: Colonial Expansion, Tropical Island Edens and the Origins of Environmentalism, 1600–1860.* Cambridge: Cambridge UP, 1995.

Guerra, Francisco. "The Influence of Disease on Race, Logistics and Colonization in the Antilles." *Journal of Tropical Medicine and Hygiene* 69 (1966): 23–35.

Haley, Bruce. *The Healthy Body and Victorian Culture.* Cambridge: Harvard UP, 1978.

Hallett, Robin. *The Penetration of Africa: European Enterprise and Exploitation, Principally in Northern and Western Africa.* London: Routledge, 1965.

———, ed. *Records of the African Association, 1788–1831.* London: Thomas Nelson, 1964.

Hamlin, Christopher. "Predisposing Causes and Public Health in Early Nineteenth-Century Medical Thought." *Social History of Medicine* 5 (1992): 43–70.

Hannaway, Caroline. "Environment and Miasmata." *Companion Encyclopedia of the History of Medicine.* Ed. W. F. Bynum and Roy Porter. London: Routledge, 1993. 1: 292–308.

Hardy, Anne. *The Epidemic Streets: Infectious Disease, and the Rise of Preventive Medicine, 1856–1900.* Oxford: Clarendon, 1993.

Harington, C. R., ed. *The Year without a Summer? World Climate in 1816.* Ottawa: Canadian Museum of Nature, 1992.

Harley, J. B. "Maps, Knowledge and Power." *The Iconography of Landscape: Essays on the Symbolic Representation, Design and Use of Past Environments.* Cambridge: Cambridge UP, 1988.

Harris, John. "Coleridge's Readings in Medicine." *Wordsworth Circle* 3 (1973): 85–95.

Harrison, Gary. *Wordsworth's Vagrant Muse: Poetry, Poverty and Power.* Detroit: Wayne State UP, 1994.

Harrison, Mark. *Public Health in British India: Anglo-Indian Preventative Medicine, 1859–1914.* Cambridge: Cambridge UP, 1994.

Hartman, Geoffrey. *The Fate of Reading and Other Essays.* Chicago: U of Chicago P, 1975.

Hartwig, Gerald W., and K. David Patterson. "The Disease Factor: An Introductory Overview." *Disease in African History: An Introductory Survey and Case Studies.* Ed. Gerald W. Hartwig and K. David Patterson. Durham: Duke UP, 1978. 3–24.

——, eds. *Disease in African History: An Introductory Survey and Case Studies.* Durham: Duke UP, 1978.

Hay, Douglas. "War, Dearth and Theft in the Eighteenth Century: The Record of the English Courts." *Past and Present* 95 (1982): 117–60.

Haydon, Benjamin Robert. *The Autobiography and Memoirs of Benjamin Robert Haydon.* Ed. Aldous Huxley. 2 vols. London: Davies, 1926.

——. *The Diary of Benjamin Robert Haydon.* Ed. Willard Bissell Pope. 5 vols. Cambridge: Harvard UP, 1960.

Hazlitt, William. *The Complete Works of William Hazlitt.* Ed. F. P. Howe. 21 vols. London: Dent, 1931.

Headrick, Daniel R. *The Tentacles of Progress: Technology Transfer in the Age of Imperialism, 1850–1940.* New York: Oxford UP, 1988.

Hearn, Lafcadio. "Youma." *Harper's Magazine* 80 (Feb. 1890): 408–25.

Heffernan, James A. W. "*Adonais*: Shelley's Consumption of Keats." *Studies in Romanticism* 23 (1984): 295–315.

Heffernan, Michael J. "Bringing the Desert to Bloom: French Ambitions in the Sahara Desert during the Late Nineteenth Century—the Strange Case of '*la Mer Intérieure.*'" *Water, Engineering and Landscape: Water Control and Landscape Transformation in the Modern Period.* Ed. Denis Cosgrove and Geoff Petts. London: Belhaven, 1990. 94–114.

Herndl, Diane Price. *Invalid Women: Figuring Feminine Illness in American Fiction and Culture, 1840–1940.* Chapel Hill: U of North Carolina P, 1993.

Hibbert, Christopher. *Africa Explored: Europeans in the Dark Continent, 1769–1889.* London: Lane, 1982.

Rev. of *Historical Account of Discoveries and Travels in Africa,* by Hugh Murray. *Quarterly Review* 17 (1817): 299–338.

"The History of the Rise, Progress, Ravages, etc. of the Blue Cholera of India." *Lancet* 19 Nov. 1831: 241–84.

Hoffmann, Frederick L. "The Decline of the Tuberculosis Death Rate, 1871–1912." *Transactions of the National Association for the Study and Prevention of Tuberculosis, 1850–1950* 9 (1913): 101–37.

Hoffmann, Friedrich. *A Dissertation on Endemial Diseases, or Those Disorders Which Arise from Particular Climates, Situations, and Methods of Living.* London: Osborne, 1746.

Hogg, Thomas Jefferson. *The Life of Percy Bysshe Shelley.* Introd. Edward Dowden. London: Routledge, 1906.

Holmes, Richard. *Shelley: The Pursuit.* London: Weidenfeld and Nicolson, 1974.

Homer. *The Odyssey.* Trans. Robert Fitzgerald. New York: Doubleday, 1963.

Howard, Thomas Phipps. *The Haitian Journal of Lieutenant Howard, York Hussars, 1796–98.* Ed. Roger Norman Buckley. Knoxville: U of Tennessee P, 1985.

Howe, George Melvyn. "Disease Mapping." *Medical Geography: Progress and Prospect.* Ed. Michael Pacione. London: Croom Helm, 1986. 35–63.

——. *Man, Environment, and Disease in Britain: A Medical Geography of Britain through the Ages.* New York: Barnes and Noble, 1972.

Hulme, Peter. *Colonial Encounters: Europe and the Native Caribbean, 1492–1797.* New York: Methuen, 1986.

Hunt, Leigh. *The Autobiography of Leigh Hunt.* Ed. J. E. Morpurgo. London: Cresset, 1948.

——. "Calendar of Nature." *Examiner* 5 Sept. 1819: 574.

——. "Distressed Seamen." *Examiner* 11 Jan. 1818: 17–18; 18 Jan. 1818: 33–34; 25 Jan. 1818: 49–52.

——. *Imagination and Fancy, or Selections from the English Poets.* London: Smith, Elder, 1844.

——. *Lord Byron and Some of His Contemporaries; with Recollections of the Author's Life, and of His Visit to Italy.* 2nd ed. 2 vols. London: Colburn, 1828.

——. *Men, Women, and Books: A Selection of Sketches, Essays, and Critical Memoirs.* New York: Harper, 1847.

——. *Poetical Works of Leigh Hunt.* London: Moxon, 1832.

Hutcheon, Linda, and Michael Hutcheon. *Opera: Desire, Disease, Death.* Lincoln: U of Nebraska P, 1996.

Hyam, Ronald. *Empire and Sexuality: The British Experience.* Manchester: Manchester UP, 1990.

Jackson, H. J. "Coleridge on the King's Evil." *Studies in Romanticism* 16 (1977): 337–47.

——. "Coleridge's Collaborator, Joseph Henry Green." *Studies in Romanticism* (summer 1982): 161–79.

Jackson, J. R. de J. *Poetry of the Romantic Period.* London: Routledge and Kegan Paul, 1980.

Jacobus, Mary. *Romanticism Writing and Sexual Difference: Essays on "The Prelude."* Oxford: Clarendon, 1989.

James, Bartholomew. *Journal of Rear-Admiral Bartholomew James, 1752–1828.* Ed. John

Knox Laughton and James Young F. Sullivan. London: Navy Records Society, 1896.

James, C. L. R. *The Black Jacobins: Toussaint l'Ouverture and the San Domingo Revolution.* 2nd ed. rev. New York: Random, 1963.

Jardine, N., J. A. Secord, and E. C. Spary, eds. *The Cultures of Natural History.* Cambridge: Cambridge UP, 1996.

Johnson, James. *The Influence of Tropical Climates on European Constitutions.* 4th ed. London: Underwood, 1827.

Johnson, Samuel. *Johnson's Dictionary: A Modern Selection.* Ed. E. L. McAdam Jr. and George Milne. London: Gallancz, 1963.

———. *Yale Edition of the Works of Samuel Johnson.* Ed. D. Greene. 15 vols. New Haven: Yale UP, 1958–.

Johnston, Kenneth, and Jonathan Barron. "The Pedlar's Guilt." *Romantic Revisions.* Ed. Robert Brinkley and Keith Hanley. Cambridge: Cambridge UP, 1992.

Jones, Elizabeth. "Keats in the Suburbs." *Keats-Shelley Journal* 45 (1996): 23–43.

———. "Suburb Sinners: The Literary Prostitution of Keats and Hunt." 1996 NASSR Conference.

Jordanova, Ludmilla J. "Earth Science and Environmental Medicine: The Synthesis of the Late Enlightenment." *Images of the Earth: Essays in the History of the Environmental Sciences.* Ed. L. J. Jordanova and Roy Porter. Chalfont St. Giles: British Society for the History of Science, 1979. 119–46.

"Journal of the Centre Division of the Army from Cawnpore." *Asiatic Journal* 6 (July 1818): 5–8.

Karlen, Arno. *Man and Microbes: Disease and Plagues in History and Modern Times.* New York: Putnam, 1995.

Kaufman, Paul. " 'The Hurricane' and the Romantic Poets." *English Miscellany: A Symposium of History, Literature, and the Arts* 21 (1970): 99–115.

Kay-Shuttleworth, James. *The Moral and Physical Conditions of the Working Classes.* 2nd ed. 1832. New York: Kelley, 1970.

Keach, William. "Cockney Couplets: Keats and the Politics of Style." *Studies in Romanticism* 25 (1986): 182–96.

———. *Shelley's Style.* New York: Methuen, 1984.

Keane, Patrick J. *Coleridge's Submerged Politics: "The Ancient Mariner" and "Robinson Crusoe."* Columbia: U of Missouri P, 1994.

Keats, John. *Complete Poems.* Ed. Jack Stillinger. Cambridge: Harvard UP, 1982.

———. *The Letters of John Keats, 1814–1821.* Ed. Hyder Edward Rollins. 2 vols. Cambridge: Harvard UP, 1958.

Kennedy, Dane. *Islands of White: Settler Society and Culture in Kenya and Southern Rhodesia, 1890–1939.* Durham: Duke UP, 1987.

———. "The Perils of the Midday Sun: Climatic Anxieties in the Colonial Tropics." *Imperialism and the Natural World.* Ed. John M. Mackenzie. Manchester: Manchester UP, 1990. 118–40.

Kennedy, James. *The History of the Contagious Cholera: With Remarks on Its Character and Treatment in England.* 3rd ed. London: Moxon, 1832.

King, A. D. *Colonial Urban Development.* London: Routledge and Kegan Paul, 1976.

King, Virginia Himmelsteib. *Another Dimension to the Black Diaspora: Diet, Disease, and Racism.* Cambridge: Cambridge UP, 1981.

Kingsley, Mary H. *Travels in West Africa, Congo Français, Corisco and Cameroons.* London: Macmillan, 1897.

Kiple, Kenneth F. "The Ecology of Disease." *Companion Encyclopedia of the History of Medicine.* Ed. W. F. Bynum and Roy Porter. London: Routledge, 1993. 1: 357–81.

——, ed. *The Cambridge World History of Human Disease.* Cambridge: Cambridge UP, 1993.

Kiple, Kenneth F., and Stephen V. Beck, eds. *Biological Consequences of European Expansion, 1450–1800.* Aldershot, Eng.: Variorum, 1997.

Klein, Herbert S. *The Middle Passage: Comparative Studies in the Atlantic Slave Trade.* Princeton: Princeton UP, 1978.

Knapp, Vincent J. *Disease and Its Impact on Modern European History.* Lewiston, NY: Mellen, 1989.

Knollenberg, Bernhard. "General Amherst and Germ Warfare." *Mississippi Valley Historical Review* 41 (Dec. 1954): 489–94.

Kolodny, Annette. *The Lay of the Land: Metaphor as Experience and History in American Life and Letters.* Chapel Hill: U of North Carolina P, 1975.

Kraut, Alan M. *Silent Travelers: Germs, Genes, and the "Immigrant Menace."* New York: Basic, 1994.

Krieg, Joann P. *Epidemics in the Modern World.* New York: Twayne, 1992.

Kristeva, Julia. *Powers of Horror: An Essay on Abjection.* Trans. Leon S. Roudiez. New York: Columbia UP, 1982.

Kupperman, Karen Ordahl. "Fear of Hot Climates in the Anglo-American Colonial Experience." *Biological Consequences of European Expansion, 1450–1800.* Ed. Kenneth F. Kiple and Stephen V. Beck. Aldershot, Eng.: Variorum, 1997. 175–202.

Lamb, Charles, and Mary Lamb. *The Letters of Charles and Mary Anne Lamb.* Ed. Edwin W. Marrs Jr. 3 vols. Ithaca: Cornell UP, 1975–78.

Lamb, F. H. "Tropical Hygiene, 1807." *Journal of the Royal Naval Medical Service* 47 (1961): 92–93.

Lamb, H. H. *Climate, History and the Modern World.* 2nd ed. London: Methuen, 1995.

Lambe, William. *A Medical and Experimental Inquiry, into the Origin, Symptoms, and Cure of Constitutional Diseases.* London: Mawman, 1805.

——. *Reports of the Effects of a Peculiar Regimen on Scirrhous Tumours and Cancerous Ulcers.* London: Mawman, 1809.

Langan, Celeste. *Romantic Vagrancy: Wordsworth and the Simulation of Freedom.* New York: Cambridge UP, 1995.

Lawrence, Christopher. "Disciplining Disease: Scurvy, the Navy, and Imperial Expansion, 1750–1825." *Visions of Empire: Voyages, Botany, and Representations of Nature.* Ed. David Philip Miller and Peter Hanns Reill. Cambridge: Cambridge UP, 1996. 80–106.

Leask, Nigel. *British Romantic Writers and the East: Anxieties of Empire.* Cambridge: Cambridge UP, 1992.

Leckie, Ross. *The Gourmet's Companion.* Edinburgh: Edinburgh Publishing, 1993.

Lee, Debbie. "Mapping the Interior: African Cartography and Shelley's *The Witch of Atlas.*" *European Romantic Review* 8.2 (1997): 169–84.

———. "Poetic Voodoo in Keats's *Lamia.*" *Times Literary Supplement* 27 Oct. 1995: 13–14.

———. "Yellow Fever and the Slave Trade: Coleridge's *The Rime of the Ancient Mariner.*" *Journal of English Literary History* 65 (1998): 675–700.

Le Roy Ladurie, Emmanuel. "A Concept: The Unification of the Globe (Fourteenth to Seventeenth Centuries)." *The Mind and Method of the Historian.* Trans. S. Reynolds and B. Reynolds. Chicago: U of Chicago P, 1981. 28–83.

———. *Times of Feast, Times of Famine: A History of Climate since the Year 1000.* Trans. Barbara Bray. New York: Farrar, 1971.

Levere, Trevor. *Poetry Realized in Nature: Samuel Taylor Coleridge and Early Nineteenth-Century Science.* Cambridge: Cambridge UP, 1981.

Levine, George. *The Realistic Imagination.* Chicago: U of Chicago P, 1981.

Levine, Philippa. "Venereal Disease, Prostitution, and the Politics of Empire: The Case of British India." *Journal of the History of Sexuality* 4 (1993–94): 579–602.

Lewis, R. A. *Edwin Chadwick and the Public Health Movement, 1832–1854.* London: Longmans, Green, 1952.

Lind, James. *Essay on Diseases Incidental to Europeans in Hot Climates.* 5th ed. London: Murray, 1792.

———. *An Essay on the Most Effectual Means of Preserving the Health of Seamen in the Royal Navy and a Dissertation on Fevers and Infection* (1759). Rpt. in *The Health of Seamen: Selections from the Works of Dr. James Lind, Sir Gilbert Blane, and Dr. Thomas Trotter.* Ed. Christopher Lloyd. London: Navy Records Society, 1965.

Linebaugh, Peter. "All the Atlantic Mountains Shook." *Labour/Le Travailleur* 10 (1982): 87–121.

———. *The London Hanged: Crime and Civil Society in the Eighteenth Century.* Harmondsworth, Eng.: Penguin, 1991.

Linebaugh, Peter, and Marcus Rediker. "The Many-Headed Hydra: Sailors, Slaves, and the Atlantic Working Class in the Eighteenth Century." *Journal of Historical Sociology* 3.3 (1990): 225–52.

Liu, Alan. *Wordsworth: The Sense of History.* Stanford: Stanford UP, 1989.

Lloyd, Christopher. *The British Seaman, 1200–1860: A Social Survey.* London: Collins, 1968.

Lloyd, Christopher, and Jack L. S. Coulter. *Medicine and the Navy, 1200–1900.* Vol. 3. *1714–1815.* Edinburgh: Livingstone, 1961.

Lockhart, John Gibson. "Letter from Z. to Leigh Hunt, King of the Cockneys." *Blackwood's Edinburgh Magazine* 3 (May 1818): 196–201.

——. "On the Cockney School of Poetry." *Blackwood's Edinburgh Magazine* 2 (Oct. 1817): 38–41; 2 (Nov. 1817): 194–201; 3 (July 1818): 453–56; 3 (Aug. 1818): 519–24.

Logan, Peter Melville. *Nerves and Narratives: A Cultural History of Hysteria in Nineteenth-Century British Prose.* Berkeley: U of California P, 1997.

Long, Edward. *The History of Jamaica, or General Survey of the Ancient and Modern State of That Island: With Reflections on Its Situation, Inhabitants, Climate, Products, Commerce, Laws and Government.* 3 vols. London: Lowndes, 1774.

Lovell, Ernest J., Jr. *Captain Medwin: Friend of Byron and Shelley.* Austin: U of Texas P, 1962.

Lowell, James Russell. "The Life of Keats." *The Poetical Works of John Keats.* Boston: Houghton, Mifflin, 1854.

Lowes, John Livingston. *The Road to Xanadu: A Study in the Ways of the Imagination.* 1927. New York: Vintage, 1959.

Lyon, George F. *A Narrative of Travels in Northern Africa, in the Years 1818, 19, and 20.* 1821. London: Cass, 1966.

MacLeod, Roy, and Milton Lewis, eds. *Disease, Medicine and Empire.* London: Routledge, 1988.

Macmichael, W. "Is the Cholera Spasmodic of India a Contagious Disease? The Questions Considered in a Letter Addressed to Sir Henry Halford, Bart." *Quarterly Review* 46 (1832): 170–212.

Macnamara, C. *A History of Asiatic Cholera.* London: Macmillan, 1876.

Magnuson, Paul. *Coleridge and Wordsworth: A Lyrical Dialogue.* Princeton: Princeton UP, 1988.

Mair, R. S. *A Medical Guide for Anglo-Indians. The European in India, or Anglo-Indian's Vade-Mecum. A Handbook of Useful and Practical Information for Those Proceeding to or Residing in the East Indies.* Ed. Edmund Hull. London: King, 1871.

Makdisi, Saree. *Romantic Imperialism: Universal Empire and the Culture of Modernity.* Cambridge: Cambridge UP, 1998.

Mani, Lata. "Contentious Traditions: The Debate on Sati in Colonial India." *Cultural Critique* 7 (1987): 119–56.

——. "Cultural Theory, Colonial Texts: Reading Eyewitness Accounts of Widow Burning." *Cultural Studies.* Ed. Lawrence Grossberg, Cary Nelson, and Paula A. Treichler. New York: Routledge, 1992. 392–408.

Manning, Peter J. "Wordsworth, Margaret and the Pedlar." *Studies in Romanticism* 15 (1976): 195–220. Rpt. in *Reading Romantics: Texts and Contexts.* New York: Oxford UP, 1990. 9–34.

Manson-Bahr, Philip. *History of the School of Tropical Medicine in London (1899–1949).* London: Lewis, 1956.

Marchand, Leslie A. *Byron: A Biography.* New York: Knopf, 1957.

Marlowe, Christopher. *"Doctor Faustus" and Other Plays.* Oxford: Oxford UP, 1995.

Marriott, Alice, and Carol Rachlin. *American Indian Mythology.* New York: New American Library, 1968.

Marshall, Henry. *Notes on the Medical Topography of the Interior of Ceylon; and on the Health of the Troops Employed in the Kandyan Provinces, during the Years 1815, 1816, 1817, 1818, 1819, and 1820; with Brief Remarks on the Prevailing Diseases.* London: Burgess and Hill, 1821.

——. "Sketch of the Geogaphical Distribution of Diseases." *Edinburgh Medical and Surgical Journal* 38 (1832): 330–52.

Marshall, P. J., and Glyndwr Williams. *The Great Map of Mankind: British Perceptions of the World in the Age of Enlightenment.* London: Dent, 1982.

Martin, Edwin Thomas. *Thomas Jefferson: Scientist.* New York: Schuman, 1952.

Martin, James Ranald. *The Influence of Tropical Climates on European Constitutions, Including Practical Observations on the Nature and Treatment of the Diseases of Europeans on Their Return from Tropical Climates.* London: Churchill, 1856.

Masefield, John. *A Sailor's Garland.* New York: Macmillan, 1928.

Mathew, G. F. Rev. of 1817 *Poems,* by John Keats. *European Magazine* 71 (May 1817): 434–37.

Mathias, Thomas James. *The Pursuits of Literature.* London: Beckert, 1798.

Matthews, G. M. *Keats: The Critical Heritage.* London: Routledge and Kegan Paul, 1971.

Matus, Jill L. *Unstable Bodies: Victorian Representations of Sexuality and Maternity.* Manchester: U of Manchester P, 1995.

Mayo, Robert. "The Contemporaneity of the 'Lyrical Ballads.' " *PMLA* 69 (1954): 486–522.

Mazzeo, Tilar J. " 'A Mixture of All the Styles': Colonialism, Nationalism, and Plagiarism in Shelley's Indian Circle." *European Romantic Review* 8.2 (1997): 155–68.

McClellan, James E., III. *Colonialism and Science: Saint Domingue in the Old Regime.* Baltimore: Johns Hopkins UP, 1992.

McClintock, Anne. *Imperial Leather: Race, Gender and Sexuality in the Colonial Contest.* New York: Routledge, 1995.

McGann, Jerome J. "Keats and the Historical Method in Literary Criticism." *The Beauty of Inflections: Literary Investigations in Historical Method and Theory.* New York: Oxford UP, 1985. 48–62.

——. "The Meaning of *The Ancient Mariner.*" *Critical Inquiry* 8 (1981): 35–67.

——. *The Romantic Ideology: A Critical Investigation.* Chicago: U of Chicago P, 1983.

McGuffie, T. H. "The Short Life and Sudden Death of an English Regiment of Foot." *Journal of the Society for Army Historical Research* 33 (1955): 16–25.

McKusick, James C. " 'That Silent Sea': Coleridge, Lee Boo, and the Exploration of the South Pacific." *Wordsworth Circle* 24 (1993): 102–6.

McNeill, John R. "The Ecological Basis of Warfare in the Caribbean." *Adapting to Conditions: War and Society in the Eighteenth Century.* Ed. Maarten Ultee. University: U of Alabama P, 1986. 26–42.

McNeill, William H. "Historical Patterns of Migration." *Current Anthropology* 20 (1979): 95–102.

———. *Plagues and Peoples.* Garden City, NY: Anchor, 1976.

Meade, Melinda S., John W. Florin, and Wilbert M. Gesler. *Medical Geography.* New York: Guilford, 1988.

Medwin, Thomas. *The Angler in Wales.* 2 vols. London: Bentley, 1834.

———. *The Life of Percy Bysshe Shelley: A New Edition.* Ed. H. B. Forman. London: Oxford UP, 1913.

———. *Oswald and Edwin, Sketches in Hindoostan, Ahasuerus.* New York: Garland, 1978.

Merchant, Carolyn. *The Death of Nature: Women, Ecology, and the Scientific Revolution.* San Francisco: Harper, 1980.

Metcalfe, Emily. *The Golden Calm: An English Lady's Life in Moghul Delhi.* Ed. M. M. Kaye. Exeter: Webb and Bower, 1980.

Meyer, Susan L. "Colonialism and the Figurative Strategy of *Jane Eyre*." *Victorian Studies* 33 (1990): 247–68.

Michael, Jennifer Davis. "Pecoriloquy: The Narrative of Consumption in the Letters of Keats." *European Romantic Review* 6 (1995): 38–56.

Millar, Richard. *Clinical Lectures on the Contagious Typhus Epidemic in Glasgow and the Vicinity during the Years 1831 and 1832.* Glasgow: Brash, 1833.

Miller, C. L. *Blank Darkness: Africanist Discourse in French.* U of Chicago P, 1985.

Miller, David Philip, and Peter Hanns Reill, eds. *Visions of Empire: Voyages, Botany, and Representations of Nature.* Cambridge: Cambridge UP, 1996.

Miller, Genevieve. "'Airs, Waters, and Places' in History." *Journal of the History of Medicine and Allied Sciences* 17 (1962): 129–40.

Milligan, Barry. *Pleasures and Pains: Opium and the Orient in Nineteenth-Century British Culture.* Charlottesville: UP of Virginia, 1995.

Mitchell, Timothy. *Colonising Egypt.* Berkeley: U of California P, 1988.

Mitchell, W. J. T. *Landscape and Power.* Chicago: U of Chicago P, 1994.

Modiano, Raimondo. "Recollection and Misrecognition: Coleridge's and Wordsworth's Reading of the 'Salisbury Plain' Poems." *Wordsworth Circle* 28 (1997): 74–82.

Montesquieu. *The Persian Letters.* Ed. George R. Healy. Indianapolis: Bobbs-Merrill, 1964.

———. *Spirit of the Laws.* Trans. Thomas Nugent. 2 vols in 1. London: Collier Macmillan, 1949.

Moore, Thomas. *The Poetical Works of Thomas Moore.* Ed. A. D. Godley. London: Oxford UP, 1929.

Moore, William. "The Constitutional Requirements for Tropical Climates, with

Especial Reference to Temperaments." *Transactions of the Epidemiological Society* 4 (1884–85): 32–51.

Morley, Henry. *Memoirs of Bartholomew Fair.* London: Routledge, 1892.

Morris, R. J. *Cholera 1832: The Social Response to an Epidemic.* London: Croom Helm, 1976.

Morton, Timothy. *Shelley and the Revolution in Taste: The Body and the Natural World.* Cambridge: Cambridge UP, 1994.

——. "Shelley's Green Desert." *Studies in Romanticism* 35 (1996): 409–30.

Moseley, Benjamin. *A Treatise on Sugar.* London: Robinson, 1799.

——. *A Treatise on Tropical Diseases; on Military Operations and on the Climates of the West-Indies.* 3rd ed. London: Robinson, 1795.

Nash, Gary B. *The Urban Crucible: Social Change, Political Consciousness, and the Origins of the American Revolution.* Cambridge: Harvard UP, 1979.

Newey, Vincent. " 'Alternate Uproar and Sad Peace': Keats, Politics, and the Idea of Revolution." *MHRA Yearbook of English Studies* 19 (1989): 265–89.

——. "Keats, History, and the Poets." *Keats and History.* Ed. Nicholas Roe. New York: Cambridge UP, 1995. 165–93.

Newton, John. *The Return to Nature, or A Defence of the Vegetable Regimen; with Some Account of an Experiment Made during the Last Three Years in the Author's Family.* London: Cadell and Davies, 1811.

"Notices in Natural History, no. 1." *Blackwood's Magazine* 2.10 (Jan. 1818): 378–81.

Notter, J. Lane. "The Hygiene of the Tropics." *Hygiene and Disease of Warm Climates.* Ed. Andrew Davidson. London: Pentland, 1893. 25–75.

Nussbaum, Felicity A. *Torrid Zones: Maternity, Sexuality, and Empire in Eighteenth-Century English Narratives.* Baltimore: Johns Hopkins UP, 1995.

"Obituary." *Lancet* 12 July 1890: 99.

Oliphant, Mrs. "John Keats." *The Literary History of England in the End of the Eighteenth and Beginning of the Nineteenth Century.* 3 vols. London: Macmillan, 1882.

Orme, Robert. *Historical Fragments of the Mogul Empire, of the Morattoes, and of the English Concerns in Indostan.* London: Wingrave, 1805.

Orton, Reginald. *An Essay on the Epidemic Cholera of India.* London: Burgess and Hill, 1831.

Park, Mungo. *Travels in the Interior Districts of Africa: Performed in the Years 1795, 1796, and 1797. With an Account of A Subsequent Mission to the Country in 1805.* 2 vols. London: Murray, 1815–16.

Patmore, Coventry. Rev. of *Life, Letters and Literary Remains of John Keats,* ed. R. M. Milne. *North British Review* 10 (Nov. 1848): 69–96.

Paulson, Ronald. *Hogarth's Graphic Works.* Rev. ed. 2 vols. New Haven: Yale UP, 1970.

——. *Representations of Revolution (1789–1820).* New Haven: Yale UP, 1983.

Pelling, Margaret. *Cholera, Fever and English Medicine, 1825–1865.* Oxford: Oxford UP, 1978.

Pernick, Martin S. "Politics, Parties and Pestilence: Epidemic Yellow Fever in Philadelphia and the Rise of the First Party System." *Sickness and Health in America.* Ed. J. Leavitt and R. Numbers. Madison: U of Wisconsin P, 1985. 241–56.

Pérouse, J. F. G. de la. *A Voyage Round the World Performed in the Years 1785, 1786, 1787, and 1788.* London: Hamilton, 1799.

Peterson, John. *Province of Freedom: A History of Sierra Leone.* London: Faber, 1969.

Petrarch, *The Triumphs of Petrarch.* Chicago: Univ. of Chicago P, 1962.

Pfister, Christian. "Climate and Economy in Eighteenth Century Switzerland." *Journal of Interdisciplinary History* 9 (1978): 223–43.

Phillips, Thomas. *Journal of a Voyage Made in the "Hannibal" of London, Ann. 1693, 1694. . . . A Collection of Voyages and Travels.* Ed. Awnsham Churchill. 6 vols. London: Churchill, 1732.

Pickstone, John V. "Dearth, Dirt and Fever Epidemics: Rewriting the History of British 'Public Health,' 1780–1850." *Epidemics and Ideas: Essays on the Historical Perception of Pestilence.* Ed. Terence Ranger and Paul Slack. Cambridge UP, 1992. 125–48.

Pluchon, Pierre, ed. *Histoire des medecins et pharmaciens de marine et des colonies.* Toulouse: Editions Privat, 1985.

Rev. of *The Poetical Works of William Wordsworth. North British Review* 13 (Aug. 1850): 473–508.

Poovey, Mary. *Making a Social Body: British Cultural Formation, 1830–1864.* Chicago: U of Chicago P, 1995.

——. *The Proper Lady and the Woman Writer: Ideology as Style in the Works of Mary Wollstonecraft, Mary Shelley, and Jane Austen.* Chicago: U of Chicago P, 1984.

Pope, Alexander. *Poetry and Prose of Alexander Pope.* Ed. Aubrey Williams. Boston: Houghton Mifflin, 1969.

Post, John D. "Meteorological Historiography." *Journal of Interdisciplinary History* 3 (1973): 721–32.

Pouchet, Georges. *The Plurality of the Human Race.* 2nd ed. Trans. and ed. Hugh J. C. Beavan. London: Longman, Green, Longman, and Roberts, 1864.

Pratt, Mary Louise. *Imperial Eyes: Travel Writing and Transculturation.* London: Routledge, 1992.

Preface. *Blackwood's Edinburgh Magazine* 19 (Jan. 1826).

Rev. of *Prometheus Unbound,* by P. B. Shelley. *Blackwood's Edinburgh Magazine* 7 (Sept. 1820): 679–87.

Radzinowicz, Leon. *A History of English Criminal Law and Its Administration from 1750.* 4 vols. London: Stevens, 1948–68.

Raleigh, Walter. *The History of the World, in Five Books.* 11th ed. 2 vols. London: Glenyers, 1736.

Ramasubban, Radhika. "Imperial Health in British India, 1857–1900." *Disease, Medicine, and Empire: Perspectives on Western Medicine and the Experience of European Expansion.* Ed. Roy McLeod and Milton Lewis. London: Routledge, 1988. 38–60.

Ramenofsky, Ann F. *Vectors of Death: The Archaeology of European Contact.* Albuquerque: U of New Mexico P, 1987.

Ranger, Terence, and Paul Slack, eds. *Epidemics and Ideas: Essays on the Historical Perception of Pestilence.* Cambridge: Cambridge UP, 1992.

Ransford, Oliver. *"Bid the Sickness Cease": Disease in the History of Black Africa.* London: Murray, 1983.

Rawley, James A. *Transatlantic Slave Trade.* New York: Norton, 1981.

Raynal, Guillaume-T.-F. *A Philosophical and Political History of the British Settlements and Trade of the Europeans in the East and West Indies.* Trans. J. O. Justamond. 8 vols. London: Strahan, 1783.

Rediker, Marcus. *Between the Devil and the Deep Blue Sea: Merchant Seamen, Pirates, and the Anglo-American Maritime World, 1700–1750.* Cambridge: Cambridge UP, 1987.

Reed, Arden. *Romantic Weather: The Climates of Coleridge and Baudelaire.* Hanover: Brown UP, 1983.

Rennell, James. *The Geographical System of Herodotus, Examined; and Explained, by a Comparison with Those of Other Ancient Authors, and with Modern Geography.* London: Bulmer, 1800.

———. *Memoir of a Map of Hindoostan; or The Mogul Empire....* London: Nicol, 1788.

Report from the Commissioners on the Supply of Water to the Metropolis (July 1828).

Richardson, Alan. "Romantic Voodoo: Obeah and British Culture, 1797–1807." *Studies in Romanticism* 32 (spring 1993): 3–28.

Richardson, Alan, and Sonia Hofkosh, eds. *Romanticism, Race, and Imperial Culture, 1780–1834.* Bloomington: Indiana UP, 1996.

Riley, James C. *The Eighteenth-Century Campaign to Avoid Disease.* Basingstoke, Eng.: Macmillan, 1987.

Ritchie, Joseph. "A Farewell to England: Departing on His Travels into the Interior of Africa." *Monthly Magazine* June 1820: 426–27.

Ritson, Joseph. *An Essay on Abstinence from Animal Food, as a Moral Duty.* London: Phillips, 1802.

Roberton, John. *Essays and Notes on the Physiology and Diseases of Women and on Practical Midwifery.* London: Churchill, 1851.

Roberts, Emma. *Notes of an Overland Journey through France and Egypt to Bombay.* London: Allen, 1841.

Roe, Nicholas. *John Keats and the Culture of Dissent.* Oxford: Clarendon, 1997.

Rollins, Hyder Edward, ed. *The Keats Circle.* 2nd ed. 2 vols. Cambridge: Harvard UP, 1965.

Rosen, George. "Leonhard Ludwig Finke, and the First Medical Geography." *Science, Medicine, and History.* Ed. Edgar Ashworth Underwood. London: Oxford UP, 1953. 186–93.

Rosenberg, Charles E. "The Cause of Cholera: Aspects of Etiological Thought in Nineteenth-Century America." *Sickness and Health in America: Readings in the*

History of Medicine and Public Health. Ed. Judith Walzer Leavitt and Ronald L. Numbers. Madison: U of Wisconsin P, 1978. 257–71.

——. *The Cholera Years*. Chicago: U of Chicago P, 1962.

——. *Explaining Epidemics and Other Studies in the History of Medicine*. Cambridge: Cambridge UP, 1992.

Rosenberg, Charles E., and Janet Golden, eds. *Framing Disease: Studies in Cultural History*. New Brunswick: Rutgers UP, 1992.

Rosner, David. *Hives of Sickness: Public Health and Epidemics in New York City*. New Brunswick: Rutgers UP, 1995.

Rothman, Sheila M. *Living in the Shadow of Death: Tuberculosis and the Social Experience of Illness in American History*. New York: Basic, 1994.

Rousseau, Jean-Jacques. *Emile, or On Education*. Introd. and trans. Allan Bloom. New York: Basic, 1979.

Rupke, Nicolaas A. "Humboldtian Medicine." *Medical History* 40 (1996): 293–310.

Rush, Benjamin. *An Account of the Bilious Remitting Yellow Fever*. Philadelphia: Dobson, 1794.

——. "An Account of the Climate of Pennsylvania, and Its Influence on the Human Body." *Medical Inquiries and Observations*. Vol. 1. 2nd ed. Philadelphia: Dilly, 1789.

——. "An Inquiry into the Causes of the Increase of Bilious and Intermitting Fevers in Pennsylvania." *Medical Inquiries and Observations*. Vol. 2. Philadelphia: Dobson, 1797. 267–76.

Ryan, Michael. *A Manual of Midwifery, and Diseases of Women and Children*. 3rd ed. London: Bloomsbury, 1841.

Rzepka, Charles J. *Sacramental Commodities: Gift, Text, and the Sublime in De Quincey*. Amherst: U of Massachusetts P, 1995.

Said, Edward. *Culture and Imperialism*. New York: Vintage, 1994.

——. *Orientalism*. New York: Pantheon, 1978.

Salmon, Thomas. *New Geographical and Historical Grammar*. 12th ed. London: Johnston, 1772.

Sargent, Frederick. *Hippocratic Heritage: A History of Ideas about Weather and Human Health*. New York: Pergamon, 1982.

Savitt, Todd L., and James Harvey Young. *Disease and Distinctiveness in the American South*. Knoxville: U of Tennessee P, 1988.

Scarry, Elaine. *The Body in Pain: The Making and Unmaking of the World*. New York: Oxford UP, 1985.

Schmidt, Arnold. "Wordsworth's Politics and the Salisbury Plain Poems." *WC* 27 (1996): 166–68.

Schnurrer, Friedrich. *Geographische Nosologie oder die Lehre von den Veränderungen der Krankheiten in den vershiedenen Gegender der Erde, in Verbindung mit physicher Geographie und Natur-Geschichte des Menschen*. Stuttgart: Steinkopf, 1813.

Schoenfield, Mark. *The Professional Wordsworth: Law, Labor and the Poet's Contract*. Athens: U of Georgia P, 1996.

Schwarz, Lewis M. *Keats Reviewed by His Contemporaries: A Collection of Notices for the Years 1816–1821*. Metuchen, NJ: Scarecrow, 1973.

Scott, H. Harold. *A History of Tropical Medicine, Based on Fitzpatrick Lectures Delivered before the Royal College of Physicians of London, 1937–38*. 2 vols. Baltimore: Williams and Wilkins, 1939.

Scrivener, Michael Henry. *Radical Shelley: The Philosophical Anarchism and Utopian Thought of Percy Bysshe Shelley*. Princeton: Princeton UP, 1982.

Shapter, Thomas. *The Climate of the South of Devon; and Its Influence upon Health*. London: Churchill, 1842.

———. *The History of Cholera in Exeter in 1832*. London: Churchill, 1849.

Sharpe, Jenny. *Allegories of Empire: The Figure of the Woman in the Colonial Text*. Minneapolis: U of Minnesota P, 1993.

Shaw, Thomas. *Travels, or Observations relating to Several Parts of Barbary and the Levant*. Oxford: Theatre, 1738.

Sheats, Paul D. *The Making of Wordsworth's Poetry, 1785–1798*. Cambridge: Harvard UP, 1973.

Shelley, Mary. *Frankenstein, or The Modern Prometheus: The 1818 Text*. Ed. James Reiger. Chicago: U of Chicago P, 1982.

———. *Journals of Mary Shelley, 1814–1844*. Ed. Paula R. Feldman and Diana Scott-Kilvert. 2 vols. Oxford: Clarendon, 1987.

———. *The Last Man*. Ed. Hugh J. Luke Jr. Introd. Anne K. Mellor Lincoln: U of Nebraska P, 1993.

———. *The Letters of Mary Wollstonecraft Shelley*. Ed. Betty T. Bennett. Baltimore: Johns Hopkins UP, 1980.

Shelley, Mary, and Percy Bysshe Shelley. *History of a Six Weeks' Tour*. Ed. Jonathan Wordsworth. Oxford: Woodstock, 1989.

Shelley, Percy Bysshe. *The Complete Works of Percy Bysshe Shelley*. Ed. Roger Ingpen and Walter E. Peck. 10 vols. London: Earnest Benn, 1926–30.

———. *Letters*. Ed. Frederick L. Jones, 2 vols. Oxford: Clarendon, 1964.

———. *Shelley: Poetical Works*. Ed. Thomas Hutchinson. Oxford: Oxford UP, 1967.

———. *Shelley's Poetry and Prose*. Ed. Donald H. Reiman and Sharon B. Powers. New York: Norton, 1977.

Shelvocke, Captain George. *A Voyage Round the World by the Way of the Great South Sea*. London: Senex, 1726.

Sheridan, Richard B. *Doctors and Slaves: A Medical and Demographic History of Slavery in the British West Indies, 1680–1834*. Cambridge: Cambridge UP, 1985.

Showalter, Elaine. *The Female Malady: Women, Madness, and English Culture, 1830–1980*. New York: Pantheon, 1985.

Shryock, Richard Harrison. *Medicine and Society in America: 1660–1860*. Ithaca: Cornell UP, 1960.

Sierra Leone Company. *Account of the Colony of Sierra Leone from Its First Establishment in 1793 [sic]*. . . . London: Philips, 1795.

Sigerist, Henry E. *Civilization and Disease.* Ithaca: Cornell UP, 1943.

Simpson, David. *Wordsworth's Historical Imagination: The Poetry of Displacement.* New York: Methuen, 1987.

Smart, Newton. "The Duty of a Christian People under Divine Visitations." *British Critic* 11 (1832): 375–90.

Smith, Bernard. "Coleridge's *Ancient Mariner* and Cook's Second Voyage." *Journal of the Warburg and Courtauld Institutes* 19 (1956): 115–54.

Smith, F. B. *The Retreat of Tuberculosis, 1850–1938.* London: Croom Helm, 1988.

Smith, Thomas Southwood. *A Treatise on Fever.* London: Longman, Rees, Orme, Brown, and Green, 1830.

Smollett, Tobias. *The Adventures of Roderick Random.* Ed. Paul-Gabriel Boucé. Oxford: Oxford UP, 1979.

——. *The Expedition of Humphry Clinker.* Ed. Thomas R. Preston. Athens: U of Georgia P, 1990.

Smyth, W. H. *The Mediterranean.* London: Parker, 1854.

Snow, John. *On the Mode of Communication of Cholera.* 2nd ed. London: Churchill, 1855.

Snowden, Frank M. "Cholera in Barletta, 1910." *Past and Present* 132 (1991): 67–103.

Sontag, Susan. *AIDS and Its Metaphors.* New York: Farrar, 1988.

——. *Illness as Metaphor.* New York: Farrar, 1977.

Southey, Robert. *The Poetical Works of Robert Southey.* London: Longman, Brown, Green, and Longmans, 1853.

——. *Selections from the Letters of Robert Southey.* Ed. John Wood Worter. 4 vols. London: Longman, 1856.

——. *Sir Thomas More, or Colloquies on the Progress and Prospects of Society.* 2 vols. London: Murray, 1831.

Spivak, Gayatri Chakravorty. "Can the Subaltern Speak? Speculations on Widow Sacrifice." *Marxism and the Interpretation of Culture.* Ed. Cary Nelson and Lawrence Grossberg. London: Macmillan, 1988. 271–313.

——. "Three Women's Texts and a Critique of Imperialism." *Critical Inquiry* 12 (1985): 243–61.

Stallybrass, Peter, and Allon White. *The Politics and Poetics of Transgression.* London: Methuen, 1986.

Stannard, David E. *American Holocaust: Columbus and the Conquest of the New World.* Oxford: Oxford UP, 1992.

——. "Disease and Infertility: A New Look at the Demographic Collapse of Native Populations in the Wake of Western Contact." *Journal of American Studies* 24 (1990): 325–50.

——. "Disease, Human Migration, and History." *The Cambridge World History of Human Disease.* Ed. Kenneth F. Kiple. Cambridge: Cambridge UP, 1993. 35–42.

Starobinski, Jean. "The Idea of Nostalgia." *Diogenes* 54 (1966): 81–103.

Staum, Martin S. *Cabanis: Enlightenment and Medical Philosophy in the French Revolution.* Princeton: Princeton UP, 1980.

Stedman, John Gabriel. *Narrative of a Five Years' Expedition against the Revolted Negroes of Surinam.* Ed. Richard and Sally Price. Baltimore: Johns Hopkins UP, 1988.

Stephens, Fran Carlock. "An Autograph Letter of S. T. Coleridge." *Review of English Studies* 33 (1982): 298–302.

Sterrenburg, Lee. "*The Last Man:* Anatomy of Failed Revolutions." *Nineteenth Century Fiction* 33 (1978): 324–47.

Stevenson, L. G. "Putting Disease on the Map: The Early Use of Spot Maps in the Study of Yellow Fever." *Journal of the History of Medicine* 20 (1965): 226–61.

Subba Reddy, D. V. "An Indo-British Medical Classic of XVIII Century, Charles Curtis on Diseases of India in the Fleet and in the Naval Hospital at Madras, in 1782–1783." *Bulletin of the Indian Institute of the History of Medicine* 4 (1974): 192–207.

Suleri, Sara. *The Rhetoric of English India.* Chicago: U of Chicago P, 1992.

Sunder Rajan, Rajeswari. *Real and Imagined Women: Gender, Culture, and Postcolonialism.* London: Routledge, 1993.

Swann, Karen. "Harassing the Muse." *Romanticism and Feminism.* Ed. Anne K. Mellor. Bloomington: Indiana UP, 1988.

Sweetser, William. *Treatise on Consumption; Embracing an Inquiry into the Influence Exerted upon It by Journeys, Voyages, and Change of Climate. . . .* Boston: Carter, 1836.

Swift, Jonathan. *Poetical Works.* Ed. Herbert Davis. London: Oxford UP, 1967.

———. *The Prose Works of Jonathan Swift.* Ed. Herbert Davis. 14 vols. Oxford: Blackwell, 1939–68.

Tetrault, Ronald. *The Poetry of Life: Shelley and Literary Form.* Toronto: U of Toronto P, 1987.

Thackeray, William Makepeace. *Vanity Fair.* Introd. John W. Dodds. New York: Holt, Rinehart and Winston, 1955.

Thompson, E. P. *The Making of the English Working Class.* London: Gollancz, 1964.

Thomson, Frederick. *An Essay on the Scurvy: Shewing Effectual and Practicable Means for Its Prevention at Sea.* London: J. Robinson, 1790.

Tillotson, Geoffrey, ed. *Eighteenth-Century English Literature.* New York: Harcourt, Brace, 1969.

Tilt, Edward John. *A Hand-Book of Uterine Therapeutics, and of Diseases of Women.* 2nd American ed. New York: Appleton, 1869.

Tindall, George Brown. *The Emergence of the New South, 1913–1945.* Baton Rouge: Louisiana State UP, 1967.

Townsend, Joseph. *A Dissertation on the Poor Laws.* Ed. Ashley Montagu. 1786. Berkeley: U of California P, 1971.

Trapham, Thomas. *A Discourse of the State of Health in the Island of Jamaica. With a Provision Therefore Calculated from the Air, the Place, and the Water: The Customs and Manner of Living; etc.* London: Boulter, 1679.

Trotter, Thomas. *Medicina Nautica: An Essay on the Diseases of Seamen.* 2nd ed. 3 vols. London: Longman, Hurst, Rees, and Orme, 1804.

———. *Observations on the Scurvy: With a Review of the Theories Lately Advanced on That Disease.* 2nd ed. London: Longman and Watts, 1792.

Tulloch, Alexander M., and Henry Marshall. "Statistical Report of the Sickness, Mortality, and Invaliding among the Troops of the West Indies." *Accounts and Papers (Parliamentary Papers),* 1837–38, 40 (417).

Twining, William. *Clinical Illustrations of the More Important Diseases of Bengal, with the Result of an Inquiry into Their Pathology and Treatment.* Calcutta: Baptist Mission, 1832.

Underwood, Edgar A. "History of Cholera in Great Britain." *Proceedings of the Royal Society of Medicine* 41 (1948): 165–78.

Vaughan, Megan. *Curing Their Ills: Colonial Power and African Illness.* Stanford: Stanford UP, 1991.

Venetz, Ignace. *Mémoires sur les variations de la température dans les Alpes de la Suisse.* Zurich: Füssli, 1833.

Vickers, Neil. "Coleridge, Thomas Beddoes and Brunonian Medicine." *European Romantic Review* 8 (1997): 47–94.

Virchow, Rudolph. "L'acclimatement." *Revue Scientifique* 3rd ser. 36.24 (12 Dec. 1885): 737–47.

Volney, Constantin-F. *The Ruins, or Meditation on the Revolutions of Empires; and The Law of Nature.* Baltimore: Black Classic, 1991.

Vrettos, Athena. *Somatic Fictions: Imagining Illness in Victorian Culture.* Stanford: Stanford UP, 1995.

Walker, Carol Kyros. *Walking North with Keats.* New Haven: Yale UP, 1992.

Walkowitz, Judith R. *Prostitution and Victorian Society: Women, Class, and the State.* Cambridge: Cambridge UP, 1980.

Wallace, Anne D. *Walking, Literature, and English Culture: The Origins and Uses of Peripatetic in the Nineteenth Century.* Oxford: Clarendon, 1993.

Wasserman, Earl R. *Shelley: A Critical Reading.* Baltimore: Johns Hopkins UP, 1971.

Welch, Henry. "Modern Views on the Etiology of Phthisis." *Practitioner* 44 (1890): 228–40.

Wells, H. G. *The War of the Worlds.* London: Heinemann, 1968.

Wells, Roger. *Insurrection: The British Experience, 1795–1803.* Gloucester, Eng.: Sutton, 1986.

Western, J. R. "Military Service as Punishment." *Journal of the Society for Army Historical Research* 32 (1954): 89.

Wilde, Oscar. *"The Importance of Being Earnest" and Other Plays.* Oxford: Oxford UP, 1995.

Williams, Michael. *Americans and Their Forests: A Historical Geography.* Cambridge: Cambridge UP, 1989.

Williams, Raymond. *The Country and the City.* New York: Oxford UP, 1973.

Wilson, Alexander. *Some Observations relative to the Influence of Climate on Vegetable and Animal Bodies.* London: Cadell, 1780.

Wiltshire, John. *Jane Austen and the Body: "The Picture of Health."* Cambridge: Cambridge UP, 1992.

Winterbottom, Thomas. *An Account of the Native Africans in the Neighbourhood of Sierra Leone to Which Is Added an Account of the Present State of Medicine among Them.* 2 vols. 1803. London: Cass, 1969.

Wise, Thomas. *The Brontës: Their Lives, Friendships and Correspondence.* 4 vols. Oxford: Shakespeare Head, 1933.

Wolfson, Susan J. "Feminizing Keats." *Critical Essays on John Keats.* Ed. Hermione de Almeida. Boston: Hall, 1990. 317–56.

——. *Formal Charges: The Shaping of Poetry in British Romanticism.* Stanford: Stanford UP, 1997.

——. "Keats Enters History." *Keats and History.* Ed. Nicholas Roe. New York: Cambridge UP, 1995. 17–45.

——. *The Questioning Presence: Wordsworth, Keats, and the Interrogative Mode in Romantic Poetry.* Ithaca: Cornell UP, 1986.

Woodring, Carl R. *Politics in the Poetry of Coleridge.* Madison: U of Wisconsin P, 1961.

Worboys, Michael. "The Emergence of Tropical Medicine: A Study in the Establishment of a Scientific Specialty." *Perspectives on the Emergence of Scientific Disciplines.* Ed. Gerard Lemaine, Roy Macleod, Michael Mulkay, and Peter Weingart. The Hague: Mouton, 1976. 75–98.

Wordsworth, Jonathan. *The Music of Humanity: A Critical Study of Wordsworth's "Ruined Cottage" Incorporating Texts from a Manuscript of 1799–1800.* London: Nelson, 1969.

Wordsworth, William. *The Letters of William and Dorothy Wordsworth.* Ed. Ernest de Selincourt. 2nd rev. ed. 6 vols. Oxford: Clarendon, 1967–82.

——. *"Lyrical Ballads," and Other Poems.* Ed. James Butler and Karen Green. Ithaca: Cornell UP, 1992.

——. *The Prelude 1799, 1805, 1850.* Ed. Jonathan Wordsworth. New York: Norton, 1979.

——. *"The Ruined Cottage" and "The Pedlar."* Ed. James Butler. Ithaca: Cornell UP, 1979.

——. *The Salisbury Plain Poems of William Wordsworth.* Ed. Stephen Gill. Ithaca: Cornell UP, 1975.

——. *William Wordsworth.* Oxford Authors. Ed. Stephen Gill. Oxford: Oxford UP, 1984.

Young, Robert C. *Colonial Desire: Hybridity in Theory, Culture and Race.* New York: Routledge, 1995.

INDEX

Denoon, Donald, 302
De Quincey, Thomas, 14, 22, 121, 186,
233, 286, 310; *Confessions,* 20–21, 154–
60, 269; on "Ruined Cottage," 121–22
Desgenettes, René, 44
Dickens, Charles: *Hard Times,* 273; *Nicholas
Nickleby,* 185
Dickson, Samuel, 237
Diet: change of, and health, 149–51, 153–
54; and colonialism, 147–60; hybridity,
154–60; imperial, 143–45, 152–53;
local, 135–38, 151–52; and nationalism,
131–32, 139–43; politics of, 131–46;
temperance, 153, 290–91; vegetarianism, 205–7
Disease: and change of diet, 149–51; control of, 30–31, 40–43, 168, 290; and dirt,
54, 249–53, 63–64, 269, 276, 293–94;
environmental causes of, 29–34; "foreign," 18–20, 260–61; framing of, 2–3;
and gender, 13, 23, 186–89, 260–62,
267–69, 273–76, 280–82, 290–91; and
hygiene, 24–26; and ideopathology,
207–9; and the Irish, 263–65, 294; and
prostitution, 104, 261–62, 269; and race,
5–6, 8, 23–26; and social breakdown,
304–7; as social phenomenon, 49–50,
208–9; and temperance, 24–26, 176–84;
traveling, 3–4, 47; and troop movements, 246, 301. *See also* Anxiety
Disease environments, colonial; analogy
between poetry and, 171–75; breakdown of boundaries, 247, 299, 302–7;
emergence of, 3–10, 17, 243–44, 248–
53; hybridity of, 48–51, 59–61, 270–73,
275–76; improvement of, 37–44, 168–
69, 211–20, 223–25; as inhibiting colonization, 37–39; as socially produced,
49–50, 209–20, 229–35, 241, 302–6
Diseases: African, 9; emerging infectious,
310; Hawaii, 105; India, 16–17, 242–53;
introduced to New World, 8; on ships,
71; sub-Saharan Africa, 10; Surinam, 92;
treated in Seamen's Hospital, 128
Dobyns, Henry F., 10
Douglas, Mary, 149, 252

Drinkwater, Maj. Thomas, 70
Dubos, René and Jean, 185
Dundas, Robert, *Sketches of Brazil,* 13, 33–
34, 281, 284
Durey, Michael, 249, 252
Dysentery, 18, 71, 74, 75, 92

East Indies, as disease environment, 38, 39–
43
Ebbatson, J. B., 99
Ecologies, colonial transformation of, 38–
44, 211–20, 233–34
Edwards, Bryan, 118
"Effects of War," 111
Elephantiasis, and P. B. Shelley, 221–22, 311
Empson, William, 103
Engels, Friedrich, 263–64, 274, 292
Equiano, Olaudah, 106
Erikson, Kai, 78
Ernst, Waltraud, 281
Evans, Richard, 251, 252, 262
Evelyn, John, 174
Everest, Kelvin, 218

Factories Enquiry Commission (1833), 272
Falconbridge, Maria, 25; *Narrative,* 153,
197–98
Farley, John, 35–36
Farr, William, 161; *Report on the Mortality of
Cholera,* 47, 275
Faucher, Leon, 274
Fawcett, Joseph, *Art of War,* 67
Fergusson, William, 79
Fever, 20, 288–89; causes, 37–38, 259; as
tropical disease, 49
Fever-nests, 50; tropicalizing of, 168, 253,
271–72
Fielding, John, 69
Fikri, Muhammad Amin, 42
Finke, Leonhard Ludwig, 29, 32
Fletcher, Charles, 79, 126
Ford, George H., 184
Fortescue, J. W., 72, 75, 76
Foucault, Michel, 32
Frank, Johann Peter, *Complete Medical
Police,* 32

Library of Congress Cataloging-in-Publication Data

Bewell, Alan, 1951–
    Romanticism and colonial disease / Alan Bewell.
        p.   cm. — (Medicine and Culture)
    Includes bibliographical references and index.
    ISBN 0-8018-6225-6 (alk. paper)
        1. Diseases—Great Britain—Colonies—History.
2. Romanticism—Great Britain.   3. Diseases in literature.
4. Colonies in literature.   5. Medicine—History—18th century.
6. Medicine—History—19th century.   I. Title.   II. Series:
Medicine & culture.
R487.B49   1999   99-33027
610'.9171'241—dc21   CIP